Introduction to
**Formulae of Traditional
Chinese Medicine**

Introduction to TCM Series

ISSN: 2335-674X

Forthcoming:

Volume 1   Fundamentals of Traditional Chinese Medicine
by Hong-zhou Wu, Zhao-qin Fang and Pan-ji Cheng
(translated by Ye-bo He)
(Shanghai University of Traditional Chinese Medicine, China)
ISBN: 978-193-813-428-9
Publication date: Summer 2013

Volume 2   Introduction to Diagnosis in Traditional Chinese Medicine
by Hong-zhou Wu, Zhao-qin Fang and Pan-ji Cheng
(translated by Chou-ping Han)
(Shanghai University of Traditional Chinese Medicine, China)
ISBN: 978-193-813-413-5
Publication date: Summer 2013

Volume 3   Introduction to Chinese Materia Medica
by Jin Yang, Huang Huang and Li-jiang Zhu
(translated by Yunhui Chen)
(Nanjing University of Chinese Medicine, China)
ISBN: 978-193-813-416-6
Publication date: Summer 2013

Volume 4   Introduction to Chinese Internal Medicine
by Xiang Xia, Xiao-heng Chen, Min Chen and Yan-qian Xiao
(translated by Ye-bo He)
(Shanghai Jiaotong University, China)
ISBN: 978-193-813-4419-7
Publication date: Summer 2013

Volume 6   Introduction to Acupuncture and Moxibustion
by Ren Zhang (translated by Xue-min Wang)
(Shanghai Literature Institute of Traditional Chinese Medicine, China)
ISBN: 978-193-813-425-8
Publication date: Winter 2013

Volume 7   Introduction to Tui Na
by Lan-qing Liu and Jiang Xiao (translated by Azure Duan)
(Shanghai University of Traditional Chinese Medicine, China)
ISBN: 978-193-813-422-7
Publication date: Winter 2013

Introduction to TCM Series - Vol. 5

Introduction to
Formulae
of Traditional
Chinese
Medicine

Jin Yang
Huang Huang
Li-jiang Zhu
Nanjing University of Chinese Medicine, China

translated by
Xiao He
Hong Li

World Century

Published by

World Century Publishing Corporation
27 Warren Street
Suite 401-402
Hackensack, NJ 07601

Distributed by

World Scientific Publishing Co. Pte. Ltd.

5 Toh Tuck Link, Singapore 596224

USA office: 27 Warren Street, Suite 401-402, Hackensack, NJ 07601

UK office: 57 Shelton Street, Covent Garden, London WC2H 9HE

Library of Congress Cataloging-in-Publication Data
Yang, Jin, 1944–
    [Yi bai tian xue kai Zhong yao fang. English]
    Introduction to formulae of traditional chinese medicine / Jin Yang, Huang Huang,
Li-jiang Zhu ; translated by Xiao Ye and Hong Li.
        p. ; cm. -- (World century compendium to TCM ; v. 5)
        ISBN 978-1-938134-10-4 (softcover : alk. paper)
        I. Huang, Huang, 1954–   II. Zhu, Lijiang, active 2013.   III. Title.
        [DNLM: 1. Drug Prescriptions.   2. Materia Medica--therapeutic use.
3. Medicine, Chinese Traditional. QV 748]

    615.1--dc23

                                            2013000746

British Library Cataloguing-in-Publication Data
A catalogue record for this book is available from the British Library.

World Century Compendium to TCM
A 7-Volume Set

INTRODUCTION TO FORMULAE OF TRADITIONAL CHINESE MEDICINE
Volume 5
Copyright © 2013 by World Century Publishing Corporation

Published by arrangement with Shanghai Scientific & Technical Publishers.

Originally published in Chinese
Copyright © Shanghai Scientific & Technical Publishers, 2005
All Rights Reserved.

All rights reserved. This book, or parts thereof, may not be reproduced in any form or by any means, electronic or mechanical, including photocopying, recording or any information storage and retrieval system now known or to be invented, without written permission from the Publisher.

For photocopying of material in this volume, please pay a copying fee through the Copyright Clearance Center, Inc., 222 Rosewood Drive, Danvers, MA 01923, USA. In this case permission to photocopy is not required from the publisher.

ISBN 978-1-938134-34-0 (Set)
ISBN 978-1-938134-10-4 (pbk)

Typeset by Stallion Press
Email: enquiries@stallionpress.com

Printed in Singapore

PREFACE

The *Learning Chinese Medicine in 100 Days* series was first published in 1996 in China and since then, 11 versions have surfaced. The contents of this series of books are arranged in such a way that profound theories and unique features of Chinese medicine are explained in a language easily comprehensible to the lay man. Hence, it is easy for learners to understand and apply the theories in clinical practice. All these versions have been reprinted multiple times, and the highest number of copies sold for one version has already reached 100,000.

From the end of the last century to the beginning of this century, the spectrum of disease has broadened greatly. And accordingly, the application scope and method of Chinese medicine in clinic have also changed. In order to ensure that readers are able to grasp the concepts of Chinese medicine and related information and technology, we have invited many experts in this field to revise this series with meticulous effort. The original format and style remain the same, but some obsolete technologies and contents have been deleted. In contrast, several other diseases and related treatments have been added. We hope that the republication of this series of books can contribute to the spread of Chinese culture and medicine around the world.

Jin Yang
Huang Huang
Li-jiang Zhu
Nanjing University of Chinese Medicine, China
May 2005

CONTENTS

INTRODUCTION

With the increasing demands on medical health care, people all over the world are gradually adopting the belief that it is not sufficient to solely depend on modern or Western medicine mainly by means of chemical products and surgeries. Instead, traditional Chinese medicine is now in the global limelight due to its many advantages in preventing and treating diseases. Many doctors and people are in favor of rectifying the whole body state, hence they are beginning to take great interest in Chinese medicine, which achieves curative effects through natural therapies such as those involving animal and plant parts. However, the theory of Chinese medicine is worlds apart from that of modern medicine, and when integrated with unique eastern philosophies and ancient terms, it becomes much more complex, deterring many who are keen to delve deeper into this highly fascinating field.

The authors of this book are heavily involved in teaching Chinese medicine in various universities, and at the same time, they are dedicated to introducing the theories and diagnostic methods of Chinese medicine to readers in a most accessible way. The book introduces the analytical method of treatment based on pattern differentiation in Chinese medicine as the key concept and then lists some common disease patterns according to medicinal formulae. It guides readers in understanding the theory of Chinese medicine and methods to prescribe Chinese medicinal formulae in a step-by-step manner. Chinese medicinal formulae have been the main technique used to treat disease in China for over two thousand years. The accordance of formula and pattern is the most specific, objective, stable, and repeatedly effective factor of treatment based on pattern differentiation.

Therefore, understanding the accordance of formula and pattern indicates that one has attained the majority of the knowledge on Chinese medicine. That is the primary focus of this book. Meanwhile, it discusses the composition of principles of formulae and integrates indispensable concepts of Chinese medicine such as basic theories, diagnostic methods, pattern differentiation, Chinese medicinals, treatment principles, and internal medicine and warm disease, opening a door for novices to understand Chinese medicine.

Study Arrangement

Study one section a day and one unit over several days. The contents of the book are for a one-hundred-day study. The reader can continue for six days a week with a day of rest. The first week is used to learn the most basic features and theories of Chinese medicine. Then, the next 13 weeks are scheduled for the study of common disease patterns and correspondingly, more than 60 medicinal formulae together with 120 additional formulae. Generally, the reader can assimilate one principal formula a day. On the last week, time can be set aside to learn some common diseases or symptoms with corresponding formulae. During the learning process of formulae and patterns, the reader can further understand related theories of Chinese medicine and the mechanisms of action of commonly used formulae. In sum, there are altogether 14 weeks for study — about one hundred days in total. At the end of this book, there is an index for formula reference as well as another for key words.

After this one-hundred-day study, though it cannot be said that one has fully mastered Chinese medicine, one must have understood the general theories of this field and rudimental methods of prescribing medicinal formulae to treat several common diseases. In addition, the method of treatment based on pattern differentiation can be ingrained in the novice's mind and serve as a foundation for further study of Chinese medicine.

Study Requirements

If the novice wishes to improve his ability to prescribe Chinese medicinal formulae, it is recommended that he proceed as follows:

(1) This book introduces its contents in an orderly and in-depth manner; hence, the reader must study the contents in order instead of in a random sequence.

(2) The contents learnt each day should be understood and memorized. Do not attempt to skim through the book, due to a lack of perseverance and diligence, for a quick study. For the contents of each day, about one hour is usually required. If possible, more time can be allocated to review and recite Chinese medicinal formulae.

(3) There are some important points in learning. For example, familiarize yourself with the main features of each disease pattern; memorize the formula's ingredients, actions, and indications; and attempt the exercises of each section to further appreciate the contents of the day to test your understanding. As for the treatment references and additional formulae in the book, they are included to supplement and extend your understanding of the contents; thus, it is up to the novice to decide if he wishes to memorize those details.

THE 1ST WEEK

CHAPTER 1

Chinese Medicine and Medicinals

DAY ONE

A Magical Formula: Why Chinese Medicinals Can Treat Diseases

Chinese medicine is the traditional medicine of China. Unlike Western medicine in both theoretical systems and therapeutic methods, it has been the rich empirical summarization of the Chinese nation in fighting against diseases for thousands of years. Treatment methods in Chinese medicine are various, among which the application of Chinese medicinals is a main approach. Chinese medicinals comprise natural products from botanical, zoological, and mineral sources instead of modern medicines such as chemicals, antibiotics, and biologicals. Chinese medicinals can be used either in a single form or in a combination of several forms, which is called a Chinese medicinal formula or prescription.

A Favorable Medicine

Chinese medicinals are vastly common in the natural world. They consist of a collection of barks, grassroots, leaves, stems, seeds, flowers, animal bodies, stones, and gravels, which have never undergone complicated processing by modern industries, and thereafter wrapped in colorful packaging. Diagnosis in Chinese medicine is largely based on several simple methods such as pulse-taking and tongue coating inspection, in contrast to the sophisticated instruments used in modern or Western medicine. That is one of the key reasons why some people remain doubtful about the efficacy of Chinese medicinals prescribed by doctors. In actual fact, the efficacy of medicine is not in direct association with the complexity of processes and purification. Concerning the diagnosis of Chinese medicine, its purpose is to study a certain state of the human body under the guidance of traditional theories of Chinese medicine and thus determine an optimal Chinese medicinal formula. It is different from that of modern medicine, which is to diagnose and determine a certain disease. From this perspective, it is wrong to judge Chinese medicine based on Western medical criteria.

What are good medicines? Medicines that can cure diseases. What are decent doctors? Doctors who can relieve the pain of patients. Surely, no one will disagree with these answers. There was a factory director in Nanjing, China, who suffered from chronic diarrhea for more than two years. Some people suggested that he should seek the aid of Chinese medicine, but he did not believe in the uses of barks and grassroots, and instead, he visited all sorts of famous doctors of Western medicine in Nanjing and was finally hospitalized in the most luxurious ward in a local hospital. He received overall and detailed laboratory tests and consumed many expensive Western medicines, but alas without alleviation. He was hospitalized for four months, and then discharged with great disappointment. In the end, he paid a visit to the TCM Hospital of Jiangshu Province. He took Chinese medicine for two weeks and, to his surprise, his ailment was completely treated. This case made him an advocator of Chinese medicine and he spoke of its good everywhere he went. This is only one example among numerous other anecdotes. For most Chinese, it is very common to seek help from doctors of Chinese medicine when they suffer from illnesses. However, for those who have no contact with or knowledge of Chinese medicine, it may seem almost magical that Chinese medicinals are able to treat diseases.

Advantages of Chinese Medicinals

Why is Chinese medicine so popular among the masses? One of the main reasons is because they possess unique features for treating diseases.

First, their curative effect is reliable. Most Chinese medicinal formulae have been in use for hundreds or even thousands of years. Doctors throughout history have accumulated great experience in managing these medicinals, such as prescribing the optimal Chinese medicinal formula for a specific disease, the administration of dosage, the modification of medicinals, and the reactions caused by these medicinals. At the same time, in the course of medical practice for thousands of years, all kinds of formulae were revised, weeding out those poor in efficacy or serious in adverse/side effects, and preserving those definite in curative effects. In such a fashion, the Chinese formulae in implementation today have withstood the test of time and are proven to be effective. If the formula is appropriately applied, the curative effect is definite. It has been shown that Chinese medicine not only treats common and chronic diseases, but also refractory and acute diseases.

Moreover, Chinese medicine is relatively safe. Most medicinals applied in Chinese medicine are mild natural medicinals without or low in toxicity. Side effects are not a primary concern unless application is not carried out under set rules. Many Chinese medicinal formulae can be administrated for a long period of time, with little cumulative effect and no drug resistance. This advantage is unparalleled as compared to chemicals and therefore, as drug-induced diseases are increasing, doctors and researchers in the medical community are shifting toward such natural medicinals. Besides, most Chinese medicinals are described for oral consumption. Although it might be a little difficult to decoct some of them, other issues such as the necessity of injection can be avoided, eliminating the risks of pain and infection. In general, Chinese medicinals are safe except for a few toxic or drastic forms. For the application of toxic medicinals, strict rules should be followed and the practitioner must be experienced. The medicinals mentioned in this book are all non-toxic, and even if some of them have certain toxicity, instructions are provided to ensure safe application.

In addition, Chinese medicine emphasizes general regulation. It has two features: holism and treatment based on syndrome differentiation. To be specific, Chinese medicine does not treat a disease by targeting at a single symptom or at a local lesion, but at the entire body. It is quite often that some patients consume Chinese medicine for treating a particular disease and incidentally, not only this disease is cured, but several other diseases as well. For example, a patient was suffering from chronic headaches for 4–5 years and cerebral hemangioma was detected by CT (computed tomography) examination. He was advised to go through an operation, but he rejected it out of fear. Thus, instead, he sought Chinese medicinals. With the application of formulae that aim to boost the liver and kidney, and to invigorate blood and dissolve stasis, his headaches were cured within half a month. He continued to take Chinese medicine for another two months and the cerebral hemangioma shrank significantly, which was shown by CT examination. On a side note, the patient told us with great pleasure that he had been impotent for more than 3 years and it was cured together with the headaches. This is in fact the result of the general regulatory effects of Chinese medicine.

The many advantages of Chinese medicine in treating diseases have aroused interest and attention in the medical community and also among the general public, and has become more and more popular in research and application worldwide.

Chinese Medicinals in Treating Diseases

Supplement the insufficiency

It is common knowledge that water quenches thirst and food relieves hunger. The various nutrients required by the body, including vitamins, trace elements, and minerals, are all absorbed from the food we consume. Similarly, many Chinese medicinals contain a vast array of nutrients and the intake of these substances can meet our body's requirements. It is similar to diet, from which the saying "Chinese medicinals and food are from the same source" is derived. In addition, modern pharmacological researches have revealed that the nutrients contained in Chinese medicinals are far richer than those in common foods. Aside from sugars, protein, fat, and vitamins, Chinese medicinals have many ingredients that are especially beneficial to the reinforcement of the human body, which cannot be replaced by common foods.

Rectify the disorder

Chinese medicinals are enriched with numerous substances such as alkaloids, glycosides, volatile oil, tannins, organic acids, fat, plant pigments, and inorganic ingredients, which can assume specialized regulation on some organs and tissues and their functions by removing or inhibiting various pathogens. Through this manner, they are able to demonstrate their curative effect. Hence, it is not incredible that Chinese medicinals can treat diseases. Many Western medicines we use in our daily life orginate from Chinese medicinals, such as ephedrine and bererine.

Theory of Chinese Medicinals in Treating Diseases

The theory of administrating Chinese medicinals in Chinese medicine differs greatly from that of Western medicine, because the medical systems of Chinese and Western medicines are completely at odds. Chinese medicine holds that, from the perspective of holism, once an individual suffers from an illness, the body is in a state of disturbed balance. There can be a certain deficiency, excess, disorder, or production of pathogenic factors, in a pathological state. This state is manifested by, in Chinese medicine terms, exuberance of cold or hot, abnormal ascent or descent, and so on. As for Chinese medicinals, it is believed that they possess natures of cold, cool, warm, heat, ascent, floating, descent, and sinking, and some of them can be used to supplement and others to purge. With these advantages, Chinese medicinals can rectify and equilibrate the abnormal state of the human body, which is why Chinese medicinals can treat diseases. For instance, if a patient experiences high fever, vexation and agitation, restlessness, and thirst, it is a disease of the heat pattern, which should be treated by Chinese medicinals with cold and cool natures; if a patient has a fear of cold, cold limbs, abdominal pain, and watery diarrhea after catching a cold, it is a disease of the cold pattern, which should be treated by Chinese medicinals with the heat nature; for diseases of vomiting, hiccups, and panting, as they belong to the pattern of abnormal qi counterflow, the medicinals used will be those with descent and sinking natures; for diseases of gastroptosis, hysteroptosis, prolonged diarrhea, and rectal prolapse, since they fall within the pattern of abnormal qi sinking, the medicinals applied will be those with ascent and floating natures.

Therefore, instead of prescribing medicine according to a deficiency of a specific nutrient or the pathology, biochemistry, immunology, or the clarification of specific pathogens, treatment by Chinese medicine primarily exploits the properties of medicinal natures to rectify the disorders of the human body, associating these medicinal natures with the body state and disease nature. This is the focal characteristic of the theory of Chinese medicine in applying medicinals to treat diseases, which is also known as "treatment according to pattern differentiation." With this critical concept in mind, it is not difficult to understand why it is unnecessary for practitioners of Chinese medicine to diagnose a definite disease before treating it and why Chinese medicine can cure the disease without the diagnosis of a definite disease. Of course, this theory of Chinese medicine is derived from numerous medical practices for thousands of years.

Daily Exercises

1. What are the advantages of Chinese medicinals in treating diseases?
2. Why are Chinese medicinal formulae able to treat diseases?

DAY TWO

General Knowledge on Chinese Medicinal Formulae

Combination of medicinals

Chinese medicinal formulae are composed of varying numbers of Chinese medicinals according to theories, which is termed medicinal combination.

The natures and actions of Chinese medicinals are different from one another and even for those used for one disease, they too have differing advantages and disadvantages. However, a proper combination can enable complementation with each other by exerting or strengthening their advantages, offsetting or making up their shortcomings, and relieving or avoiding side effects. Some Chinese medicinals are unable to treat a certain disease by themselves, but through combination, they may play an important role in treating a disease. Therefore, the overall curative effect of Chinese medicinal formula is better than that of a single medicinal.

The prescribed combination of a Chinese medicinal formula is mainly based on the analysis of a disease nature to determine the combination principle and selection of appropriate medicinals. The combination principle in Chinese medicine is called "chief, deputy, assistant, and envoy."

The chief medicinal refers to the main medicinal that takes effect on major aspects of the disease. The deputy medicinal coordinates with the chief medicinal or treats accompanying symptoms. The assistant medicinal is used to strengthen the curative effect or offset the toxicity and side effects of the chief and deputy medicinals. The envoy medicinal is used mainly to harmonize all the medicinals in a formula. For a specific formula, the chief medicinal is imperative, while others can be absent. It is not necessary to be fixated with the pattern of "chief, deputy, assistant, and envoy" in an attempt to distinguish them. In the course of combining a formula, the chief medicinal can be selected according to the main characteristics and manifestations of the disease. Thereafter, other medicinals are chosen to complement the chief component, either by strengthening its curative effect, by attenuating its toxicity and side effects, or by treating secondary pathological changes and symptoms. In this way, the combination principle of "chief, deputy, assistant, and envoy" is reflected.

Formula modification

Chinese medicinal formulae usually have fixed medicinal ingredients and dosages and most of them have names, which are termed "set formulae." More than 100,000 entries of these set formulae have been recorded throughout history. The formulae confirmed in the Han and Tang dynasties are called "classical formulae," while those confirmed after the Ming dynasty are termed "current formulae." Though the set formulae are numerous, it is not common to use an entire set formula in clinical practice. Usually, flexible modifications are applied in light of the disease condition, patient's physique, seasonal climates, geographical environments, etc. Such modifications are chiefly realized through the following three aspects: (1) modifying the medicinal ingredients, which is the addition or removal of several ingredients to or from the set formula, and most of the set formulae are derived from modifications of other set formulae; (2) modifying the medicinal dosages, in which the increase of dosages of some medicinals can strengthen the curative effect, or the reduction of dosages of other medicinals for attenuating the effect of certain aspects to avoid toxicity and side effects; (3) modifying the preparation of the formula. The commonly used preparations of Chinese medicinal formulae include decoction, pill, powder, and paste. Generally speaking, decoctions are relatively quick in exerting a strong effect, which is applicable to acute and serious diseases, and can be modified with flexibility in clinical practice. Pills have a long absorption time, but their effect is enduring, which is applicable to chronic and deficiency diseases. In addition, it is convenient to carry pills and they can be orally consumed. They can also be used in the emergency rescue of patients. Powders can be either infused directly or decocted with water, which have some advantages of both the decoction and pill, and are relatively economical among the medicinals available. Pastes are often applied to patients with a weak constitution with prolonged illness and are also convenient for usage. Therefore, a Chinese medicinal formula can be taken in the forms of decoction, pill, powder, or paste according to different disease conditions. The preparation of a number of formulae for supplementation can be modified from decoction to pill and paste.

Decoction method

The decoction method is stressed in the use of Chinese medicinal formulae. For the choice of utensil used for decoction, it is suggested to use capped ceramic or earthenware pots. Those made of metallic materials, such as iron and aluminum, are not recommended. Before decoction, the medicinals should be soaked in the pot about 3 cm below the surface of cold water for an hour. Then, as the medicinals are drenched, decoct them over fire. After the mixture has boiled, turn the fire down to mild in case of spillage of decoction or vaporizing all the water. During the process of boiling, do not lift the cap frequently so as to prevent excessive loss of medicinal odor.

Pay attention to the control of fire for decoction. Intense and strong fire is called "*wu huo*," while low and mild fire is termed "*wen huo*" in Chinese. Usually, high flame is used first and after the decoction starts to boil, low flame is applied. After 20–30 min of boiling, extract the decoction and then add cold water for re-decoction. Repeat the procedure; the only difference is to extract the decoction after it has been boiled for 15–20 min. This method is applicable to common formulae. For formulae with aromatic medicinals in chief for inducing sweating to relieve the exterior, high flame is still applied for 3–5 min after the decoction begins to boil. For formulae for supplementation or containing some toxic medicinals (*fù zǐ, cǎo wū*, etc.) and mineral ingredients (such as *cí shí, shí gāo, biē jiǎ,* and *guī bǎn*), the decoction is extracted after it has been boiled with low flame for 45–60 min and then 30 min in the repeated procedure.

Some medicinals have special requirements in the decocting process. The major ones are listed in the following:

To be decocted first

For shells and mineral products that are solid and hard, they should be smashed and boiled in water for 20–30 min before being decocted with other medicinals.

To be added later

For aromatic medicinals such as *bò he, shā rén,* and *bái dòu kòu,* they should be added and decocted for a few minutes when the decoction of other medicinals is nearly done.

To be wrapped while decocted

For medicinals such as *huá shí, chē qián zǐ, xuán fù huā,* and *chì shí zhī* that can turn the decoction turbid or trigger irritation in the throat and stomach, they should be wrapped with gauze or silk for decoction.

To be decocted separately

For some expensive medicinals such as *rén shēn, líng yáng jiǎo,* and *shuǐ niú jiǎo,* they should be decocted separately for 2 h in order to make full use of them.

To be dissolved or melted in decoction

For some water-soluble medicinals such as *máng xiāo* and *fēng mì,* they can be dissolved in the ready-done decoction, or for some colloidal medicinals such as *ē jiāo* and *lù jiǎo jiāo,* they can be melted separately in a little amount of warm water and then mixed with the ready-done decoction. This is to prevent such medicinals from sticking to the pot when they are decocted with other medicinals lest the curative effect be affected.

To be infused

For some aromatic or expensive medicinals and some powders, pellets, and juices such as *niú huáng, shè xiāng, chén xiāng* powder, *sān qī cǎo* powder, *Zǐ Xuě Dān* (Purple Snow Elixir), fresh lotus root juice, and ginger juice, they should be infused into the ready-done decoction.

Decoction to be used as water

For medicinals with a large volume or a heavy weight such as *lú gēn, zhú rú, zào xīn tǔ,* and *nuò dào gēn xū,* they can be first decocted with water separately after which the decoction that is extracted from it is used as water to be decocted with other medicinals.

Administration of medicinals

The administration of Chinese medicinals mainly involves aspects such as time and method. Generally, the medicine should be taken in the morning and evening with an empty stomach, that is, about 1 h before breakfast and 3 h after supper. However, for medicinals that are an irritant to the gastro-intestinal tract or can make the stomach uncomfortable and queasy, they can be taken after meals. Some medicinal decoctions should be taken frequently at irregular times such as when drinking tea, while others are required to be taken at specified times. For example, the decoction for malaria should be taken 2 h before the seizure and the Cock's Crow Powder (*Jī Míng Sǎn*) should be taken cold before dawn with an empty stomach. A package of Chinese medicinals is usually decocted twice. The first and the second decoctions are mixed together for oral intake in the morning and evening. Some formulae for chronic diseases can be decocted 3 times for oral intake in the morning and evening. In such a case, two packages of this formula can be consumed for 3 days, fully utilizing the ingredients. Other formulae for acute diseases can have the first and second decoctions mixed for consumption at one time, or two packages of Chinese medicinals can be decocted for consumption in a day, to allow consumption of the decoction for 4 times in a day. This is one of the ways to strengthen or maintain the potency of medicinal effects. Furthermore, some Chinese medicinal formulae can be decocted for consumption at several times and be decocted again after the first decoction. It is advisable to consume the medicinal decoction when it is warm, but for heat-striking diseases, it can be taken cold. If the patient is liable to vomit after taking the decoction, it is recommended to rub the tongue with fresh ginger slices or add some ginger juice in the decoction before consuming the decoction.

For the application of Chinese medicinal formulae, the following aspects are noteworthy. First, it is a must to understand the patient's physique and disease condition, so as to clarify the disease pattern and ascertain the "correspondence of the formula and pattern." Next, it is necessary to be familiar with the natures, actions, and dosages of Chinese medicinals and be proficient at the medicinal-combining methods and at modifying formulae. Third, practitioners must be careful when using drastic or toxic medicinals. Usually, a small dosage is gradually increased until it is effective, but the maximum should not exceed the specified dosage to avoid poisoning and inducing side effects.

Is It Difficult to Learn to Prescribe a Chinese Medicinal Formula?

To the uninitiated, the field of Chinese medicine may seem daunting due to its ancient and profound theories encompassing numerous unique features. With abundant literatures of Chinese medicine for reference, beginners feel that it is difficult to keep up with this enigmatic field, and those who are interested in Chinese medicine may find it hard to decide if it is worth pursuing. The subject of Chinese medicine covers wide fields and requires vast knowledge. Without regular study for many years in a medical college, it is hard for one to master. It is not easy to be proficient in Chinese medicine, but it is also not difficult to have a basic knowledge of it. The theories and applications of Chinese medicine can be acquired by reading literatures of Chinese medicine written by medical experts instead of delving into fully equipped laboratories, and with the knowledge from books, one can be more adept through practice in treatment and prescribing formulae. There are bountiful examples in history and at present of those who have become famous doctors through self-study. "To learn how to prescribe Chinese medicinal formulae" in this book, under the guidance of the theories of Chinese medicine in diagnosis and treatment, the reader should discern how to apply "pattern differentiation" and the action and usage of the Chinese medicinal formula based on the "pattern," thus being competent at prescribing accurate and effective formulae. From this perspective, it is realistic to be reasonably skilled at the methods of prescription of Chinese medicinal formulae in a hundred days. Certainly however, to acquire a high level of proficiency in all aspects of Chinese medicine and the prescription of formulae would require extensive reading of Chinese medicine books and many years of experience of clinical practice.

Daily Exercises

1. What do "chief, deputy, assistant, and envoy" mean?
2. What are the key points of decocting Chinese medicinals?
3. What are the key points of consuming Chinese medicinals?

CHAPTER 2

Prescribing a Formula in Accordance with the Pattern

DAY THREE

In Accordance with the Pattern

The quality of a doctor is dependent not on his age, qualifications, appearance, or manner of speech, but on the effectiveness of the formula he prescribes for his patients. With regards to Chinese medicine, the critical indicator hinges on whether the formula prescribed is in accordance with the "pattern." This chapter will be a discussion on this issue — what does it mean by "in accordance with the pattern?"

A less experienced, or quack, doctor is capable of simply prescribing Chinese medicinal formulae, but it is difficult to determine if that formula is in accordance with the pattern. Though the disease of some patients may be cured, the curative effect is not reliable in most cases. "In accordance with the pattern" is the key in prescribing a Chinese medicinal formula, in which it denotes that the nature and action of the formula should be in accordance with the disease nature, namely the pathological state of the patient. Note that "pattern" is different from "symptom." The latter refers to the specific manifestations of the disease, such as fever, headaches, coughing, and vomiting. The former refers to the overall state of the human body, which generalizes the features of the disease nature. Therefore, it is not sufficient to prescribe a formula based only on a specific symptom and by pure memorization of some formulae; more importantly, pattern differentiation should be grasped at the initial stage. For this, a novice should study the basic theories of Chinese medicine before-hand; otherwise, mastery of analyzing disease conditions and pattern differentiation will be far out of reach.

Basic Theories

The theoretic system of Chinese medicine is extremely profound. Here, we will highlight several indispensable points for analyzing the physiological state and understanding the actions of Chinese medicinals formulae.

Yin, yang, qi, blood, and fluids

In Chinese medicine, the yin–yang concept is widely applied to physiology, pathology, pattern differentiation, treatment, and many other fields. In physiology, a substance is usually yin and its function belongs to yang, both of which are in opposition to each other but still interdependent. For instance, the physiological activity of internal organs depends on nutrients for their maintenance and the production of nutrients requires the normal functioning of various organs. Yin and yang interact with each other; if either one is too excessive or too weak, a disease is resulted. For example, a yin-cold pathogen can impair yang qi; excessive yang qi causes fever and consumes yin fluids, insufficient yin fluids will lead to the hyperactivity of yang heat, and the insufficiency of yang qi can result in yin-cold symptoms. For pattern differentiation and treatment, diseases are classified under two categories: "yin pattern" and "yang pattern," while induced medicinal action is expected to rectify yin–yang imbalance.

Qi is involved in multiple functions of the human body; an example would be visceral qi. It can also refer to some nutrients, such as *ying* qi. According to different sources, qi is classified as (1) prenatal qi, which is stored in the kidney and also called true qi or source qi; (2) postnatal qi, which is derived from food; and (3) pectoral qi, which is produced by the spleen and stomach.

Blood is the red fluid in blood vessels and is produced by the spleen and stomach with the involvement of the liver and kidney. It is then distributed by the heart and lungs to nourish the entire body.

Fluids refer to the normal fluids of the organs and tissues of the human body. Clear and loose fluids are called "liquid" and thick and turbid fluids are called "humor," both of which function to moisten the body, four limbs, and orifices. Some fluids exist in the blood vessels and become a part of blood. Sweat and urine are examples of fluids discharged from the body. Fluids also stem from digested foods and are absorbed by the spleen and stomach, sharing a common source with that of blood.

Zang–fu organs; channels and collaterals

Zang–fu organs refer to the five *zang* and six *fu* organs. It is the kernel concept of physiology in Chinese medicine, which is characterized by the classification of the main functions and body parts in accordance with the five *zang* and six *fu* organs. Though the names of the five *zang* organs are literally similar to those in modern medicine, the specific content is quite different. There is a close relation among the *zang–fu* organs, a system that constitutes the organic entity of the human body.

The five *zang* organs comprise the heart, liver, spleen, lung, and kidney. The heart is responsible for blood circulation; it governs blood and vessels, and controls the mind and mental activities. The pericardium enveloping the heart can assume functions on behalf of the heart. The liver mainly takes charge of the dredging and regulating of various body functions, assists in digestion, moderates mental activities, stores blood, and nourishes tendons. The spleen is involved in digestion, nutrient transportation, and assistance in blood flow. The lung mainly controls respiration, governs interior body qi, and assists the spleen to distribute nutrients and transport water–dampness. The kidney manages reproduction and development and the essence stored in the kidney can replenish the bone marrow and brain. It also supports the production of blood and is the main organ of the urinary system.

The five *fu* organs primarily comprise the gallbladder, stomach, small intestine, large intestine, bladder, and *sanjiao*. The gallbladder assists the liver in promoting digestion and regulation of the mind. The stomach helps the spleen to digest food. The small and large intestines assist the spleen and stomach to further digest food and form urine and feces. The bladder stores urine and controls urination. The *sanjiao* is the main passage for nutrient transportation and qi flow, and is located at the region from the thorax to the abdomen. Other organs include the brain, uterus, etc.

Channels and collaterals form a net system originating from the *zang–fu* organs and distribute throughout the whole body. They can be regarded as a functional synthesis of multiple systems of the nerves, blood vessels, lymph vessels, etc. Channels and collaterals are routes of qi and blood, and they serve as a connection among all the organs and parts of the body. In this system, there are trunks and branches. The trunk channels are the 12 regular channels, which are associated with the *zang–fu* organs, namely the hand *taiyin* lung channel, the hand *jueyin* pericardium channel, the hand *shaoyang sanjiao* channel, the foot *taiyin* spleen channel, the foot *jueyin* liver channel, the foot *shaoyin* kidney channel, the hand *yangming* large intestine channel, the hand *taiyang* small intestine channel, the foot *yangming* stomach channel, the foot *shaoyang* gallbladder channel, and the foot *taiyang* bladder channel. The eight extraordinary vessels are called trunks, including *du mai, ren mai, chong mai, dai mai, yinqiao mai, yangqiao mai, yinwei mai*, and *yangwei mai*. There are numerous branches among these trunks, such as divergent collaterals, superficial collaterals, and minute collaterals.

Theories of *zang–fu* organs, channels and collaterals, as well as qi, blood, and fluids are all weaved together to form the backbone of the physiology of Chinese medicine.

Six pathogenic factors and seven emotions

The six pathogenic factors and seven emotions are the main concepts of etiology in Chinese medicine.

The six pathogenic factors are the six factors in the natural world that can cause diseases. It is doubtless that numerous diseases caused exist in the external world, including pathogenic microorganisms (bacteria, viruses, Rickettsia, protozoon, etc.), physical factors (cold, heat, light, electricity, magnetism, etc.), and chemical factors (organic or inorganic substances). However, whatever the disease may entail, the symptoms manifested share several similarities. According to these manifestations, ancient medical experts have classified causes of disease into six factors: wind, cold, summer heat, dampness, dryness, and fire. Table 1 shows a brief summary of the characteristics of each factor.

Table 1.   Characteristics of disease causes.

Pathogenic Factor	Characteristics
Wind	• Ascent
	• Effusion
	• Going outward
	• Wandering movement
	• Shaking and trembling of the limbs
Cold	• Congealing
	• Obstruction
	• Cold limbs
	• Fear of cold
	• Contraction
Summer heat	• High fever
	• Profuse sweating
	• Qi consumption
	• Occurrence in the summer
Dampness	• Heaviness
	• Turbidity
	• Stickiness
	• Swelling limbs
	• Exudates
Dryness	• Dryness
	• Fluid consumption
Fire	• Flaming upward
	• Fluid consumption
	• Local red swellings
	• Bleeding
	• Macules

The six pathogenic factors are also called externally contracted pathogens (or external pathogens), while diseases caused by such factors are called externally contracted diseases.

The seven emotions are aspects that can cause mental disorder, which include joy, anger, grief, anxiety, sorrow, fear, and fright. This concept is in fact a generalization of various long-term mental stimulations and sudden and abrupt mental traumas. The seven emotions can directly stimulate the *zang–fu* organs and result in diseases, especially disorders of the heart, liver, spleen, and stomach.

Other factors that can lead to diseases are reasons such as improper and irregular diet, preference for certain food flavors, and overstrain, all of which together with the seven emotions are called miscellaneous diseases due to internal damage (or diseases of internal damage). In addition, disease causes such as knocks, falls, injuries, and insect and animal bites are classified under external injury.

Daily Exercises

1. What are qi, blood, and body fluids? How do they come into being?
2. What are the main functions of the five *zang* and six *fu* organs?
3. What are the six pathogenic factors? What are their respective disease characteristics?
4. What are externally contracted diseases and diseases of internal damage?

DAY FOUR

The following section will introduce the diagnostics and medicinal applications of Chinese medicine.

Four Examinations and Eight Principles

The four examinations and eight principles are the basic theories and methods of Chinese medicine in diagnosing diseases and analyzing disease conditions.

The four examinations are the main techniques applied in Chinese medicine to investigate the state of the patient. This includes inspection, auscultation and olfaction, inquiry, and palpation. *Inspection* is to observe the person's spirit, vitality, appearance, tongue condition, verious secreta, excreta, etc. *Auscultation* and *olfaction* are to identify the various sounds of the patient, such as voice, breath, and hiccup, and all types of smell such as breath odor and the odor of the secreta and excreta. *Inquiry* is to ask the patient or his family members about the disease cause and course, past illnesses, family illnesses, lifestyle habits, food preferences, and chief complaints such as an aversion to cold, a fear of cold, fever, headaches, vertigo, sweating, pain, sleep, diet, thirst, urine, stool, menstruation, and vaginal discharge. *Palpation* is to feel the pulse and apply touch and pressure to detect abnormalities. Particularly, the inspection of the tongue and feeling of pulse are the key features of diagnosis in Chinese medicine.

The eight principles are the most fundamental notions of the disease location, nature and strength of healthy qi, and pathogenic factors, namely yin, yang, exterior, interior, cold, heat, deficiency, and excess. It is a diagnostic conclusion of the data collected by the four examinations, also termed "eight-principle pattern differentiation." *Exterior* and *interior* refer to the depth of disease location. At the initial stage, the disease location is usually superficial, commonly manifested as the exterior pattern. If the exterior pattern is not relieved or lasts for a long period of time, the *zang–fu* organs and qi and blood will be in obvious disorder, in which the interior pattern will then come into play. *Cold* and *heat* refer to the nature of disease. The heat pattern is usually manifested as functional hyperactivity with symptoms of fever, thirst, a flushed face and eyes, and so on. The cold pattern is often reflected by functional hypoactivity with symptoms such as cold limbs, tastelessness in the mouth without thirst, and loose stool. *Deficiency* and *excess* refer to the state of healthy qi and pathogenic factors. The deficiency pattern includes yin deficiency, yang deficiency, qi deficiency, blood deficiency, and weakness of the *zang-fu* organs, which reflects the obvious insufficiency of healthy qi. The excess pattern is described by the retention of fire–heat exuberance, phlegm–rheum, water–dampness, static blood, food accumulation, feces, etc. The above six principles can be combined into diseases characterized by both the exterior and interior, half-exterior and half-interior. exterior cold, interior cold, exterior heat, interior heat, exterior cold and interior heat, exterior heat and interior cold, upper heat and lower cold, upper cold and lower heat, true cold with false heat, true heat with false cold, deficiency–excess complex, true deficiency with false excess, true excess with false deficiency, deficiency–cold, deficiency–heat, excess–cold, and excess–heat. The principles of yin and yang are a summary of the other six principles. The exterior, heat, and excess belong to yang, while the interior, cold, and deficiency pertain to yin. Traditionally, the yang pattern refers to the excess–heat pattern and the yin pattern to the deficiency–cold pattern.

Six Channels, *Wei*, Qi, *Ying*, and Blood

The six channels, *wei,* qi, *ying*, and blood are guidelines for pattern differentiation of external contraction. In other words, they are methods to analyze and sort out various symptoms of external contraction according to the interior rules.

The six channels are the channels of *taiyang, yangming, shaoyang, taiyin, shaoyin,* and *jueyin,* which can be used to generalize the rules of development and various patterns of externally contracted diseases. *Taiyang* syndrome is an exterior pattern occurring after the invasion of an exogenous wind–cold pathogen, which is characterized by fever, an aversion to cold, a floating pulse, etc. *Yangming* syndrome occurs as the pathogens attack the interior, and the healthy qi contends severely with these foreign invaders, which is at the peak stage of struggle between exuberant pathogens and vigorous healthy qi, and is characterized by drastic heat and fluid consumption. *Shaoyang* syndrome refers to the contest between healthy qi and pathogenic qi, taking place between the exterior and interior, which causes the internal exuberance of gallbladder fire and ascending counterflow of stomach qi, and is characterized by alternating chills and fever, a bitter taste in the mouth, a dry throat, and a wiry pulse. *Taiyin* syndrome results from spleen yang deficiency and internal obstruction of cold–damp, which is characterized by abdominal fullness, vomiting, diarrhea, a pale tongue with a white coating, and a slow or moderate pulse. *Shaoyin* syndrome indicates the late stage of disease with a weak heart and kidney yang qi and poor functions, where its symptoms include cold limbs, mental fatigue, a cold appearance, clear and profuse urine, a pale tongue, and a deep and fine pulse. *Jueyin* syndrome is commonly seen also in the late stage of disease with the exhaustion of healthy qi and lingering pathogens that are manifested as a complex of cold and heat and a complex of deficiency and excess, and is characterized by thirst, a rush of rising qi to the heart, heat and pain in the heart, cold limbs and diarrhea, and vomiting.

Wei, qi, *ying*, and blood are the four main levels of warm diseases. The initial attachment of pathogenic factors on the body surface is termed *wei* level pattern. If the pathogenic factors further enter the *zang–fu* organs, they will trigger an intense struggle between the healthy qi and pathogenic factors, and exuberant heat will surface and lead to the disorder of visceral qi movement. This is termed qi level pattern. If the patient's condition deteriorates and the *ying* level and heart are influenced, rendering mental disorder and a sprinkle of macules on the skin, it is called *ying* level pattern. If the *ying* level pattern continues to worsen and becomes more serious such that macules occur in a large area and bleeding is present in the mouth, nose, urine, and stool, it is considered as a blood level pattern.

Sanjiao here refers to the classification of the *zang–fu* organs into upper, middle, and lower sections, but not as a *fu* organ. Upper *jiao* disorders include diseases of the lung and pericardium (heart), middle *jiao* disorders consist of diseases of the spleen, stomach, and large intestine, and lower *jiao* disorders comprise diseases of the liver and kidney.

Four Natures and Five Flavors

The four natures and the five flavors are important principles about the natures of Chinese medicinals.

The four natures refer to the cold, hot, warm, and cool natures of Chinese medicinals. The hot and warm natures belong to yang with the former being more drastic, while the cold and cool pertain to yin with the former being stronger. It is an important theory in Chinese medicine that the medicinal hot or cold nature is used to rectify the cold or hot state caused by the disease. The cold, hot, warm, and cool natures of medicinals are deduced from their actions on the body to rectify cold and hot states. Cold- and cool-natured medicinals are able to remedy yang exuberance or aggravate yang weakness, while warm- and hot-natured medicinals can relieve cold symptoms or activate yang qi.

The five flavors are the acrid, sweet, sour, bitter, and salty tastes of Chinese medicinals. The acrid flavor has strong dispersing and ventilating functions and is indicated for the obstruction of pores and inhibited flows of qi and blood. The bitter flavor is dry in nature and able to drain dampness, subdue fire, or bring down qi flow, which is indicated for damp retention, flaming fire, or the rising counterflow of qi. The sweet flavor is supplementary and able to relieve cramps, which is indicated for various patterns of deficiency, cramps, and pain. The sour flavor is to astringe and indicated for the outflow of fluids and qi, night sweating, spontaneous sweating, chronic coughs and diarrhea, seminal emission, and enuresis. The salty flavor softens hardness; hence, it is indicated for tumors, masses, constipation, etc. Aside from the five flavors, there are also the bland and astringent flavors. The bland flavor mainly promotes urination, while the astringent flavor is used to restrain a substance from leaking. The five flavors illustrate medicinal actions and specify the existing close relationship between flavor and action. However, medicinal action is not totally inferred from the flavor; it is generalized by its curative effect on the human body. Therefore, the action of some medicinals is not in accordance with the flavor.

A combination of the four natures and five flavors can comprehensively reflect medicinal natures and actions. For example, *huáng lián* is cold and bitter. As the cold clears heat and the bitterness dries dampness and subdues fire, it has the function of clearing heat, drying dampness, and subduing fire. Take *má huáng*, which is warm and acrid, for another example. As the warmth dispels coldness and the acridity functions to disperse and ventilate, it has the function of dispersing wind–cold and ventilating lung qi.

Ascending and Descending, Floating and Sinking

The theory of ascending and descending, floating and sinking is to illustrate the tendency of the effect of Chinese medicinals. Regardless of the disorder, there will be different disease locations in the superior, inferior, exterior, and interior as well as different disease tendencies such as rising counterflow and downward sinking. The medicinal action targets the disease to bring down rising counterflow or raise downward sinking.

Ascending refers to the medicinal effect that can lift and raise, which is indicated for gastroptosis, uterine prolapse, and rectocele due to chronic diarrhea. *Descending* refers to the medicinal effect that can promote descent and check counterflow, which is indicated for the rising counterflow of visceral qi, such as panting, vomiting, and hiccups. *Floating* denotes the medicinal effect that can flow upward and disperse, which is indicated for diseases in the exterior and upper parts of the body. *Sinking* refers to the medicinal effect that can flow downward and promote urination and defecation, which is indicated for diseases in the interior and lower parts of the body, such as constipation, inhibited urination, and edema.

The ascending and descending, floating and sinking actions of medicinals are related to their natures and textures. The ascending and floating medicinals, usually acrid, sweet, warm, and hot, are flowers and leaves with a light texture, while the descending and sinking medicinals, often bitter, sour, salty, cold, and cool, are seeds, minerals, and shells. In addition, the ascending and descending, floating and sinking actions of medicinals are related to medicinal processing. For instance, the medicinal tends to descend if processed by salt, disperse by ginger, astringe by vinegar, and float by wine.

Daily Exercises

1. What are the eight principles?
2. What are the theories of the six channels, *wei*, qi, *ying*, blood, and *sanjiao*?
3. What are the indications of the four natures, five flavors, and theory of ascending and descending, floating and sinking?

DAY FIVE

The "Pattern" in Chinese Medicine

We have mentioned in the previous section that the main characteristic of Chinese medicinals for treatment lies in "treatment according to pattern differentiation." The prerequisite to prescription is to discern the "pattern," with some pattern names also highlighted, such as the exterior cold pattern and interior heat pattern. What then is "pattern?" What is the relation between "pattern" and the effects of medicinal formulae?

"Pattern" refers to the general state of the patient, which includes pathological changes and corresponding clinical manifestations of the disease, which lead to a diagnostic conclusion to the disease nature. The pattern is the consequence of the struggle between healthy qi and pathogenic factors and is always in a dynamic state, although it may be stable at certain stages. The realm of pattern can be wide or narrow, or general or detailed. For example, the heat pattern, cold pattern, deficiency pattern, and excess pattern are general classifications, under which there may be many detailed sub-patterns. The heat pattern can be further divided into the exterior heat pattern and interior heat pattern. The interior heat pattern can be subdivided into heat exuberance in the qi level pattern, blood heat pattern, heat in the heart pattern, liver heat pattern, spleen heat pattern, lung heat pattern, kidney heat pattern, gallbladder heat pattern, stomach heat pattern, small intestine heat pattern, large intestine heat pattern, bladder heat pattern, *sanjiao* heat pattern, etc. The above patterns can be even further categorized. Take stomach heat for example. It can be classified into invisible heat exuberance (*yangming* channel syndrome) and visible heat bind (*yangming* bowel syndrome). Therefore, the classification of patterns in Chinese medicine is highly elaborate and can intricately reflect a specific disease nature.

Pattern Differentiation and Pattern

The idea of pattern differentiation is to first identify the general pattern and then further specify the most detailed. The establishment of pattern is in fact the accomplishment of the diagnosis, analysis, and exploration of the essence of the disease. As soon as the pattern is determined, the treatment principles and methods are subsequently established with the corresponding medicinal formula for administration. For example, through examination and analysis, the exuberance of stomach heat may be diagnosed as the disease pattern of a patient, thus the treatment method recommended by the practitioner would surely be to purge stomach heat and the formula applied would undoubtedly be *Bái Hǔ Tāng* (White Tiger

Decoction). From this scenario, to identify the pattern of the disease nature is the prerequisite to the application of the medicinal formula. In order to be adept at the technique of prescribing formulae, the key is to master the method of discerning patterns — the most fundamental and specific disease state of the patient. On such a basis, the beginner should be familiar with treatment methods and the corresponding actions of the formulae, and thereafter, an appropriate formula can be accurately selected to rectify the pathological condition. If the formula is not fully in accordance with the pattern, it can be modified by adding and removing medicinals as well as by increasing and decreasing dosages to fit the pattern. This is, in summary, the schematic to determine treatment based on pattern differentiation. Once achieved, one would have passed the entrance gate and gained admittance to the world of Chinese medicine.

Disease and Pattern

Patterns in Chinese medicine are tremendously complex. Clinically, each disease has several patterns. Some diseases have three to five patterns, while others have more than 10. Therefore, it is a monumental task for one to be equipped with every one of these patterns in mind. However, among the numerous patterns, some are fundamental or common, where they occur in various diseases. In other words, many diseases can present some identical patterns, indicating similar clinical manifestations and the application of treatment methods and formulae. In this book, these common patterns and related formulae will be introduced. One ought to know these patterns well, because they can be widely applied to various diseases of internal medicine, external medicine, gynecology, pediatrics, etc., thus laying a solid foundation for the further study of many clinical fields.

How to Differentiate Patterns

Pattern differentiation is the art of synthesizing and analyzing the clinical data collected by the four examinations to reveal the nature of the disease. The goal is to collect as much disease data as possible, including symptoms, disease course, previous treatment, causes, physique, living environment, lifestyle habits and addictions, and climates. Meanwhile, it is necessary to exclude false manifestations and seek the root cause by analyzing external conditions. For example, fever and thirst are symptoms of the heat pattern, but thirst without any desire for drinking or with a preference for drinking hot water, and clear and profuse urine indicate true cold with false heat. An overall analysis using the concept of holism should also be stressed in pattern differentiation. It requires grasping the primary aspect, especially for the determination of a pattern, during which attention should be given to the main symptoms. In addition, as the disease course is dynamic, the pattern of a disease is not stable. The pattern purely reveals the characteristics of the disease at a certain stage. A good example is an externally contracted febrile disease, whose change is so rapid and diverse that several patterns can emerge in a single day. The concept of the dynamic change of disease is important to the diagnosis and treatment of a disease, from which a practitioner can also improve his medical technology.

Daily Exercises

1. What are "pattern" and "symptom?"
2. What is the meaning of deciding a pattern?
3. What are the main strategies in differentiating patterns?

DAY SIX

Techniques for Prescribing a Chinese Medicinal Formula

To prescribe a formula in accordance with the disease pattern, it requires not only the correct determination of the pattern in the first place, but also several techniques.

Formulae based on treatment methods

There is a myriad of patterns in Chinese medicine and usually, several formulae can be applied to one pattern, both of which add exponentially to the difficulty in learning. A possible solution is to group these patterns and formulae. In Chinese medicine, the formulae are classified into eight groups according to their effects. This are the so-called "eight methods." There are eight treatment methods, which include sweat promotion, vomit induction, purgation, harmonization, warming, heat-clearing, dispersing, and supplementation. Sweat promotion is to induce sweating by scattering the skin and exterior, and is indicated for exterior patterns. Vomit induction is to stimulate vomiting for the elimination of phlegm–drool retained in the throat and stomach, food retention, or poisonous substances. Purgation is to promote defecation for food retention in the intestines, dry stool, biding phlegm, water retention, static blood, etc. Harmonization involves the synchronization of cold and heat in the interior and exterior, indicated for the half-exterior and half-interior pattern. Warming is to apply warm and hot medicinals for warming and supplementing yang qi, expelling pathogenic cold, and warming and unblocking channels and collaterals. Heat-clearing is to apply cold and cool medicinals for clearing pathogenic heat and restraining exuberant yang qi. Dispersing is the application of medicinals that can promote digestion, remove stagnation, resolve phlegm, move water, rectify qi, invigorate blood, and disperse masses for the elimination of masses caused by food, stagnation, phlegm, water, qi, and blood. Supplementation is to use nourishing and reinforcing medicinals for the deficiency of yin and yang, qi and blood, body fluids, *zang–fu* organs, and so on. Each of the eight methods can be further divided into more specific methods. For example, heat-clearing can be subdivided into clearing heat from the qi level, cooling the blood, clearing heart heat and opening the orifices, clearing heat and extinguishing wind, etc. Moreover, clearing heat from the qi level can be further categorized into clearing the qi level with acrid–cold medicinals and clearing the qi level with bitter–cold medicinals. These treatment methods are paired with corresponding patterns and each method has several parallel formulae for selection. Clinically, the treatment method is set according to the pattern, which is fixed. However, for the selection of formulae, medicinal ingredients, and medicinal dosage, there is great flexibility only if it is derived from the treatment method.

In addition, for the specific application of the eight methods, the methods can be interrelated. For instance, under the circumstance of cold and heat in complexity, supplementation can be combined with sweat promotion, purgation, dispersion, and clearing of heat; purgation can be combined with warming, clearing of heat, and dispersion; and warming can be combined with clearing of heat. All the medicinal formulae introduced in this book can be classified according to the eight methods. In this way, the reader is easily able to acquire and understand the main points of the formulae in study and application.

Main symptoms and main medicinals

Each pattern has a series of symptoms and each formula consists of several, or sometimes even more than 10, medicinal ingredients. Therefore, it is difficult to commit all of them to memory in a short span of time. For a novice, this book not only records verses of principal formulae for the convenience of memorization, but also stresses the main symptoms and medicinals. Though a pattern consists of many symptoms, there are some key characteristics — the main symptoms. For example, the main symptoms of the exterior excess–cold pattern are a severe aversion to cold, mild fever, and the absence of sweating and thirst; the main symptoms of the half-exterior and half-interior pattern are alternating chills and fever, a bitter taste in the mouth, and rib-side pain; and the main symptoms of the exuberant lung heat pattern are fever, cough with yellow and sticky sputum, and panting. A pattern can be easily determined according to the main symptoms observed, so it is not necessary to memorize all the symptoms of a pattern. Meanwhile, in a medicinal formula, there are certain ingredients that are of the leading role, which are primarily the main medicinals of this formula. For example, the main medicinals of *Guì Zhī Tāng* (Cinnamon Twig Decoction) are *guì zhī* and *sháo yào*; the main medicinals of *Bái Hǔ Tāng* (White Tiger Decoction) are *shí gāo* and *zhī mǔ*; and the main medicinals of *Xiǎo Chái Hú Tāng* (Minor Bupleurum Decoction) are *chái hú* and *huáng qín*. To be proficient in such main medicinals adds to the convenience of memorizing medicinal formulae, especially those containing lots of ingredients. This is also very useful in the application of formulae on the basis of main medicinals, where other medicinals can be added with flexibility according to the principles of formula composition.

Focusing on the main symptoms and medicinals is essentially the strategy to determine a pattern and the combination of medicinal ingredients.

By understanding this, one will gradually be able to apply other formulae with great dexterity.

Principles of medicinal selection

Following the determination of the pattern and formula, the practitioner can then prescribe the medicinal ingredients accordingly. Beginners usually apply established formulae mechanically and do not quite know how to modify them according to differing symptoms. They may also combine medicinals at random. Naturally, it is not absolutely wrong to use established formulae and sometimes, relatively acceptable curative effects can be achieved by administering established formulae for typical patterns. However, in most cases, the manifestations of a pattern always appear with some features, which require modification of the medicinal ingredients and dosages of the established formula so as to gear the formula toward being better in accordance with the disease condition. For those who randomly prescribe medicinal ingredients and as a result, treat patients poorly, it is due to their lack of knowledge on the nature of the disease. These haphazardly composed formulae may include only several medicinals according to some symptoms; formulae without the combination of principles and treatment centers; and formulae with dozens of medicinal ingredients even for a mild disease such as the common cold, which are not only a waste of medicinals and financial resources, but excessive randomly combined medicinals can often cause inhibition and counteraction. There are also some practitioners who blindly increase medicinal dosages for the purpose of enhancing curative effects. In actual fact, the curative effect is not definitely related to the dosage. Rather, it is dependent on the treatment according to the pattern. Usually, a low dosage of medicinals can remedy very serious diseases only if they are applied in accordance with the pattern that is accurately diagnosed. On the other hand, too low a dosage can also affect the curative effect.

Generally, it is taboo in Chinese medicine to enhance the curative effect by applying more medicinals or increasing the dosages instead of focusing on pattern differentiation. In the course of prescribing a formula, it is better to use less medicinals and to focus on the more essential aspects. On the premise of determining a pattern according to the main symptoms, the principle of composing a formula is to first select the main medicinals. A practitioner must understand that for a complicated disease, attention must be duly paid to the main pathological changes and the disease must be treated step by step, so that each medicinal can solve certain problems and attenuate other kinds of pain. It is impossible to use a single formula for all the problems of a complicated disease. While the hope is certainly to treat all of them, the reality is that nothing can be cured. Either the practitioner or the patient should know this. Indeed, for a simple and typical pattern, a novice would be able to cure the disease by applying a single formula only if pattern differentiation is correctly carried out.

Written Form of a Chinese Medicinal Formula

Traditional medicinal formulae are usually associated with specific medical cases. Medical cases are records of the following items: disease cause, symptoms, pathological analysis, diagnostic conclusion, treatment principle, formula, cautions, etc. In modern times, with the availability of medical records for noting related issues in treatment, it is only necessary to list the medicinal name, dosage, processing requirement, packs and method of preparing the decoction, and route of consumption. Other information to be recorded includes the name, gender, and age of the patient, and the date of the prescription. As for the positioning of written medicinal names, it is recommended to properly align them and add the dosages behind each name. At present, the unit for dosage is in grams (g) and sometimes, processing requirements are attached. The writing should be clear and legible. Not only does it demonstrate sincerity and whether the practitioner is serious in his occupation, but it also helps the pharmacist to collect the required medicinals efficiently.

The written form of Chinese medicinal formulae consists of two styles: the horizontal style and the vertical style. Their contents are basically similar, but the latter has a strong traditional flavor, in which numbers and dosage are written in Chinese characters. Examples of the two written forms of formulae are given below.

Horizontal style

Mr. Zhang, male, age 35.

guì zhī 3 g; *bái sháo* 12 g; *zhì gān cǎo* 4 g;

raw *mǔ lì* (crushed and decocted first) 15 g; raw *lóng gǔ* (crushed and decocted first) 12 g;

lù dǎng shēn 6 g; black *fù piàn* 5 g; *dà zǎo* 5 pieces;

shēng jiāng 2 slices.

3 packs

(Signature:)

Year/Month/Day

Vertical style

年	签 5包	大	精	木	砂	白	炙	干	党	45	女	陈
/		棗	米	香	仁	术	甘	姜	参	岁		小
月		(碎)	(干煎)	1 钱	(碎)	(焦)	草	(炮)	3 钱*			姐
/		3 片	3 钱		1钱	3 钱	1 钱	1 钱				
日												

*One 钱 (*qiǎn*) is equivalent to about 3g.

Translation (from right to left):

Ms. Chen, female, age 45.

dǎng shēn 9 g; blast-fried *gān jiāng* 3 g;

zhì gān cǎo 3 g; scorched *bái zhú* 9 g;

crushed *shā rén* (added later) 3 g; *mù xiāng* 3 g;

jīng mǐ (dry-fried until yellow) 9 g; crushed *dà zǎo* 3 pieces.

5 packs

(Signature:)

Year/Month/Day

Daily Exercises

1. What are the eight methods and the concept of prescribing "formulae based on treatment methods?"
2. What are the key points to formula composition?
3. What contents are included in an integral formula?

THE 2ND WEEK

CHAPTER 3

The Exterior Pattern

DAY ONE

The exterior pattern refers to a disease pattern manifested as exterior symptoms after an attack of exogenous pathogenic factors. It usually occurs at the initial stage of an externally contracted disease and its location and symptoms mainly reside within the body surface, while there is only very mild or no disorder in the internal organs. The external pattern is reflected on the entire body surface, which is different from local lesions such as sores and tinea.

Features of the Exterior Pattern

The symptoms of the external pattern are massive in number, but there are some special symptoms, such as fever, an aversion to cold or wind, headaches, nasal congestion, body aches, and a common tongue coating (usually thin and white). Particularly, an aversion to cold and fever are the core symptoms. In addition, the following aspects can be taken into account: quick onset, and at the initial stage, there is seldom a disorder of internal organs besides coughing or vomiting.

The Exterior Pattern and the Common Cold

It is not difficult to recognize an exterior pattern, because almost everyone would have experienced it at some point in their lives. The most common cases are the common cold and flu, symptoms of which are a reflection of the exterior pattern. However, the exterior pattern is not equivalent to the common cold, as it not only exists in the common cold, but is also at the initial stage of many acute contagious diseases, such as measles, epidemic cerebrospinal meningitis, diphtheritis, pneumonia, rheumatic fever, acute nephritis, and acute urinary tract infection. On the other hand, the common cold, especially flu, sometimes presents severe vomiting and diarrhea, and a few cases can be complicated by pneumonia, a condition that no longer belongs to a pure exterior pattern.

Although the identification of the exterior pattern is relatively easy, it is not so in the case of determining the disease that causes this pattern. Even an experienced practitioner may occasionally diagnose several acute infectious diseases as the common cold by mistake because of their similar initial symptoms. Therefore, when we encounter a patient with the exterior pattern, we should not handle the case lightly just because the symptoms are mild, and we should never unsystematically draw a diagnosis of the common cold. Instead, we should examine carefully and, when necessary, order auxiliary examinations, such as a routine blood test, urine test, stool test, or chest X-ray, for the purpose of a definite diagnosis.

Categories of the Exterior Pattern

Many diseases can present the exterior pattern and exterior patterns of a disease may also be different due to the close relation with climate and physique. Methods to classify the exterior pattern are numerous, resulting in many different names. According to the nature of external pathogenic factors, the exterior pattern can be classified as the exterior cold pattern, exterior heat pattern, exterior dampness pattern, and exterior dryness pattern. According to the strength of *wei*–yang in the body surface that functions to resist the attack of external pathogens, the exterior pattern can be classified as the exterior excess pattern and exterior deficiency pattern. If the qi of *wei*–yang is abundant, sweat pores are secure, resulting in no sweating and a forceful pulse; this belongs to the exterior excess pattern. If the qi of *wei*–yang is insufficient, sweat pores are loose, leading to profuse sweating and a slow and feeble pulse; this belongs to the exterior deficiency pattern. Combinations of the above two kinds of classifications give rise to other patterns such as exterior deficiency–cold, exterior excess–cold, exterior wind–heat, exterior cold–dampness, exterior wind–dampness, exterior cool–dryness, and exterior warm–dryness.

Although patients with the exterior pattern are not very few, in addition to the appreciation of the classification of the exterior pattern, there are many cases that are complicated with both exterior and interior patterns. In other words, some diseases not only have symptoms of the exterior pattern, but also present significant disorders in the internal organs, a pattern denoted as a disease involving both the exterior and interior.

Treatment Methods of the Exterior Pattern

The key method to treat a disease with the exterior pattern is to relieve the exterior. This is done through scattering the external pathogenic factors, stressing that the technique to treat the exterior pathogen is "to scatter." Specifically, to relieve the exterior comprises many aspects, among which the promotion of sweating is an important factor. By means of the promotion of sweating, on one hand, it can reduce the body temperature by regulating the temperature center of the body, dilating skin vessels to strengthen blood circulation of the body surface, promoting discharge of the sweat glands, and speeding up heat dissipation. On the other hand, it can boost the body's immune system to inhibit or eliminate pathogens and expel toxins. Through these processes, the disease may be very likely cured at the stage of the exterior pattern. From this perspective, the effects of stimulating sweat discharge and subduing fever through releasing the exterior are achieved via many mechanisms, which is most unlike diaphoretics and antipyretics in Western medicine.

As there are many exterior patterns, the specific method of relieving the exterior varies among them, such as by using acrid–warm medicinals to release the flesh and using acrid–cool medicinals to disperse cold, resolve dampness, and moisten dryness. For the pattern involving both the exterior and interior, methods include treating the exterior before the interior, treating the interior before the exterior, and treating the exterior and interior simultaneously.

Daily Exercises

1. Illustrate the diagnostic criteria of the exterior pattern.
2. Is the exterior pattern the same as the common cold? Why or why not?
3. What does it mean by "to relieve the exterior?" What is its function?

DAY TWO

The Exterior Excess–Cold Pattern

The exterior excess–cold pattern occurs when the obstruction of sweat pores and body surface is resulted from the attack of exogenous wind–cold pathogens. This pattern usually exists in the initial stage of the common cold, flu, lobar pneumonia, and rheumatic disease, and is especially prevalent in patients with a strong physique.

Diagnosis

The main symptoms and indications of this pattern are an aversion to cold with fever, absence of sweating, headaches, body aches, and a tight and strong floating pulse. Other observable characteristics may include lumbar pain, joint pain, shortness of breath with mild panting, coughing, chest oppression and fullness, a stuffy nose, sneezing, an runny nose, an absence of thirst, and a red tongue with a thin and white coating.

An aversion to cold is a significant and vital symptom, where the patient would usually wear thick clothes or heavy sheets, and fervently attempt to keep warm. There may be goose bumps or even chills. Fever usually occurs after the aversion to cold and is moderate, typically below 38.5°C. A classic case is that even though the patient experiences fever, he feels cold in general instead of hot. The absence of sweating is also a critical symptom, which is an important indicator of the obstruction of sweat pores. The diagnosis of an exterior excess–cold pattern will be incorrect if sweating is observed. For pain in the head, body, lumbar region, and joints, they usually manifest as tight and uncomfortable, but seldom acute and unbearable. The absence of thirst and a red tongue signifies that this is not a heat pattern and the body fluids have not been impaired, differentiating it from an exterior heat pattern as fundamental evidence. A thin and white tongue coating without grease and turbidity can be distinguished from fever, an aversion to cold, headaches, and body pains caused by pathogenic dampness within the body surface. Though the exterior excess– cold pattern is a disorder involving the body surface, Chinese medicine believes that the lung is connected to the skin and body hair. The exterior pathogen can easily influence the lung and usually enters the bronchi and lungs through the respiratory tract. Therefore, coughing is a common symptom, and sometimes even chest oppression and fullness and panting may be experienced. However, these symptoms are not serious and not characteristic, thus if they are not present, the diagnosis of an exterior excess–cold pattern may still be valid.

Treatment method

Inducing sweating to relieve the exterior.

Formula and ingredients: *Má Huáng Tāng (Ephedra Decoction)*

Má huáng (Herba Ephedrae) 9 g; *guì zhī* (Ramulus Cinnamomi) 6 g; *xìng rén* (Semen Armeniacae Amarum) 9 g; *zhì gān cǎo* (Radix et Rhizoma Glycyrrhizae Praeparata cum Melle) 3 g.

Formula verse

Use *guì zhī* in *Má Huáng Tāng*, and also *xìng rén* and *gān cǎo*. For fever, an aversion to cold, and nape pain, and also coughing and panting without sweating.

Usage

First, decoct *má huáng* in 1.8 L of water. Remove the foam on the surface and add the other ingredients when 400 mL of water have vaporized. Filter the dregs until 500 mL of the decoction are left. Take 160 mL of the decoction orally when it is warm. After that, cover the body with sheets. It is advisable to induce slight sweating all over the body. If the fever recedes and the disease is significantly relieved after perspiration, do not take the decoction again. If perspiration does not occur, take the decoction again while it is warm.

Analysis

In the formula, *má huáng*, being a principal herb, opens sweat pores, promotes sweating, and disperses cold. *Guì zhī* warms and unblocks yang qi, which can strengthen the function of *má huáng* to promote sweating and also remit body pains. *Xìng rén* diffuses and lowers lung qi, and when combined with the lung-diffusing and calming *má huáng*, it is an excellent treatment for coughing, panting, and chest fullness. *Gān cǎo* harmonizes the actions of all the medicinals in this formula, which serves to contain the dispersing property of *má huáng* and *guì zhī*, and also to reduce their dryness. Integrated as a whole, though there are only a few ingredients, the curative effect is exponential and it is a classic representative of formulae for releasing the exterior with acrid–warm medicinals.

According to modern pharmacological researches, *Má Huáng Tāng* is strong in stimulating sweating and relieving fever. *Má huáng, guì zhī*, and *gān cǎo* can inhibit the flu virus. *Má huáng* can relieve bronchial spasms to induce smooth breathing. *Guì zhī* can both enhance pain tolerance and relax blood vessels, hence it alleviates headaches and body pains. *Xìng rén* restrains the respiratory center to relieve coughing.

Treatment reference

Má Huáng Tāng is indicated for patients with a strong physique after catching a cold which presents an acute onset. Patients demonstrate an obvious aversion to cold or even chills, headaches, body pains, and an absence of sweating, or after being treated by diaphoretic and antipyretic medications with unsmooth sweating and sequential manifestations of an aversion to cold, an absence of sweating, a lack of thirst, accompanied by cough, an itchy throat, and rough urgent breathing. In addition, this formula is applicable to the exterior excess–wind–cold pattern of pneumonia at the early stage, bronchitis, bronchial asthma, and rheumatic disease. For acute rhinitis and allergic rhinitis with manifestations of nasal congestion, loose nasal discharge, frequent sneezing, an aversion to cold, headaches, and an absence of thirst, this formula can also be prescribed. This formula may also be used to treat enuresis in young children, epilepsy, conjunctivitis, and nephritis at the initial stage with facial and body edema.

In clinical practice, if the exterior pattern is mild, but coughing and panting are evident, *guì zhī* is removed from this formula, after which it becomes *Sān Ào Tāng* (Rough and Ready Three Decoction). If the clinical manifestations includes an aversion to cold with fever, fever, cold sweat, wheezing and panting, phlegm rales, a reluctance to speak, difficulty in breathing, and an inability to lie flat, add *shēng jiāng* and *bàn xià*. If coughing frequently occurs and there is whitish sputum, chest fullness, and distress, add *chuān pò*. If pain in the muscles and bones is significant due to wind–cold attacking the exterior, add *wēi líng xiān*, *xī xiān cǎo*, and *qín jiāo*.

For the exterior excess–cold pattern, several other formulae able to relieve the exterior with acrid–warm medicinals can also be applied. For example, for a few exterior excess–cold patterns, especially those of acute infectious diseases (pneumonia, bacillary dysentery, etc.), even though the initial manifestations belong to the exterior excess–cold pattern, it is not advisable to prescribe *Má Huáng Tāng*, while *Jīng Fáng Bài Dú Sǎn* (Schizonepeta and Saposhnikovia Toxin-Resolving Powder) is an option. If the exterior excess–cold pattern is mild, *Jiā Wèi Xiāng Sū Sǎn* (Supplemented Cyperus and Perilla Powder) is recommended, especially for women in their menstrual period with the common cold of the exterior excess–wind–cold pattern. For a common mild exterior excess–wind–cold pattern, *Cōng Chǐ Tāng* (Scallion and Fermented Soybean Decoction) can also be used. Besides, certain Chinese patent medicines, such as *Wǔ Shí Chá* (Noon Tea), can also be prescribed.

Cautions

Má Huáng Tāng takes effect by promoting sweating, but profuse sweating must be prevented, or yang qi will inevitably be impaired. After sweating occurs, promptly dry any moisture and avoid catching wind–cold again. Do not take raw, cold, and greasy food during the medication period. For fever of the exterior excess–wind–cold pattern, it is inappropriate to bring down the fever by using a cold compress. *Má Huáng Tāng* is potent in inducing sweating, so it is not indicated for the exterior pattern with spontaneous sweating, a weak physique, sores and ulcers, hematemesis, epistaxis, bloody stool, or a bleeding tendency. Otherwise, profuse sweating can consume excessive fluids and yang qi, resulting in harmful consequences such as the stimulation of pathogenic heat or repeated bleeding episodes.

Daily Exercises

1. How can the exterior excess–cold pattern be diagnosed?
2. What are the ingredients of *Má Huáng Tāng*? What are its indications?
3. Mr. Chen is a 31-year-old male. He drove for more than 15 km in a hurry in a blizzard yesterday evening. The next day, he showed symptoms and signs of an aversion to cold, headaches, an absence of sweating, nausea, a normal tongue with a thin and white coating, and a floating and tight pulse. Please prescribe a Chinese medicinal formula for this case.

Additional Formulae

Sān Ào Tāng (Rough and Ready Three Decoction)

Má huáng (Herba Ephedrae) without nodes; *xìng rén* (Semen Armeniacae Amarum) with skin and ends; non-fried *gān cǎo* (Radix et Rhizoma Glycyrrhizae).

The above ingredients are in equal amounts and grounded into a rough powder. Take 15 g of the mixed powder each time for decoction with 400 mL of water and 5 pieces of ginger. Remove the dregs after 250 mL of fluid are left. Take the decoction and cover the body with sheets to induce mild sweating.

Actions

Diffusing the lung and relieving the exterior.

Indications

For the common cold caused by pathogenic wind with nasal congestion, a heavy body, vague voice, headaches, dizzy vision, curled limbs, coughing, massive sputum, chest fullness, and shortness of breath.

Jīng Fáng Bài Dú Sǎn (Schizonepeta and Saposhnikovia Toxin-Resolving Powder)

Qiāng huó (Rhizoma et Radix Notopterygii); *dú huó* (Radix Angelicae Pubescentis); *chái hú* (Radix Bupleuri); *qián hú* (Radix Peucedani); *zhǐ qiào* (Fructus Aurantii); *fú líng* (Poria); *jīng jiè* (Herba Schizonepetae); *fáng fēng* (Radix Saposhnikoviae); *jié gěng* (Radix Platycodonis); *chuān xiōng* (Rhizoma Chuanxiong), 5 g, respectively; *gān cǎo* (Radix et Rhizoma Glycyrrhizae) 2 g. Add water to decoct.

Actions

Inducing sweating to relieve the exterior and resolving toxins to arrest pain.

Indications

For the initial stage of dysentery and sores with an aversion to cold with fever, absence of sweating, absence of thirst, and a thin and white tongue coating.

Jiā Wèi Xiāng Sū Sǎn (Supplemented Cyperus and Perilla Powder)

Zǐ sū yè (Folium Perillae) 5 g; *chén pí* (Pericarpium Citri Reticulatae) 4 g; *xiāng fù* (Rhizoma Cyperi) 4 g; *zhì gān cǎo* (Radix et Rhizoma Glycyrrhizae Praeparata cum Melle) 2 g; *jīng jiè* (Herba Schizonepetae) 3 g; *qín jiāo* (Radix Saposhnikoviae) 3 g; *fáng fēng* (Radix Saposhnikoviae) 3 g; *màn jǐng zǐ* (Fructus Viticis) 3 g; *chuān xiōng* (Rhizoma Chuanxiong) 1.5 g; ginger 3 pieces. Add water to decoct and after taking the decoction, cover the body with sheets to induce mild sweating.

Actions

Inducing sweating to relieve the exterior.

Indications

For the seasonal common cold with headaches, a stiff nape, nasal congestion, nasal discharge, body pain, fever, an aversion to cold or aversion to wind, an absence of sweating, a thin and white tongue coating, and a floating pulse.

Cōng Chǐ Tāng (Scallion and Fermented Soybean Decoction)

Cōng bái (Bulbus Allii Fistulosi) 3 pieces; *dàn dòu chǐ* (Semen Sojae Praeparatum) 6 g. Add water to decoct until 200 mL of fluid are left. Take the decoction warm at one time to induce sweating.

Actions

Unblocking yang and promoting sweating.

Indications

For the initial stage of external contraction of wind–cold with an aversion to cold with fever, an absence of sweating, headaches, and nasal congestion.

Wǔ Shí Chá (Noon Tea)

Huò xiāng (Herba Agastachis); *fáng fēng* (Radix Saposhnikoviae); *bái zhǐ* (Radix Angelicae Dahuricae); *chái hú* (Radix Bupleuri); *qiāng huó* (Rhizoma et Radix Notopterygii); *qián hú* (Radix Peucedani); *chén pí* (Pericarpium Citri Reticulatae); *cāng zhú* (Rhizoma Atractylodis); *zhǐ shí* (Fructus Aurantii Immaturus); *chuān xiōng* (Rhizoma Chuanxiong); *lián qiào* (Fructus Forsythiae); *shān zhā* (Fructus Crataegi); *jiāo liù qū* (Massa Medicata Fermentata Praeparata), *gān jiāng* (Rhizoma Zingiberis); *gān cǎo* (Radix et Rhizoma Glycyrrhizae), 30 g each; prepared *chuān pò* (Cortex Magnoliae Officinalis); *zǐ sū yè* (Folium Perillae) and *jié gěng* (Radix Platycodonis) 45 g, respectively; black tea 300 g.

Grind the above ingredients into powder and pack them into 13.5 g a bag, or make them into lumps and pack two lumps into a bag. Take after being infused or decocted in water, 1 bag at a time.

Actions

Dispersing wind–cold, harmonizing the stomach, and promoting digestion.

Indications

For the wind–cold common cold with internal obstruction due to food accumulation, an aversion to cold with fever, vomiting, diarrhea, etc.

DAY THREE

The Exterior Deficiency–Cold Pattern

The exterior deficiency–cold pattern is characterized by the attack of external wind–cold, causing the initially weak *wei* qi to rise in defense, and resulting in opened sweat pores and disharmony of *ying* and *wei* qi. This pattern is common in the common cold, flu, all kinds of long-term fever, rheumatic diseases, and a number of internal miscellaneous diseases, especially among patients with constitutional blood insufficiency, weak *wei* yang, and susceptibility to spontaneous sweating. The exterior deficiency–cold pattern does not mean that the general condition of the patient is poor, but compared to the exterior excess–cold pattern after being affected by wind–cold, the sweat pores are unable to close securely and sweating thus occurs, causing the normal function of *wei* qi to be relatively weak. If excessive sweating ensues due to opened sweat pores and long-term disharmony between *ying* and *wei*, it can lead to weakness of the *wei* qi, and even throughout the whole body.

Diagnosis

The main symptoms and indications of this pattern are fever, an aversion to wind, spontaneous sweating, and a floating and moderate pulse. Other symptoms may include headaches, stuffy nose, sneezing, loose and clear nasal discharge, an absence of thirst, a red tongue with a thin and white coating, and belching.

The fever occurring in this pattern is usually mild, and is related to spontaneous sweating, which expels heat from the interior. An aversion to wind is a definite symptom in this pattern, which indicates that the patient is very sensitive to wind, i.e., he feels cold when in the presence of wind and conversely when there is a lack of it. It differs from an aversion to cold only in severity, in that in the aversion to cold, the patient feels cold when there is no wind. Spontaneous sweating is a feature of this pattern, which involves the natural production of sweat without medication or other reasons. It often coexists with an aversion to wind and usually, this aversion becomes more pronounced after spontaneous sweating. Headaches in this pattern can either be stiff pain in the head and nape, or pain in the back of the head or forehead. This type of pain is generally mild. The absence of thirst and a red tongue with a thin and white coating are evident signs of no yin impairment due to exuberant heat. As for nasal congestion, sneezing, and loose and clear nasal discharge, they can occur in various wind–cold common colds, flu, and some forms of rhinitis.

The main differences of this pattern in comparison to the exterior excess–cold pattern are in the aspects of sweating and a floating and moderate pulse. For indications of *Guì Zhī Tāng* (in contrast to those of *Má Huáng Tāng*), symptoms such as coughing, panting and chest fullness can be taken into account when dispensing prescription.

Treatment method

Dispelling wind and dispersing cold; harmonizing *ying* and *wei* qi levels.

Formula and ingredients: Guì Zhī Tāng (Cinnamon Twig Decoction)

Guì zhī (Ramulus Cinnamomi) 9 g; *sháo yào* (Radix Paeoniae) 9 g; *zhì gān cǎo* (Radix et Rhizoma Glycyrrhizae Praeparata cum Melle) 6 g; *shēng jiāng* (Rhizoma Zingiberis Recens) 9 g; *dà zǎo* (Fructus Jujubae) 7 pieces.

Formula verse

Guì Zhī Tāng is indicated for exterior deficiency and wind; uses peony, licorice, ginger, and date. It relieves the flesh, diffuses the exterior, and harmonizes *ying* and *wei* levels, excellent for exterior deficiency with spontaneous sweating.

Usage

Grind the above ingredients into a rough powder, and add 1.4 L of water to decoct in low fire until 600 mL of decoction are left. Remove the dregs.

Take 200 mL of the decoction when it is warm. After some time, consume some warm porridge; this is to aid the decoction in exerting the effect of relieving muscles and the exterior. In the meantime, the patient should be covered with sheets for about 2 h. It is recommended to induce mild sweating, but not excessively. Profuse sweating may impair yang qi and body fluids and is poor for the relief of the exterior. If there is sweating and the disease is cured by the 200-mL decoction, do not take the remaining decoction. However, if there is no sweating after taking the decoction, take another 200 mL. If there is still no sweating, take the remaining 200-mL decoction as before. The intervals for taking the decoction may be shortened until the disease is cured.

Analysis

In *Guì Zhī Tāng*, *guì zhī* can disperse the exterior, warm and unblock yang qi, and promote blood flow, hence it can harmonize both *wei* yang and *ying* yin; it is the main ingredient for deficiency–cold. *Sháo yào*, especially *bái sháo*, can nourish *ying*, rectify blood, astringe fluids, and restrain the dispersing nature of *guì zhī*. The combination of *sháo yào* and *guì zhī*, whose features are dispersing and astringing, and opening and closing, respectively, can induce sweating without impairing yin and astringe yin without retaining pathogens, establishing an optimal blend for harmonizing *ying* and *wei*. *Shēng jiāng*, which is both acrid and warm, can assist *guì zhī* to disperse the pathogenic wind–cold in the exterior and also warm the stomach to check vomiting. *Gān cǎo* can calm the middle and boost qi, harmonizes the actions of all medicinals, and assist *guì zhī* to warm yang and support *sháo yào* to harmonize yin and relieve pain. *Dà zǎo* is able to fortify the spleen and stomach, harmonize *ying* blood, and assist *sháo yào* to astringe yin and relieve pain due to its sour and sweet tastes. All the medicinals as a whole function to harmonize *ying* and *wei* levels, where the wind–cold in the exterior can then be dispelled.

Modern pharmacological researches have shown that *Guì Zhī Tāng* can relieve fever, arrest pain, inhibit inflammation, calm the mind, and so on. *Guì zhī* can enhance pain tolerance, relieve vessel spasms, relax the smooth muscles of internal organs, and is superior in arresting pain. *Sháo yào* can also relieve spasms and stop pain of the smooth muscles of internal organs.

The combination of *sháo yào* and *guì zhī* exerts a greater effect in relieving pain. Both *sháo yào* and *guì zhī* can dilate blood vessels and speed up blood flow, which is similar to the function of unblocking yang qi by warming, and as a result, harmonize blood. *Gān cǎo, shēng jiāng*, and *dà zǎo* are supplementary and nourishing, and can relieve allergic reactions and promote blood circulation. Therefore, this formula has the purpose of stimulating sweating, relieving fever, restraining various pathogens, improving blood circulation, strengthening the body, relaxing spasms, and arresting pain.

Treatment reference

Guì Zhī Tāng is a commonly used formula not only for exterior patterns of external contraction, but also for miscellaneous diseases of internal damage. Modern clinical and laboratory studies have demonstrated that this formula is involved in bidirectional regulation. For instance, it is effective in relieving fever and is also able to optimize the body temperature of hypothermic patients. It can promote sweating to treat the exterior pattern, and is also used to cure spontaneous sweating. It not only induces urination for patients with symptoms of loose stool, scant urine, and even body edema caused by spleen–stomach deficiency–cold, but is also applied for the treatment of frequent urination, nocturia, and enuresis. Clearly, in order to effectively prompt its bidirectional regulation, be it for external contraction or internal damage, modification of the formula is required.

This formula can be modified to treat many diseases. For the general exterior deficiency–cold pattern of the common cold and flu, the original formula is used. For the exterior deficiency–cold pattern with a poor physique or profuse sweating, add *huáng qí*. For obvious nape stiffness and cramps, add *gé gēn* to form *Guì Zhī Jiā Gé Gēn Tāng* (Cinnamon Twig Decoction with Pueraria). For coughs and shortness of breath, add *hòu pò* and *xìng rén* to form *Guì Zhī Jiā Hòu Pò Xìng Zǐ Tāng* (Cinnamon Twig Decoction with Officinal Magnolia Bark and Apricot Kernal). For abdominal distention, fullness, and pain responding unfavorably to pressure, add *dà huáng* to form *Guì Zhī Jiā Dà Huáng Tāng* (Cinnamon Twig Decoction with Rhubarb). If the patient has a profile of the exterior deficiency–cold pattern and also manifestations such as a serious aversion to cold and wind, cold limbs with cramps, and a deep and thin pulse, it indicates the accompaniment of yang qi deficiency, which should be treated by *Guì Zhī Jiā Fù Zǐ Tāng* (Cinnamon Twig Decoction with Aconite). For a pneumonic child with low fever, sweating, dry cough, and an aversion to wind, or for postpartum women with profuse sweating, add *lóng gǔ* and *mǔ lì* to form *Guì Zhī Jiā Lóng Gǔ Mǔ Lì Tāng* (Cinnamon Twig Decoction with Keel and Oyster Shell), which is also indicated for seminal emission, sexually charged dreams, *yáng wěi* (impotence), baldness, insomnia, amnesia, mania, dizziness, etc. *Guì Zhī Tāng* is a main formula for spontaneous sweating, especially for those with signs of internal heat, such as an aversion to wind, a lack of thirst, and yellow urine. If the sweat is not ideally repressed after medicinal administration, add *huáng qí* and *nuò dào gēn xū* to strengthen its function of securing the exterior to check sweating. *Guì Zhī Tāng* is also used for mild fever, especially for those with symptoms of lingering mild fever that relapses at times, a poor appetite, an occasional aversion to wind, and sweating due to autonomic nerve functional disorder. In application, add some *huáng qí*, *dāng guī*, and *wǔ wèi zǐ*. Moreover, this formula together with *lóng gǔ*, *mǔ lì*, *fú xiǎo mài*, and *cí shí* can treat palpitations and paroxysmal tachycardia; together with *gé gēn* and *fù zǐ*, it can treat nape stiffness, spontaneous sweating, and an aversion to wind after the attack of a stroke; together with *dāng guī*, *gǒu jǐ*, and *wēi líng xiān*, it can treat arthritis caused by an inhibited flow of qi and blood. If a large dose of *sháo yào* is used, this formula becomes *Guì Zhī Jiā Sháo Yào Tāng* (Cinnamon Twig Decoction plus Peony), which is indicated for abdominal pain due to spastic constipation, various kinds of diarrhea, and dysentery.

Clinically, by exploiting *Guì Zhī Tāng*'s influence in harmonizing *ying* and *wei* levels and dredging qi and blood of the skin, various skin diseases can be treated, especially urticaria, skin pruritus, dermatitis, and chilblain occurring in the winter with manifestations of feeling cold, spontaneous sweating, and a thin and white tongue coating. For application, herbs such as *dāng guī* and *chuān xiōng* should be added to activate and nourish blood. In addition, it has a certain curative effect on erythema multiforme of the cold pattern and eczema. As *Guì Zhī Tāng* is anti-allergic, it is also used to treat allergic rhinitis with symptoms of an itchy nasal cavity, nasal congestion, sneezing, loose nasal discharge, and dizziness. For application, grind *chán tuì* and *tíng lì zǐ* into powder and take them after infusion in the *Guì Zhī Tāng* decoction.

Cautions

Though *Guì Zhī Tāng* is modest in promoting sweating and has a variety of indications, it is essentially an acrid–warm formula, which should not be used for symptoms of pathogenic heat in the exterior or internal heat. For internal damp–heat, especially for patients with an alcohol addiction, cautions should be taken while using this formula, because acrid–sweet ingredients can promote heat and generate dampness, or even cause vomiting after taking the decoction. Usually, no more than 3 doses of this formula are prescribed for treating the exterior pattern. If this decoction is still not effective, further examination is required to check if the pattern differentiation is accurate and all-rounded. This formula dispels pathogens in the exterior by relieving the flesh and promoting sweating, but the sweating should be mild instead of profuse, or the disharmony of *ying–wei* will be aggravated. After sweating occurs, dry the body at once and avoid catching wind and cold. During the medication period, do not engage in smoking or take raw, cold, greasy, difficult-to-digest, acrid, spicy, and pungent food, as well as wine.

Daily Exercises

1. What are the clinical features of the exterior deficiency–cold pattern? What are the differences between this pattern and the exterior excess–cold pattern?
2. What are the ingredients of *Guì Zhī Tāng*? When it is applied to treat spontaneous sweating, what other herbs should be added?
3. Mr. Shen is a 54-year-old male. He is highly susceptible to catching colds. Three days ago, he caught a cold and experienced symptoms of fever, an aversion to cold, and headaches. He took some aspirin on his own and thereafter, the symptoms manifested into profuse sweating, mild fever, body aches and pains, a lack of strength, sweating after exertion, an aversion to wind after sweating, headaches, a poor appetite, easily triggered palpitations, a moderate and weak pulse, and a light red tongue with a thin, white, and moist coating. Please prescribe a Chinese medicinal formula for this case.

Additional Formulae

Guì Zhī Jiā Gé Gēn Tāng (Cinnamon Twig Decoction with Pueraria)

Ingredients of *Guì Zhī Tāng*; *gé gēn* 12 g. Decoct the ingredients with water, take the decoction warm, and cover the body with sheets to promote mild sweating.

Actions

Releasing the flesh and soothing tendons.

Indications

Exterior deficiency–cold pattern with nape stiffness and cramps.

Guì Zhī Jiā Hòu Pò Xìng Zǐ Tāng (Cinnamon Twig Decoction with Officinal Magnolia Bark and Apricot Kernal)

Ingredients of *Guì Zhī Tāng*; *hòu pò* 6 g; *xìng rén* 9 g. Decoct the ingredients with water, take the decoction warm, and cover the body with sheets to promote mild sweating.

Actions

Releasing the flesh and dispersing the exterior; relieving coughing and calming panting.

Indications

Patients with coughing and increased panting who have further contracted wind–cold in the presence of the exterior deficiency–cold pattern.

Guì Zhī Jiā Dà Huáng Tāng (Cinnamon Twig Decoction with Rhuburb)

Ingredients of *Guì Zhī Tāng*; *dà huáng* 6 g; *sháo yào* 9 g. Decoct the ingredients with water and take the decoction warm.

Actions

Releasing the flesh and dispersing the exterior; purging the interior and harmonizing the middle.

Indications

Exterior deficiency–cold pattern accompanied with abdominal pain and fullness, and difficult bowel movement.

Guì Zhī Jiā Fù Zǐ Tāng (*Cinnamon Twig Decoction with Aconite*)

Ingredients of *Guì Zhī Tāng*; *fù zǐ* 9 g. Decoct the ingredients with water and take the decoction warm.

Actions

Reinforcing yang and securing the exterior; harmonizing *ying* and *wei* levels.

Indications

Patients with continuous sweating, an aversion to wind, fever, mild limb cramps with inhibited movement, inhibited urination, and a deep and thin pulse.

Guì Zhī Jiā Lóng Gǔ Mǔ Lì Tāng (*Cinnamon Twig Decoction with Keel and Oyster Shell*)

Ingredients of *Guì Zhī Tāng*; *lóng gǔ* 12 g; *mǔ lì* 12 g. Decoct the ingredients with water and take the decoction warm.

Actions

Harmonizing *ying* and *wei* levels, nourishing yin and harmonizing yang, calming the mind, and containing essence.

Indications

Chronic diseases of the deficiency pattern with symptoms of palpitations, being easily frightened, profuse sweating, seminal emission, sexually charged dreams, enuresis or postpartum sweating, and an aversion to wind.

DAY FOUR

The Exterior Heat Pattern

The exterior heat pattern manifests on the body surface and is caused by attacks of external heat. This pattern occurs in the early stage of externally contracted febrile diseases and may be accompanied by wind or dryness, which thus can be further divided into the exterior wind–heat pattern and exterior wind–dryness pattern. This section mainly discusses the diagnosis and treatment of the exterior wind–heat pattern. This pattern is commonly seen in the common cold, flu, and many acute infectious diseases at the initial febrile stage.

Diagnosis

The main symptoms and signs are fever, a mild aversion to wind–cold, and a thin and white tongue coating with a red tongue tip and edges. Other clinical manifestations include headaches, an absence of sweating or scant sweating, coughing, yellow and turbid nasal discharge, yellow sputum, red swellings and a sore throat, mild thirst, small amounts of yellow urine, and a floating and rapid pulse.

Since this is a pattern caused by pathogens invading the exterior, fever and an aversion to cold are the definite symptoms. However, as the external pathogen is heat, the fever will be relatively significant in that the patient will experience a feverish sensation and have a high body temperature, sometimes even above 39°C. The aversion to cold is usually mild. If sweat pores are obstructed and there is no sweating, the aversion to cold can be fairly serious. A febrile pathogen tends to consume fluids, hence accounting for the symptoms of mild thirst, a tongue with a red tip and edges, and small amounts of yellow urine. The heat can also boil fluids, presenting yellow and turbid nasal discharge and yellow and dense sputum. The symptoms of red swellings and a sore throat are helpful in the diagnosis of this pattern. As the lung is associated with the skin, and Chinese medicine believes that the initial attack of external pathogenic heat usually occurs at the lung, a cough often occurs in the exterior heat pattern due to the failure of the diffusion of lung qi.

Among these symptoms, if thirst is apparent and there are dry lips, nasal cavity, and throat, and a tongue lacking fluid, and the disease occurs in autumn, it usually belongs to the exterior dryness–heat pattern — a pattern with a drastic cough, scant sputum that is difficult to be coughed up, and a paroxysmal dry cough.

The main differences between the exterior heat pattern and exterior cold pattern lie in the severity of fever and the aversion to cold, as well as the presence of sweating, thirst, yellow urine, a tongue with a red tip and edges, and a rapid pulse.

As for the exterior heat pattern and interior heat pattern, they differ in the severity of the aversion to cold and the absence or presence of heat exuberance. If an aversion to cold is evident without any signs of heat exuberance impairing yin, it pertains to the exterior. If there is no aversion to cold and there are signs of heat exuberance impairing yin, such as high fever, extreme thirst, scant and brown urine, and a reddish tongue with a yellow coating, it is an interior pattern. There also exists a pattern of both exterior and interior heat, which presents exterior symptoms including an aversion to wind and cold, in alignment with the interior heat pattern.

For certain acute contagious diseases, such as epidemic encephalitis B, due to the rapid development of the disease, the exterior heat pattern at the initial stage of occurrence can be transient or atypical, which should be allocated great attention in diagnosis.

Treatment method

Dispersing exterior heat, clearing heat, and resolving toxins.

Formula and ingredients: Yín Qiào Sǎn (*Lonicera and Forsythia Powder*)

Jīn yín huā (Flos Lonicerae Japonicae) 10 g; *lián qiào* (Fructus Forsythiae) 12 g; *dàn dòu chǐ* (Semen Sojae Praeparatum) 9 g; *niú bàng zǐ* (Fructus Arctii) 9 g; *zhú yè* (Folium Phyllostachydis Henonis); *jīng jiè* (Herba Schizonepetae) 5 g; *jié gěng* (Radix Platycodonis) 5 g; *bò he* (Herba Menthae) 5 g (added later); *gān cǎo* (Radix et Rhizoma Glycyrrhizae) 5 g; *lú gēn* (Rhizoma Phragmitis) 30 g.

Formula verse

Yín Qiào Sǎn is indicated for upper *jiao* diseases. It uses *zhú yè*, *jīng niú*, and *chǐ bò he*, and also *gān jié* and *lú gēn* for releasing cool; common in treating the exterior wind–heat pattern.

Usage

Grind the ingredients into powder and decoct *lú gēn* first. After the decoction is done, add the other ingredients to boil until a strong aroma arises. Remove the dregs and consume the decoction warm. If the disease condition is serious, take the decoction 3 times in the day and once in the evening. For mild cases, take the decoction 2 times in the day and once in the evening. Do not decoct the ingredients for too long. If the disease is not relieved after taking the decoction, the dose can be doubled. If the patient does not sweat and the aversion to cold is severe, cover the body with sheets after taking the decoction and drink some hot water to promote mild sweating. If sweating is already apparent, it is not necessary to promote sweating again.

Analysis

In this formula, as both *jīn yín huā* and *lián qiào* can clear heat and resolve toxins, and are also diffusing, they are the chief ingredients. *Jīng jiè*, *bò he*, *dàn dòu chǐ*, and *niú bàng zǐ* are acrid and dispersing, which can assist *jīn yín huā* and *lián qiào* in dispelling exogenous pathogens. Though *jīng jiè* and *dàn dòu chǐ* are acrid and warm, they are not drastic and when combined with other cold and cool herbs, their warm action is restrained, while their actions of dredging the exterior and diffusing the sweat pores are retained. The combination of *niú bàng zǐ*, *jié gěng*, and *gān cǎo* can benefit the throat, diffuse the lungs, and dissolve phlegm. *Zhú yè* and *lú gēn* are sweet and cool, which can clear heat and stimulate fluids to quench thirst. *Gān cǎo* harmonizes the actions of all medicinals in the formula. As a whole, *Yín Qiào Sǎn* is a cool, acrid, and dispersing formula, which is able to dredge and disperse wind–heat in the exterior, diffuse the lung, and soothe the throat.

According to current research, this formula can inactivate various viruses, strengthen immune function, and has certain anti-microbial effects. *Jīn yín huā*, *lián qiào*, and *niú bàng zǐ* can inhibit many kinds of pathogenic bacteria. *Jīng jiè* is able to induce sweating and relieve fever by activating the sweat glands. Oral intake of *jié gěng* can promote thinning of the dense sputum in the bronchi and thus make it easy to be coughed up. *Gān cǎo* can protect the mucosal membrane of the inflamed throat and trachea by its anti-inflammatory and anti-allergy properties, thus reducing stimulation and relieving coughing. From the above, *Yín Qiào Sǎn* is indicated for the early stage of upper respiratory infection or respiratory infectious diseases.

Treatment reference

Clinically, this formula is applied to many respiratory diseases, such as the common cold, flu, acute bronchitis, the early stage of pneumonia, the early stage of measles, scarlet fever, pharyngitis, and mumps. In addition, this formula can be prescribed for the following diseases presenting the exterior heat pattern: epidemic encephalitis B, typhoid fever, leptospirosis, acute endometritis, drug eruption, and the early stages of sores and ulcers.

In practice, proper modification is required. For example, in winter, the patient may have a serious aversion to cold and does not sweat, which indicates a serious obstruction on the body surface. In such a case, the dosages of *bò he*, *dàn dòu chǐ*, and *jīng jiè* can be increased or *cōng bái*, *zǐ sū yè*, *fáng fēng*, etc. can be added. If the exterior heat pattern occurs in summer or the patient sweats profusely, *jīng jiè* can be removed from the formula. If there are secondary manifestations such as chest oppression, stomach cavity *pǐ*, a white and greasy tongue coating, or nausea, it indicates the presence of further pathogenic dampness, and *huò xiāng*, *pèi lán*, and *dà dòu juǎn* are recommended to be added. For extreme thirst, add *tiān huā fěn*. For a severe sore throat and even swellings and pain in the nape, add *mǎ bó*, *xuán shēn*, *jiāng cán*, *shè gān*, and *bǎn lán gēn*. For nasal bleeding, remove *jīng jiè* and *dàn dòu chǐ*, while adding *bái máo gēn*, *qiàn cǎo gēn*, *cè bǎi yè*, and charred *zhī zǐ*. If fever is serious, add *huáng qín*, *pú gōng yīng*, and *yā zhí căo*. For the convenience of oral intake, *Yín Qiào Săn* has been made into patented medicines, examples of which include *Yín Qiào Jiĕ Dú Piàn* (Lonicera and Forsythia Toxin-Removing Tablet), to be taken 4 tablets at a time, 2 times a day; *Yín Qiào Jiĕ Dú Wán* (Lonicera and Forsythia Toxin-Removing Pill), to be taken 1–2 pills a time, 2 times a day for honey pills weighing 15 g each, and 9 g at a time, 2 times a day for water pills; and *Yín Qiào Săn Pào Jì* (Lonicera and Forsythia Infusion Granule), to be taken 1 bag at a time after infusion with water, 2 times a day. Among these different forms, it has been shown that the infusion granule has the optimal curative effect. Further, for the common cold with wind–heat in the exterior, *Găn Mào Tuì Rè Chōng Jì* (Common Cold and Fever-Relieving Infusion Granule) is applicable. For the wind–heat exterior pattern with a severe cough, add *xìng rén*, *pí pá yè*, *qián hú*, and *zǐ wăn* to *Yín Qiào Săn*. If the cough is severe but the exterior pattern is mild, prescribe *Sāng Jú Yĭn* (Mulberry Leaf and Chrysanthemum Beverage), which is moderate in releasing the exterior and clearing heat, but is strong in relieving coughing and dissolving phlegm. If the exterior heat pattern has obvious signs of dryness, apply *Sāng Xìng Tāng* (Mulberry Leaf and Apricot Kernel Decoction) to moisten and relieve the exterior by its acrid and cool nature.

Cautions

For the application of *Yín Qiào Săn*, the induction of sweating depends on the state of sweat pores. If the aversion to cold is serious and there is no sweating, the formula should be combined with some acrid–warm herbs to disperse instead of the use of cold–cool ingredients, as otherwise, the exterior cannot be relieved. If the pattern belongs to exterior cold, do not prescribe this formula.

In addition, many acute infectious diseases present the exterior heat pattern at the early stage, which can be treated by *Yín Qiào Săn* when the pathogens are in the exterior. However, close observation is required to prevent the pathogenic factors from entering the interior and mutating into other patterns. If disease transmission and change have occurred, the formula should be promptly modified.

Daily Exercises

1. How is the exterior heat pattern diagnosed? What is the treatment principle of this pattern?
2. What are the ingredients of *Yín Qiào Sǎn*? What are its indications?
3. Ms. Shen is a 31-year-old female. She exhibited sweating after overstraining herself and caught a cold when she removed her clothes. The next day, she suffered from fever, a mild aversion to wind, headaches, a sore throat with cough, but without any sweating. A physical examination revealed a body temperature of 39.1°C, a thin and white tongue coating with a reddish tip, and a floating and rapid pulse. Please prescribe a Chinese medicinal formula for this case.

Additional Formulae

Gǎn Mào Tuì Rè Chōng Jì (*Common Cold and Fever-Relieving Infusion Granule*)

Dà qīng yè (Folium Isatidis) 30 g; *bǎn lán gēn* (Radix Isatidis) 30 g; *cǎo hé chē* (Rhizoma Paridis) 15 g; *lián qiào* (Fructus Forsythiae) 15 g. These ingredients are made into infusion granules.

Dosage

18 g for each bag.

Usage

One bag at a time, 3 times a day. If the body temperature is above 38°C, take 2 bags a time, 4 times a day.

Actions

Clearing heat and resolving toxins.

Indications

The common cold or flu presenting fever, a mild aversion to cold, and a sore throat.

Sāng Jú Yǐn (Mulberry Leaf and Chrysanthemum Beverage)

Sāng yè (Folium Mori) 7.5 g; *jú huā* (Flos Chrysanthemi) 3 g; *xìng rén* (Semen Armeniacae Amarum) 6 g; *lián qiào* (Fructus Forsythiae) 5 g; *bò he* (Herba Menthae) 2.5 g; *jié gěng* (Radix Platycodonis) 6 g; *gān cǎo* (Radix et Rhizoma Glycyrrhizae) 2.5 g; *lú gēn* (Rhizoma Phragmitis) 6 g. Add water to decoct.

Actions

Scattering wind and clearing heat; diffusing the lung and relieving coughing.

Indications

Exterior wind–heat presenting cough, moderate fever, mild thirst, a reddish tongue tip, a thin and white tongue coating, and a floating and rapid pulse.

Sāng Xìng Tāng (Mulberry Leaf and Apricot Kernel Decoction)

Sāng yè (Folium Mori) 6 g; *xìng rén* (Semen Armeniacae Amarum) 9 g; *shā shēn* (Radix Adenophorae seu Glehniae) 12 g; *zhè bèi mǔ* (Bulbus Fritillariae Thunbergii) 6 g; *xiāng dòu chǐ* (Semen Sojae Praeparatum) 6 g; skin of *zhī zǐ* *(Radix et Rhizoma Glycyrrhizae)* 6 g; pear skin 6 g. Add water to decoct.

Actions

Releasing the exterior by clearing and diffusing with its cool and moist natures.

Indications

Dryness–heat invading the exterior presenting fever, a mild aversion to wind and cold, headaches, thirst, a dry cough, or a cough with scant and sticky sputum, a tongue with white coating lacking moisture, a reddish tongue tip and edges, and a floating and rapid pulse.

DAY FIVE

The Exterior Dampness Pattern

The exterior dampness pattern occurs when exogenous pathogenic dampness accumulates on the body surface, resulting in the obstruction of *wei* yang. The pathogenic dampness usually acts in combination with wind–cold or wind–heat to invade the exterior. Aside from the exterior manifestations of this pattern, there are two outcomes: one features as a disorder of the joints and the other is characterized by gastrointestinal complications. The exterior dampness pattern reviewed in this section refers to dampness in accompaniment with wind–cold, which means that after the invasion of pathogenic wind, cold, and dampness, not only the exterior pattern occurs, but there are also apparent symptoms of dampness encumbering the spleen and stomach. Joint pain caused by pathogenic dampness will be discussed later in Chapter 12 (i.e., the wind–damp pattern). Here, this pattern is frequently seen in the common cold in summer and autumn, together with diarrhea, acute gastroenteritis, toxic dyspepsia, virus hepatitis, etc.

Diagnosis

The main symptoms and indications are fever, an aversion to cold, chest and gastric fullness and oppression, nausea, vomiting, diarrhea, and a white and greasy tongue coating. Other symptoms and signs include headaches, body heaviness, gastric and abdominal pain, borborygmus, distressed limbs, and a soggy and slow pulse.

When pathogenic dampness invades the body, healthy qi is triggered in defense. However, the dampness with wind–cold obstructs the qi of *wei* yang, presenting fever, an aversion to cold, and a lack of sweating in most cases. Dampness belongs to yin and it is heavy, greasy, and sticky. When it impedes the body surface, it causes the inhibited flows of qi and blood, hence the patient feels body heaviness and distressed limbs. When it encumbers the spleen and stomach, it leads to the associated disorders of these organs, presenting chest and gastric fullness and oppression, gastric and abdominal pain, nausea, vomiting, borborygmus, and diarrhea. Usually, the contents of the vomit consist of indigested food in the stomach and for diarrhea, the stool is loose or yellow and watery but without pus, blood, a strong smell, or a hot sensation around the anus. These symptoms can help to differentiate this pattern from dysentery and diarrhea of the pattern of internal accumulation of damp–heat. Therefore, cholera with rinsed rice-like stool is a completely different type of illness.

In conclusion, the features of this pattern are exterior symptoms, including fever, an aversion to cold, absence of sweating, and gastrointestinal disorder symptoms, such as vomiting and diarrhea. This pattern has no obvious heat signs and often occurs in summer and autumn, as in these seasons, people tend to sleep in cool places, and coupled with the overconsumption of raw and cold food and a moist climate, the pattern is hence easily triggered.

Treatment method

Releasing the exterior and removing dampness; dissipating cold and harmonizing the middle.

Formula and ingredients: Huò Xiāng Zhèng Qì Sǎn (Agastache Qi-Correcting Powder)

Huò xiāng (Herba Agastachis) 9 g; *zǐ sū yè* (Folium Perillae) 6 g; *bái zhǐ* (Radix Angelicae Dahuricae) 6 g; *dà fù pí* (Pericarpium Arecae) 9 g; *fú líng* (Poria) 9 g; *bái zhú* (Rhizoma Atractylodis Macrocephalae) 9 g; *chén pí* (Pericarpium Citri Reticulatae) 6 g; *bàn xià qū* (Rhizoma Pinelliae Fermentata) 9 g; ginger juice-prepared *hòu pò* (Cortex Magnoliae Officinalis) 6 g; *jié gěng* (Radix Platycodonis) 6 g; *zhì gān cǎo* (Radix et Rhizoma Glycyrrhizae Praeparata cum Melle) 3 g; fresh ginger 3 pieces; jujube 2 pieces.

Formula verse

Huò Xiāng Zhèng Qì contains *fù pí sū* and also *gān jié chén líng zhú pò*; together with *xià qū bái zhǐ*, ginger and jujubes, it dispels wind, cold, and dampness.

Usage

Grind the ingredients into a fine powder. Take 6 g each time to boil with water, fresh ginger, and jujubes. Consume the decoction warm As there are many aromatic herbs in this formula, do not decoct it for too long in case it diminishes the curative effect. If the patient does not sweat, cover the body with sheets. If the disease is not relieved after taking the decoction, take the decoction again. At present, 1 dose of these ingredients is usually decocted with 1.2 L of water for consumption. Twelve hours later, these ingredients are again decocted for consumption.

Analysis

Huò Xiāng Zhèng Qì Sǎn mainly uses acrid–warm and aromatic *huò xiāng* to release wind–cold in the exterior and remove damp–turbidity in the spleen and stomach. *Zǐ sū yè* and *bái zhǐ* are also acrid–warm and aromatic, both of which can assist *huò xiāng* to remove dampness via their aromatic nature. *Jié gěng* serves to diffuse the lung and soothe the throat; *hòu pò* to move qi, remove dampness, loosen the chest, and relieve fullness; *dà fù pí* to drain dampness and move qi; *chén pí* to dry dampness and regulate qi; and *bàn xià* to dry dampness, direct qi downward, harmonize the stomach, and arrest vomiting, all of which can dispel dampness by unblocking inhibited qi movement. *Fú líng* and *bái zhú* have the function of fortifying the spleen to promote circulation, removing dampness, and promoting urination. Fresh ginger and jujubes harmonize the spleen and stomach, while *gān cǎo* harmonizes the actions of all medicinals in the formula.

It has been found that *huò xiāng* has an inhibitory effect on various viruses and bacteria, and can promote the secretion of stomach juices to strengthen the digestive system, being a principal herb for treating the common cold complicated by a gastrointestinal disorder. *Hòu pò* also enjoys a broad-spectrum antibiotic effect, and is able to relax the flesh and activate the intestines and bronchi. *Fú líng* can promote urination and has a certain curative effect on gastrointestinal damage and inflammation. *Zǐ sū yè* can relieve fever to some extent; *jié gěng* dispels phlegm, calms the mind, and inhibits inflammation; *bái zhǐ* has antibiotic actions; *gān cǎo* relaxes spasms of the smooth muscles; and ginger can promote blood circulation and activate the intestines. Overall, this formula is indicated for fever, infection, and digestive and respiratory diseases.

Treatment reference

Huò Xiāng Zhèng Qì Sǎn is a common formula for treating externally contracted diseases. It is often applied in summer and autumn to treat flu, acute gastroenteritis, typhoid fever of the intestines at the early stage,

child diarrhea, infectious hepatitis, etc. Clinically, by exploiting its beneficial effect of removing dampness, dissipating cold, warming the middle,
rectifying qi, and eliminating stagnation, this formula can be applied to
treat chronic gastritis, peptic ulcers, adaptive colitis, all types of dyspepsia,
chronic hepatitis, and chronic nephritis with symptoms of cold in the
middle of the body, dampness obstruction, and qi stagnation. Its curative
effect is favorable and it has since been applied beyond the realm of
externally contracted diseases.

For convenience, this formula has been made into pills, an example of
which is *Huò Xiāng Zhèng Qì Wán* (Agastache Qi-Correcting Pill) for oral
intake, 6–9 g at a time, 2 times a day. It has also been made into a liquid
form, namely *Huò Xiāng Zhèng Qì Shuǐ* (Agastache Qi-Correcting Liquid)
for oral intake at 10 mL at a time, 2–3 times a day. In practice, proper modification according to the disease state is required. If the exterior pathogen is
so serious that there are palpable symptoms of an aversion to cold, an
absence of sweating, and joint and muscle aches and pain, *xiāng rú* should
be added to induce sweating to relieve the exterior, remove dampness, and
harmonize the middle. If there are accompanying symptoms such as food
stagnation, gastric and abdominal distending pain, and a pungent smell arising from the contents of vomit, add *shén qū* and *lái fú zǐ* to promote digestion
and guide food stagnation out of inactivity. If diarrhea is severe and the stool
is mainly yellow and watery, add *yì yǐ rén*, *chē qián zǐ*, and *zé xiè* to fortify
the spleen, promote urination, and relieve diarrhea. In addition, for internal
damage caused by summer damp–heat and external damp–cold due to the
obstruction of the exterior, which is in turned caused by resting in a cool
place and excessive intake of cold food in the summer, symptoms such as
fever, an aversion to cold, an absence of sweating, joint pain, body cramps,
vexation, thirst, and a reddish tongue with a white and greasy coating are
manifested. In this case, prescribe *Xīn Jiā Xiāng Rú Yǐn* (Newly Supplemented
Mosla Beverage). In summer and autumn, if pathogenic damp–heat initially
attacks the body surface where heat signs are insignificant and there are only
manifestations of dampness encumbering the body surface, spleen, and
stomach, such as fever, a mild aversion to cold, fatigue, a lack of thirst, chest
oppression, a sticky and greasy feeling in the mouth, a thin, white, and a
mildly greasy tongue coating, and a soggy and moderate pulse, prescribe
Huò Pò Xià Líng Tāng (Agastache, Magnolia, Pinellia, and Poria Decoction).

Cautions

Although *Huò Xiāng Zhèng Qì Sǎn* is usually applied to treat the common cold with gastrointestinal disorders in the summer and autumn, as well as several other acute infectious diseases at the early stage, the pathogenic dampness in the exterior can linger for a long time and transform into the interior dampness pattern or damp–heat pattern, which should not be neglected. *Huò Xiāng Zhèng Qì Sǎn* is warm and mildly dry in nature, so it is not advisable to apply this formula to treat damp–heat either in the exterior or in the interior. For interior summer heat symptoms, even if there are signs of damp–cold, herbs that can clear summer heat must be added or *Xīn Jiā Xiāng Rú Yǐn* should be used instead.

Daily Exercises

1. What is the exterior dampness syndrome? What are its clinical manifestations?
2. What are the ingredients of *Huò Xiāng Zhèng Qì Sǎn*? What are its indications?
3. Mr. Wang is a 22-year-old male. One night, he slept in the open air on a summer evening, and the next morning, he suffered from an aversion to cold, discomfort, and fever. In the afternoon, he experienced nausea, vomiting, abdominal pain, and yellow and watery stool 4 times. A physical examination showed his body temperature to be at 39.1°C, with normal heart and lungs, a flat and soft abdomen with mild tenderness and without rebound tenderness, a thin, white, and mildly greasy tongue coating, an absence of taste in the mouth, and a lack of thirst. Please prescribe a Chinese medicinal formula for this case.

Additional Formulae

Xīn Jiā Xiāng Rú Yǐn (Newly Supplemented Mosla Beverage)

Xiāng rú (Herba Moslae) 6 g; *jīn yín huā* (Flos Lonicerae Japonicae) 9 g; fresh *biǎn dòu huā* (Flos Lablab Album) 9 g; *hòu pò* (Cortex Magnoliae Officinalis) 6 g; *lián qiào* (Fructus Forsythiae) 6 g.

Add 5 cups of water to decoct until 2 cups of decoction are left. Take 1 cup of decoction first. If sweating occurs, discard the remaining decoction. If sweating does not occur, take the decoction once more.

Actions

Releasing the exterior, removing dampness, and dispelling summer heat.

Indications

Contraction of summer heat and exterior obstruction of damp–cold presenting fever, an aversion to cold, an absence of sweating, body heaviness, headaches, vexation, thirst, and a reddish tongue with a thin and greasy coating.

Huò Pò Xià Líng Tāng (Agastache, Magnolia, Pinellia, and Poria Decoction):

Huò xiāng (Herba Agastachis) 6 g; *bàn xià* (Rhizoma Pinelliae) 4.5 g; *chì fú líng* (Poria Rubra) 9 g; *xìng rén* (Semen Armeniacae Amarum) 9 g; raw *yì yǐ rén* (Semen Coicis) 12 g; *bái kòu rén* (Fructus Amomi Rotundus) 2 g; *zhū líng* (Polyporus) 4.5 g; *dàn dòu chǐ* (Semen Sojae Praeparatum) 9 g; *zé xiè* (Rhizoma Alismatis) 4.5 g; *hòu pò* (Cortex Magnoliae Officinalis) 3 g. Add water to decoct.

Actions

Releasing the exterior and removing dampness.

Indications

Damp–warm diseases at the initial stage presenting fever, an aversion to cold, fatigue, chest oppression, a greasy taste in the mouth, a tongue with a thin and white coating, and a soggy and moderate pulse.

CHAPTER 4

The Half-Exterior and Half-Interior Pattern

DAY SIX

In the half-exterior and half-interior pattern, the external pathogen is neither on the body surface nor in the internal organs. This pattern is diagnosed purely from the disease manifestations, which is different from the exterior pattern as well as the interior pattern. It often occurs in externally contracted diseases and its location is neither in the exterior nor in the interior.

Features of the Half-Exterior and Half-Interior Pattern

Manifestations of the half-exterior and half-interior pattern are extensive. The most common symptom is the repeated alternation of fever and an aversion to cold, in that the patient feels cold for a moment, after which the feeling of cold disappears, and a feverish sensation, or even red eyes, a flushed face, and thirst with a compulsion for drinking, are experienced. It is often called "alternating chills and fever." Still, there are many similar manifestations of alternating chills and fever. For example, some manifest as a paroxysmal aversion to cold and paroxysmal feverish sensation that can be repeated several times in a day. Others manifest as a mild aversion to cold in the afternoon and feeling feverish in the evening, though the body temperature is normal. There are also some patients who display an initial aversion to cold or even continual chills, resulting in the urge to cover the body with sheets or more drastically, gravitate toward the heating stove. But later, the aversion to cold fades away, and a feverish sensation builds up, causing the patient to feel like he is on fire and consequently, thirst for iced beverages. Following that, as profuse sweating occurs and fever remits, other symptoms gradually disappear. However, on the second day or a couple of days later, all of the above symptoms relapse. This type of manifestation can also be observed in patients who contract malaria, which is known as timely chills and fever. In contrast, the time of onset of such symptoms in the half-exterior and half-interior pattern is irregular. The classic alternating characteristic of the half-exterior and half-interior pattern is evident as a co-existence of fever and chills, though sometimes fever may be significant, while the aversion to cold is palpable at other times, which sets it apart from the exterior pattern and interior pattern.

If the half-exterior and half-interior pattern occurs in an externally contracted disease, the disease is usually at the early stage and a few cases can be at convalescence. Several febrile diseases, such as malaria and relapsing fever, are mainly characterized by alternating chills and fever. Some diseases of internal damage can also present the half-exterior and half-interior pattern, but patients may only experience mild fever and an aversion to cold or there are only several self-felt symptoms, such as certain types of nerve dysfunction and chronic cholecystitis, while high fever may be triggered in other patients, usually remittent fever and an aversion to cold, such as some rheumatic diseases, systemic lupus erythematosus, and acute leukemia. Whatever the disease, only if there are symptoms of alternating chills and fever or cases likewise, it usually provides an important key indicator for the diagnosis and administration of medicine.

Categories of the Half-Exterior and Half-Interior Pattern

Besides the shared symptom of alternating chills and fever among all types of half-exterior and half-interior patterns, there are many secondary symptoms, according to which this pattern can be further subcategorized. A common classification is based on the disease location, such as pathogens invading the *shaoyang*, lurking in the pleuro-diaphragmatic interspace (*mó yuán* 膜原), or lingering in the *sanjiao*. The *shaoyang*, pleuro-diaphragmatic interspace, and *sanjiao* mentioned here are different locations of the half-exterior and half-interior pattern. *Sanjiao* specifically refers to one of the six *fu* organs (see Chapter 2), which is an organ responsible for the flow and distribution of water–dampness, but not the three sections of the location of *zang–fu* organs. Another type of classification is based on the nature of different pathogens, such as damp–heat in the gallbladder channel pattern, *shaoyang* with the exterior pattern (namely the *shaoyang taiyang* pattern), *shaoyang* with the bowel excess pattern (namely the *shaoyang yangming* pattern), the *shaoyang* phlegm–heat pattern, and the *shaoyang* fluid retention channel pattern. Various pathogens of these different sub-patterns will be reviewed in this section.

Treatment Methods of the Half-Exterior and Half-Interior Pattern

The main treatment method of the half-exterior and half-interior pattern is to harmonize the exterior and interior. Harmonization refers to the technique of diffusing outward and clearing in the interior to remove the pathogens in the affected half-exterior and half-interior regions. Therefore, such a method includes medicinals that can either diffuse the exterior or clear the interior. The typical medicinals for diffusing the exterior are *chái hú* and *qīng hāo*, while for clearing the interior, it is *huáng qín*. Harmonization encompasses multiple curative effects, by not only relieving fever and possessing antibacterial and anti-inflammatory properties, but also soothing the liver, promoting gallbladder functions, and rectifying digestive disorders.

As there are many sub-patterns of the half-exterior and half-interior pattern, the application of the harmonization technique in practice varies under different specific circumstances. This method can be further broken down into harmonizing *shaoyang*, clearing and discharging damp–heat from the *shaoyang* level, opening the pleuro–diaphragmatic interspace, and dispersing ills from the *sanjiao*. If patterns of the exterior such as bowel excess, phlegm–heat, and water retention, are also observed, harmonization should be combined with releasing the exterior, unblocking the interior, clearing and dissolving hot phlegm, and warming and dissolving water retention.

Since the indications of the harmonization method are relatively precise, the cases are usually not difficult to handle. However, if erroneously used to treat the exterior pattern, it will cause the pathogens to invade the interior. Similarly, if it is applied to treat the interior pattern by mistake, it will be too feeble to dispel interior pathogens and will prolong recovery as the correct treatment is delayed. In addition, qi and blood deficiencies may also present the intermittent feeling of cold and heat, which cannot be treated by harmonization.

Daily Exercises

1. What is the half-exterior and half-interior pattern? Illustrate its diagnostic criteria.
2. What are the main sub-patterns of the half-exterior and half-interior pattern?
3. What is the "harmonization" treatment method? What are its main curative effects?

THE 3RD WEEK

DAY ONE

The *Shaoyang* Pattern

The *shaoyang* pattern is resulted from the invasion of external pathogens in the *shaoyang* channel with manifestations of struggle between healthy qi and pathogenic qi between the interior and exterior. This pattern can either be developed from the exterior pathogen or from the direct attack of the external pathogen on the *shaoyang* level. It is commonly seen in externally contracted diseases, and certain diseases of internal damage such as the common cold, malaria, tonsillitis, mumps, acute viral hepatitis, acute pancreatitis, acute cholecystitis, acute pleuritis, postpartum infection, and septicemia can also present similar manifestations of this pattern.

Diagnosis

The main symptoms and signs of this pattern are alternating chills and fever, and chest and rib-side distending pain. Other indications include vexation, vomiting, loss of appetite, a bitter taste in the mouth, a dry throat, and blurred vision.

The gallbladder channel, which is neither in the exterior nor in the interior (hence called half-exterior and half-interior), is the location of the struggle between healthy qi and invading pathogens. If the pathogens are in dominance, yang qi will be checked, thus giving rise to an aversion to cold. If the yang qi is strong enough, the aversion to cold can be relieved as a high body temperature is observed. However, *wei* yang circulates throughout the body only at certain times, hence manifesting as alternating chills and fever or an aversion to cold and fever. The *shaoyang* gallbladder channel runs along the chest and rib sides, so pathogens in the *shaoyang* level are able to inhibit the flow of channel qi, leading to chest and rib-side distention and fullness or pain, though the symptoms can either be on one side or both. The gallbladder channel is derived from its namesake, the gallbladder, so pathogens in the gallbladder channel can cause gallbladder qi to attack the stomach, thus adversely causing stomach qi to rise, which will result in vomiting and a lack of appetite. If heat is present in the gallbladder channel, the fire can upset the upper part of the body, triggering vexation, a bitter taste in the mouth, and blurred vision.

Generally, the pathogen in *shaoyang* level is heat, but sometimes, it can be heat–dampness, especially the external contraction of damp–heat pathogens, whose symptoms are chills and fever that are similar to malaria, a mild aversion to cold, high fever, a bitter taste in the mouth, chest oppression, vomiting, hiccups, and a white and greasy tongue coating. Its pathological features are moderately severe gallbladder heat and internal obstruction of phlegm–dampness, which also indicate the presence of damp–heat symptoms.

The clinical manifestations of pathogens in the *shaoyang* level are various, but for diagnosis, the conclusion can be made according to one or two main symptoms instead of evaluating every possible symptom.

Treatment method

Harmonizing the exterior and interior and regulating the spleen and stomach.

Formula and ingredients: Xiǎo Chái Hú Tāng (Minor Bupleurum Decoction)

Chái hú (Radix Bupleuri) 12 g; *huáng qín* (Radix Scutellariae) 9 g; *rén shēn* (Radix et Rhizoma Ginseng) 9 g; *bàn xià* (Rhizoma Pinelliae) 9 g; *zhì gān cǎo* (Radix et Rhizoma Glycyrrhizae Praeparata cum Melle) 6 g; sliced *shēng jiāng* (Rhizoma Zingiberis Recens) 9 g; jujube 4 pieces.

Formula verse

Xiǎo Chái Hú Tāng is used for harmonization; includes *bàn xià*, *rén shēn* and *gān cǎo*; and also *huáng qín*, ginger and jujubes; being a classic formula for *shaoyang* diseases.

Usage

Add 2.4 L of water to decoct until 1.2 L are left. Remove the dregs and decoct it again until 600 mL are left. Take 200 mL of the decoction warm each time, 3 times a day.

Analysis

In the formula, *chái hú* is the chief ingredient. It is light and dispersing, which has the effect of venting pathogens outward and dredging qi stagnation. *Huáng qín*, bitter and cold, serves to clear heat accumulation in the *shaoyang* channel, which removes the pathogens from the interior. The combination of these two ingredients can harmonize *shaoyang*. As there is an ascending counterflow of stomach qi caused by the disharmony of the gallbladder and stomach, *bàn xià* and *shēng jiāng* are used to harmonize the stomach and direct the counterflow downward. *Rén shēn*, *gān cǎo*, and jujubes can boost qi and fortify the spleen, which on the one hand, prevent interior transmission and development of pathogens, and on the other hand, expel pathogens outward. The ingredients as a whole can harmonize *shaoyang*, fortify the middle, boost healthy qi, relieve the stomach, and arrest vomiting.

Aside from its fever-relieving property, *Xiǎo Chái Hú Tāng* can also protect hepatic cells, promote bile secretion, etc. *Chái hú* acts by calming the mind, relieving coughing, protecting the liver, and diminishing inflammation. *Huáng qín* not only has bacteriostatic and antiviral effects, but can also reduce inflammation, boost immunity, lower capillary permeability, and so on. The combination of the two above-mentioned herbs can relieve fever, promote gallbladder functions, and relieve spasms of smooth muscles. *Rén shēn* strengthens body resistance to various harmful stimulations, relieves fatigue, activates the central nervous system, and improves digestive functions when combined with *gān cǎo* and *shēng jiān*. *Bàn xià* relieves vomiting and coughing. In conclusion, *Xiǎo Chái Hú Tāng*'s curative effect targets many different regions of the body, such as the digestive system, the nervous system, and immunity.

Treatment reference

Clinically, *Xiǎo Chái Hú Tāng* is indicated for many diseases, including the common cold, flu, intestinal typhoid, acute pleuritis, acute and chronic heptitis, acute and chronic cholecystitis, acute pyelonephritis, postpartum infection, septicemia, intercostal neuralgia, malaria, and chronic eczema.

It can be used as long as there are *shaoyang* symptoms, such as alternating chills and fever, a bitter taste in the mouth, and a dry throat.

In practice, proper modification is required. For patients with heat bind in the intestines presenting as aggravated fever in the afternoon and constipation, *máng xiāo* is added and the prescription is thus changed to *Chái Hú Jiā Máng Xiāo Tāng* (Bupleurum Decoction with Sulfas). If *Xiǎo Chái Hú Tāng* is combined with *Píng Wèi Sǎn* (Stomach-Calming Powder), it becomes *Chái Píng Jiān* (Bupleurum Stomach-Calming Decoction), which is used to treat dampness in malaria with general body pains, body heaviness, a severe aversion to cold, moderate fever, and a soggy pulse; for some *shaoyang* patterns with the internal accumulation of phlegm–damp; or for chronic cholecystitis with abdominal pain, low fever, nausea, vomiting, abdominal distention, loose stool, etc. If *Xiǎo Chái Hú Tāng* is combined with *Sì Wù Tāng* (Four Substances Decoction), it can treat prolonged deficiency–consumption and mild alternating chills and fever, and is indicated for tuberculosis, stubborn hepatitis, and scant or delayed menstruation. If *zhǐ qiào, jié gěng, chén pí*, and green tea are added, *Xiǎo Chái Hú Tāng* becomes *Chái Hú Zhǐ Jiè Tāng* (Bupleurum Decoction plus Bitter Orange and Platycodon), which is used to treat *shaoyang* patterns presenting alternating chills and fever and chest and gastric fullness. Currently, *chái hú, huáng qín, bàn xià, mù xiāng, yù jīn, chē qián zǐ, chuān mù tōng, zhī zǐ, yīn chén*, and raw *dà huáng* have been blended into *Chái Hú Lì Dǎn Tāng* (Bupleurum Gallbladder-Benefiting Decoction), which is indicated for acute and chronic cholecystitis, pancreatitis, gallbladder stones, and suppurative cholangitis presenting alternating chills and fever, distending right rib-side pain, a bitter taste in the mouth, a dry throat, yellowish eyes, yellow and turbid urine, constipation, a reddish tongue with a yellow and greasy coating, and a wiry pulse. If *Xiǎo Chái Hú Tāng* is used together with *dāng guī, dān shēn, yì mǔ cǎo*, and *jīng jiè tàn*, it can treat postpartum body weakness further contracted with external pathogens that invade the *shaoyang* level, presenting alternating chills and fever and a persistent flow of lochia. *Xiǎo Chái Hú Tāng* together with *shēng dì, dāng guī, táo rén, hóng huā*, and *mǔ dān pí* can treat external pathogenic attacks during menstrual periods, which presents alternating chills and fever, abdominal pain, and even unconscious ravings. *Xiǎo Chái Hú Tāng* can also be applied to many diseases without apparent alternating chills and fever, such as bile reflux gastritis, mammary tumors, and renal colic, which indicates that this formula has a promising future for medical application.

For pathogens in the *shaoyang* level that induces relatively serious gallbladder heat and internal obstruction of phlegm–damp, where manifestations such as alternating chills and fever, malaria-like symptoms, mild chills and high fever, a bitter taste in the mouth, chest oppression, belching or spitting of sticky saliva, and a red tongue with a greasy coating are observed, *Hāo Qín Qīng Dǎn Tāng* (Sweet Wormwood and Scutellaria Gallbladder-Clearing Decoction) is prescribed. In this formula, bitter–cold and aromatic *qīng hāo* replaces *chái hú* and is combined with *huáng qín* to clear the heat of *shaoyang*. *Qīng hāo* has the effect of removing dampness and clearing heat, applicable to patients with high fever and phlegm–damp.

Cautions

The pathogens of the *shaoyang* pattern resides in the half-exterior and half-interior, hence methods of inducing sweating, promoting vomiting, and purgation should not be used, otherwise healthy qi, blood, and body fluids will be impaired, and the *shaoyang* pattern might mutate into the interior pattern. Therefore, close observation is required in clinical practice so as to modify the treatment method when the need arises.

Daily Exercises

1. What are the main clinical manifestations of the *shaoyang* pattern?
2. What are the ingredients of *Xiǎo Chái Hú Tāng*?
3. Ms. Shen is a 41-year-old female. She has had fever and an aversion to cold for 5 days. The fever is mild in the morning, but in the afternoon after the occurrence of an aversion to cold, her body temperature peaked at 39.4°C. Other symptoms are a lack of strength, a bitter taste in the mouth, nausea, poor appetite, and right rib-side distending pain. A physical examination shows an enlarged liver 3 cm below the rib cage, soft and tender. Please prescribe a Chinese medicinal formula for this case.

Additional Formulae

Chái Hú Jiā Máng Xiāo Tāng (Bupleurum Decoction with Sulfas)

Chái hú (Radix Bupleuri) 9 g; huáng qín (Radix Scutellariae) 6 g; rén shēn (Radix et Rhizoma Ginseng) 6 g; zhì gān cǎo (Radix et Rhizoma Glycyrrhizae Praeparata cum Melle) 6 g; shēng jiāng (Rhizoma Zingiberis Recens) 3 g; bàn xià (Rhizoma Pinelliae) 6 g; dà zǎo (Fructus Jujubae) 4 pieces; máng xiāo (Natrii Sulfas) 6 g infused. Add water to decoct.

Actions

Releasing shaoyang to the exterior and purging heat bind in the interior.

Indications

Alternating chills and fever, or aggravated fever in the afternoon, a bitter taste in the mouth, chest and rib-side distention and fullness, constipation, a dry tongue with a yellow coating, and a slow and wiry pulse.

Chái Píng Jiān (Bupleurum Stomach-Calming Decoction)

Chái hú (Radix Bupleuri) 5 g; huáng qín (Radix Scutellariae) 6 g; rén shēn (Radix et Rhizoma Ginseng) 12 g; bàn xià (Rhizoma Pinelliae) 6 g; zhì gān cǎo (Radix et Rhizoma Glycyrrhizae Praeparata cum Melle) 3 g; chén pí (Pericarpium Citri Reticulatae) 6 g; hòu pò (Cortex Magnoliae Officinalis) 6 g; cāng zhú (Rhizoma Atractylodis) 6 g; shēng jiāng (Rhizoma Zingiberis Recens) 3 g; jujube 3 g. Add water to decoct.

Actions

Harmonizing shaoyang and the stomach and dispelling dampness.

Indications

Dampness malaria presenting body pains and heaviness, relatively serious chills, low fever, and a soggy pulse.

Chái Hú Zhǐ Jiè Tāng *(Bupleurum Decoction Plus Bitter Orange and Platycodon)*

Chái hú (Radix Bupleuri) 4 g; *zhǐ qiào* (Fructus Aurantii) 4.5 g; *jiāng bàn xià* (Rhizoma Pinelliae Praeparatum) 4.5 g; fresh *shēng jiāng* (Rhizoma Zingiberis Recens) 3 g; fresh *huáng qín* (Radix Scutellariae) 4 g; *jié gěng* (Radix Platycodonis) 3 g; *chén pí* (Pericarpium Citri Reticulatae) 4.5 g; *yǔ qián chá* (Folium Theae) 3 g.

Actions

Harmonizing and venting the exterior, and soothing the chest and diaphragm.

Indications

Alternating chills and fever, bilateral upper head pain, deafness, dizzy vision, chest and rib-side fullness and pain, a white and greasy tongue coating, and a wiry pulse.

Hāo Qín Qīng Dǎn Tāng *(Sweet Wormwood and Scutellaria Gallbladder-Clearing Decoction)*

Qīng hāo (Herba Artemisiae Annuae) 6 g; *zhú rú* (Caulis Bambusae in Taenia) 9 g; *bàn xià* (Rhizoma Pinelliae) 5 g; *chì fú líng* (Poria Rubra) 9 g; *huáng qín* (Radix Scutellariae) 6 g; raw *zhǐ qiào* (Fructus Aurantii) 5 g; *guǎng chén pí* (Pericarpium Citri Reticulatae) 5 g; *Bì Yù Sǎn* (Jasper Jade Powder) 1 bag (9 g). Add water to decoct.

Actions

Clearing the gallbladder and draining dampness; harmonizing the stomach and dissolving phlegm.

Indications

Chills and fever similar to malaria, relatively mild chills and high fever, a bitter taste in the mouth, chest oppression, vomiting of sour and bitter liquids or yellow and sticky drool, or even dry vomiting, hiccups, chest and rib-side distending pain, a red tongue with a white and variegated coating, and a rapid pulse (right: slippery and left: wiry).

DAY TWO

The *Shaoyang Yangming* Pattern

The *shaoyang yangming* pattern is the *shaoyang* pattern complicated with heat bind in the stomach and intestines. This pattern can be seen either in externally contracted diseases or in diseases of internal damage, especially those of the digestive system, such as acute and chronic biliary infection, acute pancreatitis, acute ulcer perforation, and hepatitis.

Diagnosis

The main symptoms and signs of this pattern are alternating chills and fever, and distress and pain or fullness and pain aggravated upon pressing the region below the heart. Other indications, in addition to manifestations of the *shaoyang* pattern, include fullness and discomfort in the chest and rib sides, a bitter taste in the mouth, a dry throat, mild vexation, constipation, or loose and smelly stool with a hot sensation, vomiting, jaundice, a yellow tongue coating, and a wiry and rapid pulse. The manifestation of pain when pressure is applied on the area below the heart in fact originates from the stomach, intestines, liver, gallbladder, pancreas, etc. It is due to local muscular tension and pain, usually tenderness, which is evident when the patient responds unfavorably to pressure or experiences rebound pain if the hand pressing the painful region is suddenly removed. This region can either be on one side or both sides below the heart. According to the theory of Chinese medicine, fullness, pain, and hardness below the heart, constipation or diarrhea with a hot sensation, a yellow tongue coating, and a wiry and rapid pulse are signs that pathogens have been in *yangming* level and there is heat bind in *yangming*. Therefore, this pattern is termed as the *shaoyang yangming* pattern.

Treatment method

Harmonizing *shaoyang* and purging heat bind in the interior.

Formula and ingredients: Dà Chái Hú Tāng
(Major Bupleurum Decoction)

Chái hú (Radix Bupleuri) 15 g; *huáng qín* (Radix Scutellariae) 9 g; *sháo yào* (Radix Paeoniae) 9 g; *bàn xià* (Rhizoma Pinelliae) 9 g; dry-fried *zhǐ shí* (Fructus Aurantii Immaturus) 9 g; *dà huáng* (Radix et Rhizoma Rhei) 6 g; *shēng jiāng* (Rhizoma Zingiberis Recens) 15 g; *dà zǎo* (Fructus Jujubae) 5 pieces.

Formula verse

Dà Chái Hú Tāng uses *dà huáng* and *zhǐ qín xià sháo zǎo shēng jiāng*; for diseases both in *shaoyang* and *yangming*, by harmonization and purgation as a favorable method.

Usage

Add 2.4 L of water to decoct until 1.2 L are left. Remove the dregs and decoct it again until 600 mL are left. Take 200 mL of the decoction warm each time, 3 times a day.

Analysis

Dà Chái Hú Tāng is based on *Xiǎo Chái Hú Tāng* by removing *rén shēn* and *gān cǎo*, and adding *dà huáng*, *sháo yào*, and *zhǐ shí*. In the formula, *chái hú* and *huáng qín* together can harmonize *shaoyang*. *Dà huáng* and *zhǐ shí* together can purge heat bind in the *yangming* level, which is blended with the function of *Xiǎo Chéng Qì Tāng* (Minor Purgative Decoction). For this reason, this formula can also be regarded as the combination of *Xiǎo Chái Hú Tāng* and *Xiǎo Chéng Qì Tāng*. For the other ingredients, *sháo yào* relaxes cramps, relieves pain, and harmonizes blood flow; *bàn xià* directs counterflow downward and arrests vomiting, and when it is combined with *shēng jiāng*, it becomes more effective in arresting vomiting; the combination of *shēng jiāng* and *dà zǎo* can harmonize *ying* and *wei* levels and protect stomach qi. The reason for *rén shēn* and *gān cǎo* being removed from *Xiǎo Chái Hú Tāng* to treat the *shaoyang yangming* pattern by *Dà Chái Hú Tāng* is that due to heat bind in the *yangming* level, it is inappropriate to apply sweet and warm ingredients, in case of promoting heat to impair yin. All the ingredients as a whole can harmonize, relieve fever, cramps, and pain, direct counterflow downward, arrest vomiting, relax bowels, and resolve heat bind.

Dà Chái Hú Tāng is excellent in promoting gallbladder functions and decreasing sphincter tone. *Dà huáng* and *sháo yào* can act synergistically to enhance gallbladder functions. The combination of *dà huáng* and *zhǐ shí* is able to strengthen intestinal peristalsis and relax bowels. *Dà huáng* and many other ingredients have antibiotic, anti-inflammatory, analgesic, and anti-pyretic effects. Therefore, this formula is effective in treating inflammation of the digestive system.

Treatment reference

The application of *Dà Chái Hú Tāng* in clinical practice is widespread, as it is often used for acute epigastric diseases. This formula is frequently indicated for treating various acute gallbladder infections, gallbladder stones, acute pancreatitis, gastric and duodenal perforation, acute and chronic hepatitis, and so on. For some cases, this formula is even able to spare patients from undergoing surgery. Moreover, as this formula can also regulate blood circulation, eliminate toxins, and improve internal metabolism, it works well in rectifying hypertension, stroke, nasosinusitis, chronic eczema, diabetes, and gout.

For application, if yellowish eyes, skin, and urine are observed, add *yīn chén* and *zhī zǐ*; for high fever, thirst, vexation, and a reddish tongue, add *pú gōng yīng*, *jīn yín huā*, *lián qiào*, and *bǎn lán gēn*. If there is lingering fever, an aversion to cold, and heat bind in the intestines (which belongs to the *shaoyang yangming* pattern, but the interior *yangming* pattern is more significant), apply *Hòu Pò Qī Wù Tāng* (Officinal Magnolia Bark Seven Substances Decoction). For gallbladder stones, this formula can be used with modifications to promote gallbladder functions and expel stones, such as *Dǎn Dào Pái Shí Tāng* (Gallbladder Stone-Expelling Decoction).

Cautions

In practice, it is important to know which pattern dominates — the *shaoyang* pattern or the *yangming* pattern. If the *shaoyang* pattern is more serious, harmonization should be applied; if the interior *yangming* excess pattern is more significant, the treatment method is chiefly to purge interior heat bind. The *shaoyang yangming* pattern is usually severe and develops quickly, so close observation is required and the patient may be hospitalized in case of further complications.

Daily Exercises

1. What are the indications of *Dà Chái Hú Tāng?* What are its key points of pattern differentiation?
2. What are the ingredients of *Dà Chái Hú Tāng?*
3. Mr. Feng is a 30-year-old male. He has had severe paroxysmal epigastric pain for 3 days and there is local tenderness. Other manifestations are nausea, vomiting of yellowish-green sour fluids, a bitter taste in the mouth, thirst, a dry throat, no defecation since yesterday, yellow and scant urine, a red tongue with a yellow and greasy coating, and a wiry, slippery, and rapid pulse. Tests show counts of WBC at 15.6×10^9/L, NEU 91%, LYM 9%, and UAMY 1,024 U/L. Please prescribe a Chinese medicinal formula for this case.

Additional Formulae

Hòu Pò Qī Wù Tāng
(Officinal Magnolia Bark Seven Substances Decoction)

Hòu pò (Cortex Magnoliae Officinalis) 15 g; *gān cǎo* (Radix et Rhizoma Glycyrrhizae) 6 g; *dà huáng* (Radix et Rhizoma Rhei) 9 g; *zhǐ qiào* (Fructus Aurantii) 9 g; *guì zhī* (Ramulus Cinnamomi) 6 g; *dà zǎo* (Fructus Jujubae) 5 pieces; *shēng jiāng* (Rhizoma Zingiberis Recens) 12 g. Add water to decoct.

Actions

Releasing the flesh and dispersing the exterior; moving qi and relaxing bowels.

Indications

Lingering exterior pattern with the formation of interior excess presenting abdominal fullness, fever, constipation, and a floating and rapid pulse.

Dǎn Dào Pái Shí Tāng (Gallbladder Stone Expelling Decoction)

Yīn chén (Herba Artemisiae Scopariae) 30 g; *jīn qián cǎo* (Herba Lysimachiae) 30 g; *hēi shān zhī* (Fructus Gardeniae Nigrum) 12 g; *chái hú* (Radix Bupleuri) 6 g; *dān shēn* (Radix et Rhizoma Salviae Miltiorrhizae) 12 g; *zhǐ qiào* (Fructus Aurantii) 6 g; *chì sháo* (Radix Paeoniae Rubra) 6 g; *bái sháo* (Radix Paeoniae Alba) 6 g; *guǎng mù xiāng* (Radix Aucklandiae) 9 g; raw *dà huáng* (Radix et Rhizoma Rhei) 6 g. Add water to decoct.

Actions

Clearing heat, promoting gallbladder functions, and expelling stones.

Indications

Resolving gallbladder stones, hepatic duct stones, residual stones after operation, etc.

DAY THREE

The *Shaoyang* Phlegm–Heat Pattern

The *shaoyang* phlegm–heat pattern involves phlegm–heat obstruction in the *shaoyang* gallbladder channel. Since the liver and gallbladder are located close to each other in an exterior–interior relation, and phlegm–heat often affects the heart spirit, this pattern is related to the liver and heart. Clinically, diseases of the nervous system such as mania, nervous prostration, schizophrenia, and some kinds of vertigo often pertain to this pattern.

Diagnosis

The main symptoms and signs are chest and rib-side fullness and oppression, and mental disorder (including vexation, paranoia, anxiety, depression, delirium, and even unconsciousness, mania, etc.). Other indications include occasional fever or alternating chills and fever, body heaviness, inhibited urination, dizziness, tinnitus, insomnia, a bitter taste in the mouth, a reddish tongue with a yellow or greasy coating, and a wiry, rapid, or slippery pulse.

Two main causes of this pattern are: (1) external pathogens entering the *shaoyang* level due to a deficiency of healthy qi as the presence of the exterior pattern still lingers, or (2) from *zang–fu* deficiency and internal obstruction of phlegm–heat due to diseases of internal damage affecting the gallbladder channel, heart, and liver. As the pathogens are in the *shaoyang* channel and are in conflict with healthy qi in the chest and rib-side regions, chest and rib-side fullness and oppression are thus observed. In addition, the obstruction of the liver and gallbladder or the clouding of the heart spirit by pathogens gives rise to the various symptoms of mental disorder. These are the primary characteristics to diagnose the *shaoyang* phlegm–heat pattern. Furthermore, if this pattern is a result of an externally contracted febrile disease, because the pathogen remains in the exterior *taiyang* or *shaoyang* channel or enters the interior *yangming* channel, there will be different fever types. On the contrary, if this pattern arises from diseases of internal damage, the symptom of fever may not occur. As there are pathological changes of a lingering exterior pattern, impaired healthy qi, and pathogen obstruction in channels, body heaviness or even difficulty in turning the body may be experienced. As pathogens obstruct the *shaoyang* channel, qi movement is inhibited, affecting the transportation and distribution of body fluids and manifesting as decreased volumes of urine or inhibited urination. Phlegm–heat disrupting the upper part of the body causes dizziness, tinnitus, and a bitter taste in the mouth. A reddish tongue with a yellow or greasy coating and a wiry, rapid, or slippery pulse are also signs of phlegm–heat.

For the identification of this pattern, aside from the main symptoms and signs, its close relation to gallbladder channel can also be taken into account. For example, Meniere's syndrome is associated with a ear disorder of the *shaoyang* channel; some mania patients usually experience chest and rib-side distention and oppression before the attack, which is related to the course of the *shaoyang* channel.

Treatment method

Harmonizing *shaoyang*, clearing and dissolving hot phlegm, and calming the mind with heavy sedatives.

*Formula and ingredients: Chái Hú Jiā Lóng Gǔ Mǔ Lì Tāng
(Bupleurum Decoction with Keel and Oyster Shell)*

Chái hú (Radix Bupleuri) 9 g; *lóng gǔ* (Fossilia Ossis Mastodi) 15 g; *huáng qín* (Radix Scutellariae) 6 g; *shēng jiāng* (Rhizoma Zingiberis Recens) 6 g; *shēng tiě luò* (Frusta Ferri) 30 g; *rén shēn* (Radix et Rhizoma Ginseng) 6 g; *guì zhī* (Ramulus Cinnamomi) 6 g; *fú líng* (Poria) 9 g; *bàn xià* (Rhizoma Pinelliae) 6 g; *dà huáng* (Radix et Rhizoma Rhei) 6 g; calcined *mǔ lì* (Concha Ostreae) 15 g; *dà zǎo* (Fructus Jujubae) 3 pieces.

Formula verse

Chái Hú Jiā Lóng Gǔ Mǔ Lì Tāng, huáng qín tiě luò rén shēn jiāng; qín xià dà huáng guì zhī zǎo, clears heat and calms fright effectively.

Usage

Add 1.6 L of water to decoct until 800 mL are left. Then, add chess piece-sized *dà huáng* to decoct again. Take 200 mL of the decoction each time while warm, 3 times a day.

Analysis

Chái Hú Jiā Lóng Gǔ Mǔ Lì Tāng (Bupleurum Decoction with Keel and Oyster Shell) is based on *Xiǎo Chái Hú Tāng*. In the formula, the combination of *Xiǎo Chái Hú Tāng* and *guì zhī* can expel pathogens in the *shaoyang* level. *Gān cǎo* is removed from the *Xiǎo Chái Hú Tāng* formula because it is sweet and warm, which is not favorable for the elimination of phlegm–heat. *Lóng gǔ, mǔ lì*, and *shēng tiě luò* are heavy and sinking, which can suppress fright and calm the mind. *Dà huáng* purges heat and *fú líng* promotes urination and calms the mind, both of which contribute to the elimination of phlegm–heat.

Research has shown that this formula is effective for treating disorders of the nervous system. *Lóng gǔ* and *mǔ lì* can regulate the central nervous system and relax the mind. *Xiǎo Chái Hú Tāng* in this formula has a certain calming effect, and this effect is strengthened when combined with *lóng gǔ, mǔ lì, and shēng tiě luò*. Therefore, this formula is particularly pertinent to disorders of the nervous system.

Treatment reference

Chái Hú Jiā Lóng Gǔ Mǔ Lì Tāng is a formula that implicates warm and cold, purgation and supplementation, and ascending and descending. It is commonly applied to treat various nervous disorders such as mania, schizophrenia, neurosis, and traumatic brain syndrome presenting restlessness, headaches, a flustered state, susceptibility to fright, depression, or even insanity. In addition, it is also used to treat hyperthyroidism presenting low fever, constipation, insomnia, and irritability, as well as to treat some cases of hypertension presenting dizziness, headaches, dysphoria, a bitter taste in the mouth, and tinnitus with its function of inhibiting liver yang. Due to its properties in clearing phlegm–heat and calming the mind, it is also prescribed to treat postpartum profuse sweating with vertigo, dizziness, and palpitations.

In clinical application, if there are symptoms of internal obstruction by static blood, such as chest and rib-side pain, dark stool, and a dark purple tongue, add *táo rén*, *hóng huā*, *chuān xiōng*, and *tǔ biē chóng*. For internal exuberance of heat presenting a flushed face and red eyes, constipation, brown, and scant urine, add *lóng dǎn cǎo* and *zhī zǐ*, while removing *rén shēn*, *guì zhī*, *shēng jiāng*, *and dà zǎo*. For serious phlegm–heat presenting severe dizziness, massive sputum, and a thick greasy tongue coating, add *méng shí*, *chén xiāng*, and *shí chāng pú*. For dysphoria, add *zhū shā*, *yè jiāo téng*, and *suān zǎo rén*. For patients with a weak constitution, reduce the doses of *dà huáng* and *shēng tiě luò*. For serious phlegm–heat, reduce the dose of *rén shēn*.

Cautions

The composition of this formula is relatively complex. The main symptoms and signs in clinical practice need to be accurately identified. If there is no sign of the *shaoyang* pattern, remove *chái hú* from the formula. As symptoms of phlegm–heat are usually not obvious, the practitioner can prescribe this formula as a treatment for 2–3 days. If there is no curative effect, other therapies may be used as alternatives. In the original formula, *shēng tiě luò* is replaced by *qiān dān* (the former can suppress fright and dispel phlegm, but it is cold and toxic, so it is not applied). However, for diseases that can be treated by this formula, it is not always appropriate to use this formula.

That is because according to the theory of Chinese medicine, only diseases with the *shaoyang* phlegm–heat pattern are the indications. If the pattern pertains to pure deficiency or fire–heat, this formula is not suitable.

Daily Exercises

1. What are the main symptoms and signs of the *shaoyang* phlegm–heat pattern?
2. What are the ingredients of *Chái Hú Jiā Lóng Gǔ Mǔ Lì Tāng*?
3. Ms. Huang is a 26-year-old female. Seven years ago, she suffered from mania. Her condition has since worsened, and in recent months, an attack has been occurring 2–3 times a day. Clinical manifestations include a flushed face, vertigo, constipation, occasional nausea, chest and epigastric oppression and discomfort, a red tongue tip with a greasy tongue coating, and a wiry and rapid pulse. Please prescribe a Chinese medicinal formula for this case.

DAY FOUR

The *Shaoyang* Fluid Retention Pattern

The invasion of exogenous pathogens in the *shaoyang* half-exterior and half-interior together with internal water retention constitutes the *shaoyang* fluid retention pattern. It is commonly observed in the common cold, tuberculosis, pleuritis, hepatitis, cholecystitis, mania, neurosis, acute nephritis, and hyperplasia of the breast glands. Fluid retention may be originally present in the body, or can be a result of fluid distribution disorder due to qi blockage after the invasion of exogenous pathogens into the *shaoyang* level.

Diagnosis

The main symptoms and signs of this pattern are alternating chills and fever, chest and rib-side fullness and oppression, and inhibited urination. Other indications include vexation, thirst, no vomiting, an absence of sweating except from the head, a thin and white tongue coating, and a deep and wiry pulse.

This pattern is in fact a variant of the pattern treated by *Xiǎo Chái Hú Tāng*, so it has the primary symptoms and signs of the *shaoyang* pattern, such as alternating chills and fever, chest and rib-side distending pain, and vexation. However, since it is accompanied by fluid retention obstructing the *shaoyang* channel, the blockage of qi is more severe, manifesting as relatively serious chest and rib-side distention and fullness (even with the sensation of feeling something hard on the inside). With internal water retention, the flow of fluids becomes abnormal, so there is inhibited urination. The binding of pathogenic heat in the *shaoyang* channel and water retention causes an upward flow of the constrained heat, manifesting as an absence of sweating except from the head. Thirst as a result of this pattern is caused by the consumption of fluids by the constrained heat and the abnormal distribution of fluids after the obstruction of water retention in the middle. A thin and white tongue coating and a wiry pulse are signs of pathogen invasion in the *shaoyang*. Internal fluid retention usually manifests as a deep pulse.

Treatment method

Harmonizing *shaoyang*, and warming and removing fluid retention.

Formula and ingredients: Chái Hú Guì Jiāng Tāng (Bupleurum, Cinnamon Twig, and Dried Ginger Decoction)

Chái hú (Radix Bupleuri) 15 g; *guì zhī* (Ramulus Cinnamomi) 9 g; *gān jiāng* (Rhizoma Zingiberis) 6 g; *tiān huā fěn* (Radix Trichosanthis) 12 g; *huáng qín* (Radix Scutellariae) 9 g; *mǔ lì* (Concha Ostreae) 6 g; *zhì gān cǎo* (Radix et Rhizoma Glycyrrhizae Praeparata cum Melle) 6 g.

Formula Verse

Chái Hú Guì Jiāng Tāng; use *tiān huā qín lì cǎo*.

Usage

Add 2.4 L of water to decoct until 1.2 L are left. Remove the dregs and decoct it again until 600 mL are left. Take 200 mL of the decoction warm each time, 3 times a day. There will be mild vexation at the beginning after taking the decoction. Take the decoction again and the disease can be cured after perspiration.

Analysis

Chái Hú Guì Jiāng Tāng is a variant of *Xiǎo Chái Hú Tāng*. In this formula, *chái hú* and *huáng qín*, if used together, can harmonize *shaoyang*. *Guì zhī*, *gān jiāng*, and *gān cǎo* are warm and hot, which can unblock yang and eliminate water retention by warming. Both *tiān huā fěn* and *mǔ lì* can dissipate masses and expel water retention. Further, *tiān huā fěn* can also clear heat and promote fluid production and when it is combined with *huáng qín*, it can purge the constrained heat in the interior. *Bàn xià* used in *Xiǎo Chái Hú Tāng* has been removed because this pattern does not induce vomiting. *Rén shēn* and *dà zǎo* are removed as well; as there is water retention in this pattern, supplementary products are inappropriate. All ingredients as a whole can harmonize and clear heat, warm and remove fluid retention, promote fluid production to quench thirst, release the pathogens in the *shaoyang* from the exterior, and resolve fluid retention in the interior.

Gān jiāng and guì zhī can activate the vascular center and sympathetic nervous system, dilate blood vessels, and improve blood circulation. *Guì zhī* can also promote urination and relieve fever, which are functions related to this formula's effect in clearing heat and eliminating fluid retention. The modern research work involving *chái hú*, *huáng qín*, *mǔ lì*, and *gān cǎo* has been introduced in the previous section.

Treatment reference

The clinical application of *Chái Hú Guì Jiāng Tāng* is similar to *Xiǎo Chái Hú Tāng*. The only difference is that the former is more effective in treating fairly serious heat constraint in the *shaoyang* level with internal water retention or water retention affecting the upper part of the body, in which manifestations include eye congestion, an itching scalp, eczema in the head or upper part of the body, and eye and ear pain. Certainly, these symptoms do not solely pertain to water retention affecting the upper part of the body, but if there are also other manifestations of water retention in the *shaoyang* level, or other pathological changes have been excluded, this formula can be applied. This formula is applicable to malaria, acute pyelonephritis, tuberculosis, pleuritis, hepatitis, cholecystitis, mania, neurosis, coronary disease, and hyperplasia of the breast glands presenting the *shaoyang* water retention pattern.

In practice, if this pattern is accompanied with body fluid deficiency and a dry cough, add *tiān dōng* and *yù zhú*. For heat deficiency and night sweat, add *huáng qí* and *biē jiǎ*. For dizziness due to severe water retention, add *zé xiè*, *fú líng*, and *bái zhú*. For palpitations and insomnia, add *suān zǎo rén*, *yuǎn zhì*, *lóng chǐ*, and *yè jiāo téng*.

Cautions

This formula is applied mainly for the treatment of the *shaoyang* pattern together with internal water retention or water retention affecting the upper part of the body. If signs of water retention and constrained heat are absent, do not use *guì zhī* and *gān jiāng*. This formula can assist healthy qi to expel pathogens outward, resulting in feelings of mild vexation. However afterwards, the yang qi of the interior and exterior would be unblocked and sweating would occur. This mechanism of sweating is different from that of the exterior-releasing formulae.

Daily Exercises

1. What are the key points of pattern differentiation in the *shaoyang* water retention pattern?
2. What are the ingredients of *Chái Hú Guì Jiāng Tāng*?
3. Mr. Jin is a 46-year-old male. He has complaints of right chest and rib-side pain for a week, especially during inhalation. Other manifestations are a fear of cold, fever in the afternoon, sweating in the evening, headaches, dizziness, a mild cough, brown and scant urine, a deep and wiry pulse, and a white and greasy tongue coating. A chest X-ray shows acute pleuritis. Please prescribe a Chinese medicinal formula for this case.

CHAPTER 5

The Cold Pattern

DAY FIVE

The cold pattern is typically manifested as the hypofunction of the whole body due to yang qi obstruction or yang qi deficiency after the patient has contracted an exogenous cold pathogen or suffers from exuberance of yin cold such as water–dampness and phlegm–turbidity.

The cold pattern is divided into the exterior cold pattern and interior cold pattern. The exterior excess–cold pattern and exterior deficiency–cold pattern learnt in Chapter 3 both belong to the exterior cold pattern. The interior cold pattern is further subdivided into the interior excess–cold pattern and the interior deficiency–cold pattern. The former mainly manifests as pathogenic cold obstructing yang qi, while the latter is chiefly due to yang qi deficiency.

Features of the Interior Cold Pattern

All categories of interior cold patterns have the common manifestation of body hypofunction, hence there are several similar symptoms between the interior excess–cold pattern and interior deficiency–cold pattern. However, some differences still remain. Manifestations of the interior excess–cold pattern include cold limbs, a fear of cold, abdominal pain which hurts when pressed, constipation or massive sputum, panting, a white, thick, and greasy tongue coating, and a deep and hidden pulse or a wiry and tight pulse. On the other hand, in the interior deficiency–cold pattern, commonly observed signs are cold limbs, a fear of cold, abdominal pain in favor of pressure, dispiritedness, loose stool, clear and profuse urine, feeble or deep, a slow, and weak pulse. In this section, the diagnosis and treatment of the interior deficiency–cold pattern will be discussed, but these can also be a form of reference in the case of the interior excess–cold pattern.

The common clinical manifestations of all interior deficiency–cold patterns have been listed above, but as the disorders may involve varying combinations of *zang–fu* organs and channels, the specific symptoms are different, which will be discussed in detail later.

Formation of the Interior Deficiency–Cold Pattern

The interior deficiency–cold pattern often results from the deterioration of yang qi. Yang qi can warm the whole body, promote the normal functions of *zang–fu* organs, and support the sustenance of life. If yang qi is in decline, "cold" signs of body hypofunction will emerge. Moreover, yang qi deficiency leads to hypofunction of the spleen and kidney converting and transporting food and water–dampness, presenting abdominal pain, diarrhea, water retention or internal retention of cold–damp, etc.

The interior deficiency–cold pattern usually occurs at the late stage of acute diseases or long after chronic diseases. It may also be caused by deficiencies in body systems. Therefore, the severity of the different diseases with this pattern spreads across a large scale. Examples of varying manifestations are a fear of cold, cold limbs, immediate diarrhea caused by the intake of raw and cold food or by catching a cold (which belong to a mild interior deficiency–cold pattern), while others can be a pale complexion, dispiritedness, or even profuse cold sweating, a feeble pulse, and death due to yang qi collapse (which pertain to a serious interior deficiency–cold pattern).

Clinically, this pattern can be observed in acute and chronic enteritis, chronic nephritis, chronic gastritis, chronic bronchitis, certain types of neurosis, and also various acute infectious diseases presenting peripheral circulatory failure, heart failure, and kidney failure.

Categories of the Interior Deficiency–Cold Pattern

Clinical manifestations of the interior deficiency–cold pattern are very complex. This is primarily due to the close relationship of this pattern with yang qi. The severity of yang qi deficiency, and more importantly, the location of yang qi deficiency affect what kind of symptoms will emerge. Yang qi exists in all *zang–fu* organs, channels, and collaterals. If deficiency of yang qi occurs and body functions deteriorate, there will be specific clinical manifestations. This provides substantiation for the classification of the interior deficiency–cold pattern into further sub-patterns. There are two main kinds of classification: (1) based on the six channels, including the *taiyin* deficiency–cold pattern, the *shaoyin* deficiency–cold pattern, the *jueyin* deficiency–cold pattern, etc; and (2) based on the *zang–fu* organs, including the heart yang deficiency pattern, the spleen yang deficiency pattern, and the kidney yang deficiency pattern. However, the six channels are closely associated with the *zang–fu* organs, so the *taiyin* deficiency–cold pattern is actually the spleen–stomach deficiency–cold pattern; the *shaoyin* deficiency–cold pattern corresponds to the heart–kidney yang deficiency pattern; and the *jueyin* deficiency–cold pattern is similar to the liver–gallbladder deficiency–cold pattern. Apart from above lists, the interior deficiency–cold pattern also includes the lung deficiency pattern, the large intestine deficiency–cold pattern, the small intestine deficiency–cold pattern, and the bladder deficiency–cold pattern. This section will discuss the diagnosis and treatment of the *taiyin* deficiency–cold pattern, the *shaoyin* deficiency–cold pattern, and the *jueyin* deficiency–cold pattern, which are the most common among all interior deficiency–cold patterns.

Treatment Methods of the Interior Deficiency–Cold Pattern

Warming the interior is the key component in treating this pattern, which involves the application of acrid–warm or acrid–hot medicinals to warm and supplement yang qi, and warm and unblock channels. As various cold symptoms are caused by yang qi deficiency of the interior cold pattern, these signs will wane spontaneously when yang qi is restored. The interior-warming medicinals can also expel pathogenic cold (exterior cold), which is also the reason why some formulae that treat the interior deficiency–cold pattern can also be applied to the excess–cold pattern. The specific purpose of warming the interior is to activate related functions of the *zang–fu* organs, such as improving the endocrine system, strengthening blood circulation, dilating blood vessels, enhancing blood pressure, boosting appetite, fortifying heart contractions, and regulating the immune system.

Since the severity and disease location of the interior deficiency–cold pattern are different for every case, the method of warming the interior is further divided into: warming the center to dissipate cold, warming and supplementing yang qi, restoring yang to prevent from desertion, warming the kidney, warming the spleen, warming the stomach, warming the liver, and warming the lung.

The interior-warming formulae are warm and hot, so improper application can assist pathogenic heat in impairing yin, which should be avoided. In addition, the ingredients should never be used in excessive doses. The medicinal decoction should be withdrawn immediately after the disease has been cured. For patients with yin deficiency, be cautious when applying warming formulae. In hot summer days, the doses of interior warming formulae should be relatively smaller.

Daily Exercises

1. What are the cold, interior cold, and interior deficiency–cold patterns?
2. What are the clinical features of the interior deficiency–cold pattern?
3. What is the main treatment principle for the interior deficiency–cold pattern? Which aspects should be paid attention to?

DAY SIX

The *Taiyang* Deficiency–Cold Pattern

The *taiyang* deficiency–cold pattern is an interior deficiency pattern due to spleen yang deficiency in that the spleen fails to transport and convert food into usable substances and warm the extremities. As the spleen belongs to the *taiyin* channel, it is also termed as the *taiyin* deficiency–cold pattern. This pattern is frequently seen in several diseases of the digestive system such as acute and chronic enteritis, gastroduodenal ulcers, and chronic gastritis; infectious diseases such as cholera, intestinal typhoid, and chronic hepatitis; and also chronic diseases of the respiratory system such as pulmonary heart disease and chronic bronchitis, presenting obvious symptoms of disorders of the spleen and stomach. This pattern is especially common among patients with spleen yang deficiency, and after undergoing serious and prolonged illnesses.

Diagnosis

The main symptoms and signs of this pattern are distending abdominal pain in favor of warmth and pressure, vomiting, diarrhea, thirst, and a pale tongue. Other indications include a reduced appetite, aggravated abdominal distention after food intake, a thirst for hot beverages, vomiting of loose drool, a white and mildly greasy tongue coating, and a thin and feeble pulse.

The spleen governs the transportation and conversion of food and raises clear yang. If the spleen and stomach are functioning abnormally or if the patient consumes raw and cold food excessively, spleen yang will be impaired, leading to failure of the spleen to perform its activities at its optimum and also to a disorder of "ascending and descending." Therefore, vomiting (upper region of the body) and diarrhea (lower region of the body) are resulted. Internal exuberance of cold and inhibited yang qi manifest as abdominal fullness and pain, a lack of thirst, a white and greasy tongue coating, and a thin and weak pulse. Abdominal pain in favor of warmth and pressure are one of the characteristics of the interior deficiency–cold pattern, which can be differentiated from the abdominal pain of the interior heat and excess–cold patterns. Patients with this pattern can sometimes feel thirsty, but prefer only hot drinks, as they may dispel interior cold. For this pattern, the contents of vomit are usually loose drool or gastric contents without any pungent odor. The diarrhea is manifested as loose or watery stool with clear and profuse urine, which is significantly different from the diarrhea due to damp–heat.

If the spleen and stomach are suddenly infected with external cold that obstructs the spleen yang, symptoms similar to the interior deficiency–cold pattern will occur. Although one is a deficiency pattern and the other is an excess pattern, spleen yang obstruction can also be associated with yang deficiency. Therefore, each of the pattern's treatment and diagnosis can serve as a reference to the other.

Treatment method

Warming the center and fortifying the spleen.

Formula and ingredients: Lǐ Zhōng Tāng (Center-Regulating Decoction)

Gān jiāng (Rhizoma Zingiberis) 5 g; *rén shēn* (Radix et Rhizoma Ginseng) 6 g; *bái zhú* (Rhizoma Atractylodis Macrocephalae) 9 g; *zhì gān cǎo* (Radix et Rhizoma Glycyrrhizae Praeparata cum Melle) 6 g.

Formula verse

Lǐ Zhōng Tāng is for warming center yang; with *rén shēn bái zhú cǎo gān jiāng*.

Usage

Add 2.4 L of water to decoct until 1.2 L are left. Remove the dregs and decoct it again until 600 mL are left. Take 200 mL of the the decoction warm each time, 3 times a day.

About 30 min after taking the decoction, consume about 200 mL of loose warm porridge and cover the body with sheets to keep warm in case of contracting a cold. These four ingredients can also be made into pills with honey, called *Lǐ Zhōng Wán* (Center-Regulating Pill). The pills are 6–9 g each, and at one time, 1 pill should be taken by chewing with warm water, 3 times in the day and 2 times in the evening. If a warm sensation in the abdomen still does not arise, increase the dosage. This formula has also been made into water pills the size of firmiana seeds, 6–9 g each, and taken 3 times a day.

Analysis

In the formula, the acrid–warm *gān jiāng*, as the main medicinal, warms and fortifies the spleen and stomach yang qi to dispel interior cold and restore the descending and ascending functions of the spleen and stomach. *Rén shēn* is combined to supplement qi and strengthen the spleen to assist in conversion and transportation; *bái zhú* is used to fortify the spleen and dry dampness; *zhì gān cǎo* is for boosting qi and harmonizing the middle. These four ingredients as a whole can warm center yang, improve the middle *jiao*, dispel cold in the middle, raise the clear and direct turbid yang downward, promote transportation, and remove dampness.

Gān jiāng has effects of fortifying the stomach and improving blood circulation. *Rén shēn* can strengthen gastrointestinal functions, activate the nervous system, and improve metabolism. *Gān cǎo* is able to reduce spasms of intestinal smooth muscles, inhibit the secretion of gastric acids, and protect the gastrointestinal membrane and lining. Therefore, this formula is typically applied for the regulation of the digestive system and the normal functioning of the whole body.

Treatment reference

Lǐ Zhōng Tāng is a common formula for warming the middle and fortifying the spleen. It has a wide clinical application so all spleen–stomach deficiency–cold patterns caused by spleen–stomach deficiency–cold or other factors can be treated by this formula. It is indicated for acute and chronic gastroenteritis, gastroduodenal ulcers, gastric prolapse, edema, chronic bronchitis, severe malnutrition in children, and profuse menstruation presenting signs of spleen–stomach deficiency–cold. For chronic diarrhea and abdominal pain, it is very important to recognize the features of spleen–stomach deficiency–cold; aside from the main symptoms and signs mentioned above, the following symptoms can be taken into account: dull pain aggravated during hunger and remission after having food, and aggravated after overstrain or catching a cold. In addition, a patient with a physique of spleen–stomach deficiency–cold provides some diagnostic values.

In practice, modification of the formula is required and many similar formulae are derived from it. For severe vomiting, add *wú zhū yú* and *jiāng bàn xià*. For severe diarrhea, increase the dosage of *bái zhú* or add *cāng zhú* and *fú líng*. For profuse menstruation, spitting of blood, and bloody stool belonging to spleen–stomach deficiency–cold, replace *gān jiāng* with *páo jiāng*, and add *zhì huáng qí*, charred *qiàn cǎo*, and *ǒu jié*. If deficiency–cold is serious and the extremities are cold, add *fù zǐ*, becoming *Fù Zǐ Lǐ Zhōng Wán* (Aconite Center-Regulating Pill). For middle *jiao* deficiency–cold with constrained heat presenting acid regurgitation, abdominal pain, and loose stool, add *huáng lián*, becoming *Lián Lǐ Tāng* (Coptis-Regulating Decoction). For spleen–stomach deficiency–cold accompanied by the *taiyang* exterior cold pattern, add *guì zhī*, becoming *Guì Zhī Rén Shēn Tāng* (Cinnamon Twig and Ginseng Decoction). For spleen–stomach deficiency–cold accompanied by phlegm–rheum retention, add *bàn xià* and *fú líng*, becoming *Lǐ Zhōng Huà Tán Wán* (Center-Regulating and Phlegm-Transforming Pill). For spleen–stomach deficiency–cold accompanied with water–damp retention, add *Wǔ Líng Sǎn* (Five Substances Powder with Poria), which becomes *Lǐ Líng Tāng* (Regulating with Poria Decoction).

Moreover, if the symptoms and signs of spleen yang deficiency are dull abdominal pain that are relieved by warmth or pressure, a lusterless complexion, fatigue, palpitations, and a light red tongue with a white coating, *Lǐ Zhōng Tāng* will be too warm and dry a formula, and this can be changed to *Xiǎo Jiàn Zhōng Tāng* (Minor Center-Fortifying Decoction). This modified formula consists of *Guì Zhī Tāng* with *yí táng* (Saccharum Granorum) and a doubled dose of *sháo yào* (Radix Paeoniae), thus being able to warm the interior, relieve cramps, fortify middle qi, and boost the spleen and stomach.

Cautions

Lǐ Zhōng Tāng is very effective for the interior deficiency–cold pattern, but it is warm and hot, and hence cannot be applied for a long period of time. For spleen–stomach deficiency–cold with pathogenic heat, heat-clearing medicinals should be added. If this formula is applied to treat various kinds of bleeding, pattern differentiation must be accurate, or the warm–hot nature of this formula can drive frenetic flow of blood and worsen the bleeding. In addition, blood-arresting methods should also be combined if bleeding is massive, and close observation may be required when using this formula, in case of further complications.

Daily Exercises

1. What are the key points of pattern differentiation of the *taiyin* deficiency–cold pattern?
2. What are the ingredients of the *Lǐ Zhōng Tāng*? Can you list three modified formulae derived from this formula?
3. Mr. Ha is a 54-year-old male. He has a history of chronic gastritis. Two days ago, he suffered from dull gastric pain that can sometimes be acute after having cold and raw food. He feels comfortable when his abdomen is pressed by hot water bags. Other clinical manifestations are a pale complexion, four extremities lacking warmth, a bland taste in the mouth, a lack of thirst, loose stool thrice a day, a pale tongue with a thin and white coating, and a thin and weak pulse. Please prescribe a Chinese medicinal formula for this case.

Additional Formulae

Fù Zǐ Lǐ Zhōng Wán (Aconite Center-Regulating Pill)

Gān jiāng (Rhizoma Zingiberis); *rén shēn* (Radix et Rhizoma Ginseng); *bái zhú* (Rhizoma Atractylodis Macrocephalae); *zhì gān cǎo* (Radix et Rhizoma Glycyrrhizae Praeparata cum Melle); *fù zǐ* (Radix Aconiti Lateralis Praeparata); 30 g each.

The ingredients are ground into a fine powder, fried with honey, and make into pills. Take a pill 6–9 g each time with warm water before meals, times a day.

Actions

Warming yang, dispelling cold, boosting qi, and fortifying the spleen.

Indications

Spleen–kidney deficiency–cold presenting cold abdominal pain, vomiting, diarrhea, a lack of warmth in the extremities, and a deep and slow pulse.

Lián Lǐ Tāng (Coptis Regulating Decoction)

Ingredients of *Lǐ Zhōng Tāng* plus *huáng lián* (Rhizoma Coptidis) and *fú líng* (Poria). Add water to decoct.

Actions

Warming the center, dispelling cold, and clearing constrained heat.

Indications

Spleen–stomach deficiency–cold with summer heat after consuming raw and cold food, presenting diarrhea, vomiting with acidic juices, and a red tongue, coating, tip, and edges.

Guì Zhī Rén Shēn Tāng (Cinnamon Twig and Ginseng Decoction)

Gān jiāng (Rhizoma Zingiberis) 6 g; *rén shēn* (Radix et Rhizoma Ginseng) 9 g; *bái zhú* (Rhizoma Atractylodis Macrocephalae) 9 g; *zhì gān cǎo* (Radix et Rhizoma Glycyrrhizae Praeparata cum Melle) 9 g; *guì zhī* (Ramulus Cinnamomi) 12 g added later. Decoct the ingredients with water and take the decoction warm.

Actions

Warming the interior and releasing the exterior.

Indications

Disorder of both the interior and exterior with a lingering exterior pattern, and impaired spleen yang presenting dull pain, diarrhea, a hard and stuffy sensation below the heart, headaches, and an aversion to cold.

Lǐ Zhōng Huà Tán Wán (Center-Regulating and Phlegm-Transforming Pill)

Gān jiāng (Rhizoma Zingiberis); *rén shēn* (Radix et Rhizoma Ginseng); dry-fried *bái zhú* (Rhizoma Atractylodis Macrocephalae); *zhì gān cǎo*

(Radix et Rhizoma Glycyrrhizae Praeparata cum Melle); *fú líng* (Poria); *bàn xià* (Rhizoma Pinelliae) prepared by ginger.

The ingredients are made into powder and fried with water to make pills the size of firmiana seeds. Take 40–50 pills each time with water.

Actions

Boosting qi and fortifying the spleen; warming and removing phlegm–drool.

Indications

Spleen–stomach deficiency–cold and internal retention of phlegm–drool, presenting vomiting, poor appetite, loose stool, indigestion, and spitting of sputum and drool.

Lǐ Líng Tāng (Regulating with Poria Decoction)

Gān jiāng (Rhizoma Zingiberis) 5 g; *rén shēn* (Radix et Rhizoma Ginseng) 6 g; *bái zhú* (Rhizoma Atractylodis Macrocephalae) 9 g; *gān cǎo* (Radix et Rhizoma Glycyrrhizae) 5 g; *zhū líng* (Polyporus) 9 g; *zé xiè* (Rhizoma Alismatis) 15 g; *fú líng* (Poria) 9 g; *guì zhī* (Ramulus Cinnamomi) 5 g. Decoct the ingredients with water and take the decoction warm.

Actions

Fortifying the spleen and promoting urination.

Indications

Weak spleen and stomach presenting a poor appetite, loose stool, inhibited urination, and body and facial edema.

Xiǎo Jiàn Zhōng Tāng (Minor Center Fortifying Decoction)

Guì zhī (Ramulus Cinnamomi) 9 g, *sháo yào* (Radix Paeoniae) 18 g, *zhì gān cǎo* (Radix et Rhizoma Glycyrrhizae Praeparata cum Melle) 6 g, *shēng jiāng* (Rhizoma Zingiberis Recens) 10 g, *dà zǎo* (Fructus Jujubae) 4 pieces; *yí táng* (Saccharum Granorum) 30 g.

Add 1.4 L of water to decoct the first five ingredients until 600 mL are left. Remove dregs and add *yí táng* to decoct in low fire. Take the decoction warm, 200 mL each time, 3 times a day.

Actions

Warming the center and supplementing the deficiency; harmonizing the middle and suppressing urgency.

Indications

Deficiency–consumption with abdominal urgency, presenting occasional abdominal pain relieved by warmth and pressure, a thin, wiry, and moderate pulse, palpitations, restlessness, a lusterless complexion, aching extremities, vexing heat in the palms and soles, and a dry throat and mouth.

THE 4TH WEEK

DAY ONE

The *Shaoyin* Deficiency–Cold Pattern

The *shaoyin* deficiency–cold pattern is marked by heart–kidney yang deficiency and internal exuberance of yin cold. As the heart and kidney belong to the hand *shaoyin* channel and foot *shaoyin* channel, respectively, it is thus called the *shaoyin* deficiency–cold pattern. This pattern is commonly seen in the course of various acute infectious diseases, such as encephalitis, epidemic hemorrhagic fever meningitis, intestinal typhoid, pneumonia, severe hepatitis, measles, and diphtheria, among which some are in the pre-shock, shock, or heart failure stage. In addition, some can exist in several chronic diseases, such as coronary heart disease, chronic nephritis, and autonomic cephalalgia. The formation of this pattern is sometimes caused by the direct invasion of external cold in the heart and kidney, which inhibits and further impairs yang qi, or by heart–kidney yang qi impairment and internal engendering of deficiency–cold in the course of diseases.

Diagnosis

The main symptoms and signs of this pattern are cold limbs or even body chills, an aversion to cold, mental fatigue, a tendency to sleep, a pale tongue, and a slight thin pulse. Other indications include vomiting, a lack of thirst, diarrhea with undigested food in the stool, a white and slippery tongue coating, a pale complexion, cool breath from the nose and mouth, abdominal urgency and pain, vexation, and so on.

This pattern is triggered by heart–kidney qi deficiency. In Chinese medicine, the spleen is the postnatal root, and the kidney is the prenatal root. Spleen yang relies on the assistance of kidney yang, while kidney yang requires the supplementation of spleen yang. The spleen yang and kidney yang have synergistic effects on warming limbs, and converting and transporting food substances. If kidney yang is deficient, spleen yang wanes consequently, presenting internal exuberance of yin cold, failure of food transportation and conversion, and fluid retention. Spleen–kidney yang declination fails to warm the extremities, showing symptoms of cold limbs, or even a body without warmth, and an aversion to cold and a tendency to huddle. Additionally, this pattern comprises heart yang deficiency, which results in the heart yang being unable to promote blood flow and may aggravate the symptoms of deficiency–cold, leading to a a slight thin pulse, or even a pulse that cannot be felt. As yang qi is deficient, it fails to warm and convert water–damp and food, presenting vomiting, diarrhea, or undigested food in the stool, and a white and slippery tongue coating. Yang qi deficiency together with the internal exuberance of yin cold show abdominal urgency and pain, a pale complexion, and cool breath from the nose and mouth. Heart yang insufficiency leads to a mal-nourished heart spirit, presenting vexation and restlessness.

If this pattern further develops, it will be difficult to maintain yang qi internally and it will float outward due to both severe yang deficiency and extreme exuberance of yin cold, presenting signs of true cold with false heat, such as coldness of the hands and feet, vomiting, diarrhea, and an aversion to cold (signs of deficiency–cold), and fever or a flushed face (signs of false heat). This is a highly critical case, which demands great attention.

Since this pattern is usually serious and requires timely treatment, it is necessary to detect manifestations of heart–kidney yang deficiency as soon as possible, some of which include dispiritedness, a thin and weak pulse, and a lusterless complexion. An examination of blood pressure levels and an ECG can be performed for a more accurate diagnosis.

This pattern is similar to the *taiyin* deficiency–cold pattern, both of which pertain to deficiency–cold patterns. However, the *taiyin* deficiency pattern is limited at the spleen and stomach and yang deficiency of the whole body is relatively mild, while the *shaoyin* deficiency–cold pattern lies in deficiency of both heart and kidney yang qi, with obvious yang deficiency of the whole body, where signs of dispiritedness, a tendency to lie, an aversion to cold, cold limbs, and an extremely thin pulse can be observed.

Treatment method

Restoring yang to rescue from desertion.

Formula and ingredients: Sì Nì Tāng (Frigid Extremities Decoction)

Zhì fù zǐ (Radix Aconiti Lateralis Praeparata) 9 g; *gān jiāng* (Rhizoma Zingiberis) 6 g; *zhì gān cǎo* (Radix et Rhizoma Glycyrrhizae Praeparata cum Melle) 6 g.

Formula verse

Sì Nì Tāng uses *fù cǎo jiāng,* effective for yang deficiency with cold limbs.

Usage

Add 600 mL of water to decoct until 240 mL are left. Remove the dregs and take it warm, 2 times a day.

Analysis

In this formula, *fù zǐ* is very acrid and hot, which can invigorate heart--kidney yang and dispel yin cold, being a chief ingredient. *Gān jiāng* is used mainly to warm the middle *jiao* for the benefit of spleen–stomach qi, and assists *fù zǐ* to warm and supplement yang qi of the whole body. When yang qi is restored, the cold sensations felt by the extremities will fade, thus lending the formula the name "Frigid Extremities Decoction." *Gān cǎo* boosts qi and harmonizes the spleen and stomach. It can assist *gān jiāng* and *fù zǐ* to restore yang and prevent desertion, and reduce their acrid, hot, and dry natures. *Gān cǎo* also lessens the toxicity of *fù zǐ.* Though there are only three ingredients in the formula, their combined effect of warming yang is still pronounced.

Sì Nì Tāng can improve the cardiovascular system, strengthen blood circulation, and increase the blood pressure of animals in shock. Both *fù zǐ* and *gān cǎo* have functions similar to adrenocortical hormones, which can improve capillary permeability and reduce inflammatory exudation. *Fù zǐ* and *gān cǎo* can temporarily trigger heart contraction. Research has indicated that the combined decoction of *fù zǐ, gān jiāng,* and *gān cǎo* can significantly enhance the effect of strengthening the heart and reducing toxicity. This formula also has a bidirectional regulation on the body temperature; for high fever, it brings down the body temperature, while for low body temperature, it adjusts the body temperature back to normal. Moreover, *Sì Nì Tāng* can rectify gastrointestinal abnormalities. Judging from the above, the pharmacological actions of this formula appear to be fairly complicated.

Treatment reference

Sì Nì Tāng is a common formula for critical diseases, such as acute heart failure, shock or pre-shock stages, myocardial infarction, acute and chronic gastroenteritis with severe vomiting and diarrhea, acute profuse sweating, infantile diarrhea (*huáng lián* can be added), gastroptosis, and chronic intestinal spasms. After the application of this formula, vomiting and diarrhea are arrested and cold limbs will be warmed after a short while.

In practice, proper modification is required. If this pattern is accompanied by edema and leukorrhea caused by spleen–kidney deficiency–cold and internal retention of water–dampness, add *dǎng shēn*, *fú líng*, *zé xiè*, *chē qián zǐ*, and so on. For joint pain caused by cold–damp, add *guì zhī*, *bái zhú*, and *cāng zhú*. If this formula is applied with *rén shēn*, it becomes *Sì Nì Jiā Rén Shēn Tāng* (Frigid Extremities Decoction plus Ginseng), which can boost innate qi and strengthen the effect on restoring yang and preventing abandonment. If the dosage of *fù zǐ* is increased, it becomes *Tōng Mài Sì Nì Tāng* (Channel-Unblocking for Frigid Extremities Decoction), which is applied to treat heart–kidney yang deficiency and floating deficient yang with false heat signs like a flushed face. If *gān jiāng* and *gān cǎo* are removed from this formula, and *rén shēn* is added, it becomes *Shēn Fù Tāng* (Ginseng and Aconite Decoction), which is for the sudden desertion of yang qi with symptoms of cold limbs, sweating, and a fine pulse. If this formula is used with *rén shēn*, *shú dì huáng*, and *dāng guī*, it becomes *Liù Wèi Huí Yáng Yǐn* (Six-Ingredient Yang-Returning Decoction), which is a supplementary formula for qi desertion of both yin and yang.

Cautions

To be specific, the cold limbs treated by this formula are caused by the reversal counterflow cold of the four limbs (cold distal extremities with cold moving proximally; *sì zhī jué nì*, 四肢厥逆), or briefly, cold syncope. It is triggered by extreme yang qi deficiency of the heart and kidney However, the reversal counterflow cold of the four limbs can also be caused by internal constraint of heat, termed heat syncope. In this situation, interior heat signs are definitely present, some of which are chest and abdominal burning heat, constipation, yellowish-brown urine, thirst, a rapid pulse, and a reddish tongue. All these demonstrate true heat with false cold, to which this formula should never be applied. Also, when the pathogenic cold stays in the exterior, presenting an aversion to cold and cold limbs, it can never be deemed as yang deficiency, hence this formula should not be erroneously applied. In addition, *fù zǐ* in this formula is toxic, so it is recommended to lower its dosage, and decoction for a long duration or decoction prior to other herbs is encouraged to reduce its toxicity.

Daily Exercises

1. What is the *shaoyin* deficiency–cold pattern? Illustrate its defining characteristics.
2. What are the ingredients of *Sì Nì Tāng*? What are its indications?
3. Ms. Han is an 8-year-old female child. She complained of diarrhea after catching a cold and consuming raw and cold food. She has taken berberine twice without any curative effect. The next day, she suffered from continuous diarrhea 4 times with watery stool. Other symptoms and signs were dispiritedness, a pale complexion, cold hands and feet, occasional abdominal pain and nausea, a pale red tongue with a white and greasy coating, and a thin and feeble pulse. Please prescribe a Chinese medicinal formula for this case.

Additional Formulae

Sì Nì Jiā Rén Shēn Tāng (Frigid Extremities Decoction plus Ginseng)

Rén shēn (Radix et Rhizoma Ginseng) 3 g; *fù zǐ* (Radix Aconiti Lateralis Praeparata) 9 g; *gān jiāng* (Rhizoma Zingiberis) 6 g; *zhì gān cǎo* (Radix et Rhizoma Glycyrrhizae Praeparata cum Melle) 6 g.

First, add water to decoct the *fù zǐ* for 1 h, and then together with the other ingredients; or decoct *rén shēn* separately and then mix both decoctions.

Actions

Restoring yang and boosting qi to rescue from desertion.

Indications

Deterioration of yang and original qi, presenting reversal cold counterflow of the four limbs, an aversion to cold, huddling, a feeble pulse, and diarrhea which has already been relieved, but with no improvement for other symptoms.

Tōng Mài Sì Nì Tāng (Channel-Unblocking for Frigid Extremities Decoction)

Fù zǐ (Radix Aconiti Lateralis Praeparata) 15 g; *gān jiāng* (Rhizoma Zingiberis) 9 g; *zhì gān cǎo* (Radix et Rhizoma Glycyrrhizae Praeparata cum Melle) 6 g. Add water to decoct and take the decoction warm 2 times.

Actions

Restoring yang and unblocking channels.

Indications

Shaoyin deficiency–cold pattern, presenting diarrhea with undigested food in the stool, cold hands and feet, an extremely thin pulse, no aversion to cold, and a flushed face.

Shēn Fù Tāng (Ginseng and Aconite Decoction)

Rén shēn (Radix et Rhizoma Ginseng) 12 g; *fù zǐ* (Radix Aconiti Lateralis Praeparata) 9 g. Add water to decoct.

Actions

Restoring yang and boosting qi to rescue from desertion.

Indications

Exreme deficiency of innate qi and sudden desertion of yang qi, presenting cold hands and feet, sweating, feeble breathing, and a slight thin pulse.

Liù Wèi Huí Yáng Yĭn (Six-Ingredient Yang-Returning Decoction)

Rén shēn (Radix et Rhizoma Ginseng) 15 g; *shú dì huáng* (Radix Rehmanniae Praeparata) 15 g; *dāng guī* (Radix Angelicae Sinensis) 9 g; *zhì fù zĭ* (Radix Aconiti Lateralis Praeparata) 6 g; *páo jiāng* (Rhizoma Zingiberis Praeparatum) 6 g; *zhì gān căo* (Radix et Rhizoma Glycyrrhizae Praeparata cum Melle) 3 g. Add water to decoct.

Actions

Supplementing both yin and yang, with immediate rescue from desertion.

Indications

Exhaustion of yang qi and desertion of yin due to consumption of fluids in the course of acute febrile diseases.

DAY TWO

The *Jueyin* Deficiency–Cold Pattern

The *jueyin* deficiency–cold pattern is a pattern of yin exuberance and yang declination due to pathogenic cold invading the liver channel or yang qi deterioration in the liver channel. As the liver channel belongs to *jueyin*, it is thus called the *jueyin* deficiency–cold pattern. Since the liver is closely associated with the stomach, and the liver channel runs along the head and the external genitalia, this pattern often manifests as an ascending counterflow of stomach qi, with symptoms related to the head and external genitalia. This pattern is often observed among hypertensive headaches, nervous vomiting, pernicious vomiting during pregnancy, and auditory vertigo. For diseases of the external genitalia, refer to the pattern of qi stagnation in Chapter 9.

Diagnosis

The main symptoms and signs are vomiting or dry belching, cold gastric pain, swallowing of acid, epigastric upset, headaches located at the top of the head, and spitting of drool and saliva. Other indications include chest and diaphragm fullness and oppression, a lack of warmth in hands and feet, diarrhea, a bland taste in the mouth, a lack of thirst, a pale and moist tongue with a white and slippery coating, and a wiry and slow pulse.

When yang qi of the liver channel is inhibited or deficient, deficiency–cold signs are engendered in the interior, which invades the stomach and leads to the ascending counterflow of stomach qi, manifesting as vomiting or dry belching. Pathogenic cold then runs along the liver channel to attack the head, producing headaches at the top. Deficiency–cold in the stomach gives rise to cold gastric pain, spitting of drool and saliva, and sometimes swallowing of acids, and epigastric upset. The internal obstruction of cold and inhibited qi movement lead to chest and diaphragm fullness and oppression. Stomach cold is reflected as diarrhea, a bland taste in the mouth, a lack of thirst, and a pale tongue with a white slippery coating. A lack of warmth in the hands and feet is often a sign of severe liver and stomach deficiency–cold. The clinical manifestations of this pattern are often aggravated at midnight and remitted at dawn.

It should be noted that vomiting will occur in deficiency–cold patterns of *taiyin*, *shaoyin*, and *jueyin*, so in diagnosis, secondary symptoms should be taken into account to distinguish between these three patterns. Generally, vomiting that occurs in the *jueyin* deficiency–cold pattern is accompanied by spitting of saliva and drool and headaches. Diseases such as migraines, intracranial inflammation, and space-occupying lesions often manifest as vomiting or dry belching together with headaches.

Although the *jueyin* deficiency–cold pattern can be manifested in externally contracted diseases, it is more frequent in diseases of internal damage, especially those concerning the digestive and nervous systems.

Treatment method

Warming the liver and stomach, arresting vomiting, and directing counterflow downward.

Formula and ingredients: Wú Zhū Yú Tāng (Evodia Decoction)

Wú zhū yú (Fructus Evodiae) 9 g; *rén shēn* (Radix et Rhizoma Ginseng) 9 g; *shēng jiāng* (Rhizoma Zingiberis Recens) 18 g; *dà zǎo* (Fructus Jujubae) 4 pieces.

Formula verse

Wú Zhū Yú Tāng uses *shēn zǎo jiāng*, effective for liver–stomach deficiency–cold; also for stomach cold, vomiting, and spitting of drool and saliva, and *jueyin* headaches.

Usage

Add 1.4 L of water to decoct until 400 mL are left. Remove the dregs and take 140 mL warm each time, 2–3 times a day.

Analysis

In the formula, *wú zhū yú*, the principal ingredient, is acrid, bitter, dry, and hot, which can warm the stomach and disperse cold, diffuse constraints and stagnation, and direct qi and turbidity downward. *Rén shēn* is used as a powerful supplement for innate qi, warming the center, and nourishing the stomach. *Shēng jiāng* is used in large doses to warm the stomach and dissipate cold, and assist *wú zhū yú* to counteract deficiency, direct counterflow downward, and arrest vomiting. *Dà zǎo* is sweet and warm, which can support *wú zhū yú* and *rén shēn* to warm the stomach and counteract deficiency. As a whole, the ingredients can warm the liver and stomach, direct counterflow downward, and arrest vomiting.

  Wú zhū yú can relax spasms of smooth muscles, arrest vomiting, relieve pain, reduce blood pressure, inhibit inflammation, and promote the secretion of digestive juices. *Rén shēn* can simulate the nervous system and pituitary–adrenocortical system, and enhance body resistance to harmful external stimuli. *Shēng jiāng* is able to strengthen blood circulation and arrest vomiting. *Dà zǎo* is nutritive.

Treatment reference

This formula is indicated for the *jueyin* deficiency–cold pattern, but as this pattern is related to the stomach, kidney, heart, and spleen, it is not only applied to treat acute gastroenteritis, gastroduodenal ulcers, nervous vomiting, pyloric spasms, nervous headaches, and Meniere's syndrome, but also to deficiency–cold eye diseases presenting dilated pupils, blurred vision, glaucoma, and headaches due to hypertension.

In practice, proper modification is required. For the pattern with serious yang deficiency and significant cold signs, add blast-fried *fù zǐ*, *gān jiāng*, or *gāo liáng jiāng*. For numbness or aches in hands and feet, add *guì zhī*. For severe vomiting, add *jiāng bàn xià*, *shā rén*, and *dài zhě shí*. For severe headaches, add *chuān xiōng*, *gé gēn*, and *quán xiē*. For epigastric upset and swallowing of acid, add *hǎi piāo xiāo*, *bì bá*, and calcined *wǎ léng zǐ*. For chronic gastritis and peptic ulcers of the stomach deficiency–cold, add *gāo liáng jiāng*, *dīng xiāng*, *bái dòu kòu*, and *bái hú jiāo*.

Cautions

This formula is acrid and hot, so improper application will result in additional heat causing damage to yin. It should never be applied to dizziness, headaches, nausea, vomiting, and abdominal pain caused by ascendant hyperactivity of liver yang or exuberant stomach heat. A few patients may experience temporary gastric discomfort or aggravated dizziness after consuming the decoction of this formula, but they will fade soon after.

Daily Exercises

1. What are the clinical manifestations of the *jueyin* deficiency–cold pattern?
2. What are the ingredients of *Wú Zhū Yú Tāng*? What are its indications?
3. Ms. Zhou is a 45-year-old female. She has been complaining for several years of dull stomach pain aggravated by catching a cold or consuming cold food. Other clinical manifestations are spitting of saliva and drool, migraines, a lusterless complexion, a pale tongue with a white coating, a deep and wiry pulse. Please prescribe a Chinese medicinal formula for this case.

CHAPTER 6

The Heat Pattern

DAY THREE

The heat pattern is typically manifested as hyperactivity of the whole body due to yang qi exuberance in the course of diseases. This pattern can be seen either in externally contracted diseases, especially externally contracted febrile diseases, or in diseases of internal damage. The heat pattern of externally contracted febrile diseases is mostly caused by excited yang qi when resisting external pathogens, while the heat pattern of internal damage is often due to an imbalance of yin and yang with relative preponderance of yang qi, namely yang exuberance causing heat.

The heat pattern is classified into the exterior heat pattern and interior heat pattern. The former has been discussed in Chapter 3. The interior heat pattern is further categorized into the interior excess–heat pattern (reviewed in this chapter) and interior deficiency–heat pattern. Since the interior deficiency–heat pattern is caused by insufficiency of body fluids, its diagnosis and treatment will be discussed later in yin deficiency patterns in Chapter 13.

Features of the Interior Heat Pattern

The interior heat pattern presents hyperactive manifestations, such as fever, a preference for thin clothing, thirst for cold beverages, a flushed face, red eyes, vexation and agitation, constipation or diarrhea with hot and pungent loose stool, a red and dry tongue, and a rapid pulse. Most cases of acute febrile diseases at the late stage, or a long period for time after chronic or prolonged disease presenting low fever, night sweat, emaciation, vexing heat in the five centers (chest, palms, and soles), a dry mouth and throat, a red tongue with a scant coating, a thin and rapid pulse, pertain to the interior deficiency–heat pattern.

Heat Pattern, Body Temperature, and Inflammation

The heat pattern is different from an increase in body temperature, because causes for the latter are various. Even certain cold patterns can present fever, so not all kinds of fever belong to the heat pattern. The heat pattern generally gives rise to fever, but in some cases, the patient only experiences a feverish sensation though the body temperature is not high, especially for some heat patterns of internal damage. Therefore, the diagnosis of the heat pattern is mainly based on heat signs, but not the body temperature. The heat signs refer to several manifestations of heat, such as a flushed face, red eyes, thirst for cold beverages, and scant and brown urine. The heat pattern is also different from inflammation from the perspective of modern medicine. Most cases of inflammation may present the heat pattern, but only a few cases of inflammation can manifest as the deficiency pattern or the cold pattern. In addition, some cases of the heat pattern are not caused by inflammation; hence, these two concepts must not be confused with each other.

Clinically, the heat pattern is the most common pattern in numerous infectious and epidemic diseases. Among diseases of internal damage, all five *zang* and six *fu* organs will display the fire–heat pattern. The heat pattern also exists in following diseases: hypertension, dysfunction of the autonomic nervous system, certain rheumatic or rheumatoid diseases, and diabetes.

Categories and Treatment Methods of the Heat Pattern

The heat pattern is a very comprehensive category in Chinese medicine, in which almost all patterns are either heat patterns or cold patterns. For the interior excess heat pattern, which we will introduce in this chapter, there are many sub-patterns and corresponding treatment approaches.

Categories of the interior excess–heat pattern

The interior excess heat pattern is caused by various pathogenic factors and manifests as the exuberance of fire–heat. It is commonly seen at the feverish stage of externally contracted febrile diseases, and also exists in diseases of internal damage. According to the classification of *zang–fu* disorders, examples of such patterns are: the lung heat pattern, stomach heat pattern (including the *yangming* qi heat pattern and *yangming* bowel excess pattern), liver heat pattern (including the liver yang exuberance pattern and liver fire flaming upward pattern), heart heat pattern, intestine heat pattern, bladder heat pattern, and gallbladder heat pattern. Heat patterns can be categorized in two different ways: (1) according to the classification of *wei*, qi, *ying*, and blood levels, where there are heat patterns at the qi level, *ying* level, and blood level; and (2) according to the heat nature, where there are the toxic heat pattern, damp–heat pattern, heat binding pattern, phlegm–heat pattern, and static heat pattern.

The interior excess–heat pattern is unlike the deficiency–heat caused by insufficient body fluids, but as pathogenic heat tends to consume and impair such fluids, the interior excess–heat pattern often presents symptoms of insufficient body fluids, generating a complex of excess and deficiency. However, for the interior excess pattern, the insufficiency of body fluids is secondary.

Treatment methods of the interior excess–heat pattern

The principle of treatment is to rectify the interior excess–heat pattern by clearing heat, which refers to the clearance of exuberant heat from the body. This method is largely applied to the interior excess–heat pattern, while for fevers caused by yin deficiency, the aim of treatment is to nourish yin in chief and clear deficiency–heat as supplementation. In practice, clearing heat should be applied in accordance to the heat nature. It is especially important to take accompanying pathogens into account. If the pathogenic heat is purely hyperactive and exuberant, it is called invisible pathogenic heat, which should be treated by clearing heat, purging heat, and resolving toxins. If the pathogenic heat is mixed with dry stool in the intestines, water–dampness, phlegm–turbidity, static blood, and stagnation, it is termed visible heat bind, which should be treated by clearing heat together with methods of eliminating visible pathogens, such as purgation, promoting urination, resolving dampness, dispelling phlegm, removing stasis, promoting digestion, and so on.

Approaches to clearing heat are not only to relieve fever, but also exert very complex effects, which include the inhibition and inactivation of bacteria and viruses, elimination and neutralization of bacterial and various toxins in the course of the disease, the improvement of body immunity, the calming of the mind, the protection of tissues and organs, and the regulation of the nervous system. Therefore, the approach of clearing heat is not equivalent to relieving fever.

Clinically, techniques of clearing heat vary according to different disease natures, degrees, and regions, such as treatment by acrid–cold medicinals, purgation, diffusing the lung to clear heat, purging fire by bitter–cold medicinals, cooling blood, cooling the *ying* level, removing dampness, and clearing heat from the *zang–fu* organs.

The formulae and medicinals administered in clearing heat are cool and cold, which are clearly contraindicated for the cold pattern and are also unsuitable for the deficiency–heat pattern. Since heat-clearing products damage the stomach qi quite easily, they should not be applied in excess. When necessary, this method can be combined with spleen-fortifying and stomach-harmonizing products to minimize its shortcomings.

Daily Exercises

1. What are the heat pattern, interior heat pattern, and interior excess–heat pattern?
2. What are the diagnostic criteria of the heat pattern?
3. Does the heat pattern absolutely indicate fever or an inflammatory disease?
4. What is the main treatment principle for the heat pattern? What aspects should be paid attention to?

DAY FOUR

The *Yangming* Qi Level Heat Pattern

The *yangming* qi level heat pattern is manifested through the six channels and the *wei*, qi, *ying*, and blood levels. It refers to the qi level heat pattern of exuberant heat in the *yangming* (stomach) channel, and thus is also called the *yangming* channel syndrome or exuberant stomach heat pattern. This pattern comes under an interior excess–heat pattern caused by invisible pathogenic heat, and is commonly seen among various infectious and epidemic diseases at the feverish stage, examples of which include epidemic encephalitis B, lobar pneumonia, leptospirosis, and epidemic hemorrhagic fever.

Diagnosis

The main symptoms and signs of this pattern are high fever, extreme thirst with a compulsion for drinking, profuse sweating, and a large, surging, and strong pulse. Other indications include vexation, a dry mouth and tongue, a flushed face and red eyes, an aversion to heat, coarse breath, and a rough yellow tongue coating or dry dark coating with pricks.

For externally contracted febrile diseases, if the pathogens in the exterior penetrate the interior, yang qi of the whole body will be activated to resist these external invaders. Thus, it becomes yang heat exuberance of the interior excess–heat pattern. As the excess–heat is exuberant in the qi level, there would be high fever, a flushed face, an aversion to heat instead of cold, and a reluctance to wear clothes and cover sheets over the body. Exuberant interior heat drives body fluids outward, so there is profuse sweating. The pathogenic heat consumes and impairs fluids, making the patient feel extremely thirsty and dry in the mouth. A surging, large, and strong pulse and a rough yellow or dry darkish tongue coating with pricks are signs of exuberant interior heat.

These signs can be summarized into four main symptoms, namely high fever, extreme thirst, profuse sweating, and a surging and large pulse. However, in clinical practice, diagnosis should not be limited to these four manifestations. For instance, externally contracted febrile diseases usually trigger profuse sweating aligned with high fever, extreme thirst, and a surging and large pulse, but in some cases, it may not present sweating due to blockage of sweat pores. In certain scenarios of internal damage, though there are signs of extreme thirst and a surging pulse without profuse sweating and high fever, they are also diagnosed as the stomach heat exuberance pattern. Moreover, if this pattern is accompanied by an unrelieved exterior pattern, it may also present a mild aversion to wind and an absence of sweating. If there is also profuse sweating where the sweat pores are loosened and yang qi is relatively insufficient, there will also be manifestations of an aversion to wind and cold or a mild aversion to cold in the back of the patient. Therefore, the diagnosis of this pattern should be based on the comprehensive entirety of symptoms and signs observed throughout the whole body.

This pattern may also give rise to cold hands and feet due to pathogenic heat obstruction in the interior (prevented from traveling outward), but definite excess heat signs will be observed, such as burning heat in the chest and abdomen, vexing thirst with a compulsiveness for drinking, a yellow or dry dark coating, and a surging and strong pulse. Such a symptom of cold hands and feet is called heat syncope, which belongs to the nature of true heat with false cold.

Treatment method

Clearing heat to preserve fluids by acrid and cold medicinals.

Formula and ingredients: Bái Hǔ Tāng (White Tiger Decoction)

Crushed *shí gāo* (Gypsum Fibrosum) 30 g; *zhī mǔ* (Rhizoma Anemarrhenae) 10 g; *zhì gān cǎo* (Radix et Rhizoma Glycyrrhizae Praeparata cum Melle) 3 g; *jīng mǐ* (Oryza Sativa L.) 15 g.

Formula Verse

Bái Hǔ Tāng uses *shí gāo zhī, gān cǎo*, and *jīng mǐ*; applicable to *yangming* profuse sweating with vexing thirst, by its heat-clearing and fluid-producing functions.

Usage

Add 2 L of water to decoct until *jīng mǐ* (rice) is cooked. Remove the dregs when about 600 mL of decoction are left. Take the decoction warm, 200 mL each time, 3 times a day. If the condition is acute and severe, take the decoction once every 2 or 3 h. As *shí gāo* is difficult to be dissolved in water, its dose can be a little larger, e.g., 250 g when necessary.

Analysis

Bái Hǔ Tāng is an important formula for treating invisible heat exuberance at the qi level. The pathogenic heat of the *yangming* qi heat pattern is manifested at the exterior where there are symptoms of high
fever, profuse, steam-like sweating, a flushed face, and red eyes. In the
formula, *shí gāo*, acrid, sweet, and cold, is used to vent and discharge
heat, being the chief ingredient. *Zhī mǔ*, bitter, cold, and moist, assists
shí gāo to clear heat and conserve fluids. *Jīng mǐ* and *zhì gān cǎo* can
fortify the stomach and harmonize the center, preventing ingredients
with an extreme cold nature from impairing spleen and stomach yang.
All ingredients as a whole can clear heat without being overly cold
(which will damage the spleen and stomach), and simultaneously dispel pathogens while conserving fluids. Therefore, this formula is simple yet effective.

  Bái Hǔ Tāng can relieve fever, but if *shí gāo* is absent, this effect will
not be achieved. It has been proven that *shí gāo* acts rapidly on relieving
fever, and if combined with *zhī mǔ*, this effect will be more lasting. *Zhī
mǔ* also harbors certain antibacterial properties. *Gān cǎo* can protect the
stomach mucosa as well as has functions similar to adrenocortical hormones. It is also anti-inflammatory and anti-allergic, and can relieve
spasms, arrest pain, and eliminate toxins.

Treatment reference

The applications of *Bái Hǔ Tāng* in clinical practice are widespread. For
example, various infectious diseases at the advanced feverish stage with
yangming qi level heat and without other visible excess–heat can usually
be treated by this formula. In addition, it is applicable to some diseases of
internal damage, such as diabetes, hypertension, acute rheumatic diseases,
and summer heat syndrome or summer heat stroke with extreme thirst,
profuse sweating, or high fever.

  This formula can be modified into many other variants. If *rén shen* is
added, it becomes *Bái Hǔ Jiā Rén Shēn Tāng* (White Tiger Decoction
plus Ginseng), which is used to treat the *yangming* qi heat pattern with
serious yin damage, presenting vexing thirst, profuse sweating, a mild

aversion to cold in the back, and a floating, large, and weak pulse. If *guì zhī* is added, it becomes *Bái Hǔ Jiā Guì Zhī Tāng* (White Tiger Decoction plus Cinnamon Twig), which is applied to treat high fever, sweating, and joint pain and swellings. If *cāng zhú* is added, it becomes *Bái Hǔ Jiā Cāng Zhú Tāng* (White Tiger Decoction plus Atractylodes), which is applied to treat the *yangming* qi heat pattern with pathogenic dampness encumbering the spleen and stomach, presenting high fever, thirst, sweating, chest and gastric stuffiness and fullness, and head heaviness. For the *yangming* qi heat pattern comprising the exterior pattern and an aversion to cold, add *hé yè*, *bò he*, and *zhú yè*, becoming *Xīn Jiā Bái Hǔ Tāng* (Newly Supplemented White Tiger Decoction). If this formula is used for treating encephalitis (all types), cephalomeningitis, septicemia, and pneumonia, add *jīn yín huā* and *lián qiào* to enhance the strength of clearing heat and removing toxins.

Cautions

Bái Hǔ Tāng is a famous formula for clearing heat, but clinically it is only applicable when there are severe signs of *yangming* qi level heat. It should never be administered when fever appears in any case. For some patients with the exterior pattern in which the aversion to cold has not been relieved and the body temperature is high, or with an extreme deficiency of yang qi (floating outward), presenting true cold with false heat, such as fever, a flushed face, cold feet, a preference for hot drinking, a slight thin pulse, or a scattered, large, and weak pulse, this formula should never be prescribed. Furthermore, if pathogenic heat is bound with visible excess pathogens, such as dry stool, phlegm–rheum, static blood, and water–dampness, do not apply this formula solely for clearing heat, because it is not sufficient to achieve the expected curative effect.

Daily Exercises

1. What is the *yangming* qi level heat pattern?
2. What are the ingredients of *Bái Hǔ Tāng*? What are its main modified formulae in clinical practice?

3. Mr. Guo is a 28-year-old male. He has been complaining of fever for 3 days. His body temperature has gradually increased to 39.8°C, with other clinical manifestations such as a flushed face, eye congestion, profuse sweating all over the body, thirst with a compulsiveness to drink, headaches, vexation, scant and brown urine, normal defecation, a reddish tongue with a yellow and dry coating, and a surging and rapid pulse. Please prescribe a Chinese medicinal formula for this case.

Additional Formulae

Bái Hǔ Jiā Rén Shēn Tāng (White Tiger Decoction plus Ginseng)

Rén shēn (Radix et Rhizoma Ginseng) 9 g; crushed *shí gāo* (Gypsum Fibrosum) 30 g; *zhī mǔ* (Rhizoma Anemarrhenae) 10 g; *zhì gān cǎo* (Radix et Rhizoma Glycyrrhizae Praeparata cum Melle) 6 g; *jīng mǐ* (Oryza Sativa L.) 15 g. Add water to decoct until rice is cooked. Remove the dregs and take the decoction warm.

Actions

Clearing heat, boosting qi, and producing body fluids.

Indications

The *yangming* qi heat pattern presenting a surging, large, and weak pulse, and a mild aversion to cold in the back.

Bái Hǔ Jiā Guì Zhī Tāng (White Tiger Decoction plus Cinnamon Twig)

Ingredients of *Bái Hǔ Tāng* plus *guì zhī* (Ramulus Cinnamomi) 9 g. Add water to decoct.

Actions

Clearing heat, unblocking collaterals, and harmonizing *ying–wei* levels.

Indications

Fever without an aversion to cold, acute joint pain or swelling pain, coarse breath, vexation, thirst, a white or yellow and dry tongue coating, and a wiry and rapid pulse.

Bái Hǔ Jiā Cāng Zhú Tāng (White Tiger Decoction plus Atractylodes)

Ingredients of *Bái Hǔ Tāng* plus *cāng zhú* (Rhizoma Atractylodis) 9 g. Add water to decoct.

Actions

Clearing heat and dispelling dampness.

Indications

The *yangming* qi heat pattern accompanied by dampness obstruction in the middle *jiao*, presenting high fever, chest and gastric stuffiness and full-ness, profuse sweating, thirst, a reddish tongue with a yellow or white greasy coating, and a rapid pulse.

Xīn Jiā Bái Hǔ Tāng (Newly Supplemented White Tiger Decoction)

Bò he (Herba Menthae) 1.5 g; raw *shí gāo* (Gypsum Fibrosum) powder 24 g; a piece of fresh lotus leaf; long-term stored rice 9 g; *zhī mǔ* (Rhizoma Anemarrhenae) 12g; *Yì Yuán Sǎn* (Original Qi-Boosting Powder) wrapped 9 g; fresh bamboo leaf 30 pieces; tender mulberry twig 65 cm cut into 3cm each.

First decoct fresh reed rhizome 60 g, *dēng xīn cǎo* (Medulla Junci) 1.5 g, and gypsum powder and the use the decoction to decoct with other ingredients.

Actions

Clearing the liver and stomach; cooling the heart and lung.

Indications

Stomach heat exuberance presenting high fever, vexing thirst, scant and brown urine with a hot sensation, coughing of blood, and so on.

DAY FIVE

The *Yangming* Bowel Excess Pattern

The *yangming* bowel excess pattern is a combination of pathogenic heat and dry stool in the intestines with heat exuberance and consumption of body fluids. "*Yangming*" essentially signifies the *yangming* stomach, so this pattern also belongs to the stomach excess–heat pattern. However, *yangming* here mainly refers to the hand *yangming* large intestine and thus, it can be deemed as the large intestine excess–heat pattern. This pattern is often seen in various acute infectious diseases at the advanced feverish stage as well as in diseases of internal damage, such as ileus and schizophrenia of the digestive and nervous systems.

Diagnosis

The main symptoms and signs are abdominal fullness and pain, and constipation. Other indications include fever without an aversion to cold, thirst, vexation, sweating, unconsciousness, ravings, a yellow and dry or even dark grey and dry tongue coating with fissures, and a deep, slippery, and forceful pulse.

The binding of pathogenic heat and dry stool in the intestines is called heat bind, which obstructs the intestines and causes failure of the intestines to conduct food residues. Together with dry stool, which is a visible pathogen, there will be abdominal fullness, distention and pain, and constipation. As the heat bind is in the interior, the pathogenic heat is unable to move outward and will manifest its exuberance internally. Therefore, there is fever without an aversion to cold, and in some cases, the fever worsens between 3 pm and 5 pm, which is known as late afternoon tidal fever. The steaming interior heat drives body fluids outward, so there is sweating, which in some cases is mainly in the hands and feet, and in other cases the whole body. If the pathogenic heat disrupts the heart spirit, there will be restlessness, or even unconsciousness or delirium. Pathogenic heat burning and impairing body fluids are manifested as thirst. A yellow and dry or dark grey tongue coating with fissures is a sign of heat exuberance impairing yin. As the dry stool obstructs the intestines, qi movement is inhibited, manifesting as a slippery and forceful pulse that is usually deep and not floating.

For the diagnosis of this pattern, constipation is an important indicator. However, some cases manifest as diarrhea, because stool cannot be defecated due to dry stool obstruction in the intestines. Furthermore, as the fluids in the intestines flow outward along the sides of the dry stool, watery stool with a pungent odor will result and a hot sensation around the anus will be felt, which is termed heat retention with watery discharge. Nevertheless, this phenomenon is rare in clinical practice.

This pattern usually comprises fever, but it may not be the case in some diseases of internal damage. Moreover, since there is binding of pathogenic heat and dry stool, it tends to drive heat retention in the interior, giving rise to cold extremities, which belongs to the category of heat syncope.

Treatment method

Purging heat bind in the intestines.

Formula and ingredients: Tiáo Wèi Chéng Qì Tāng (Stomach-Regulating and Purgative Decoction)

Skinless *dà huáng* (Radix et Rhizoma Rhei) washed with pure wine 12 g; *zhì gān cǎo* (Radix et Rhizoma Glycyrrhizae Praeparata cum Melle) 6 g; *máng xiāo* (Natrii Sulfas) 12 g.

Formula verse

Tiáo Wèi Chéng Qì uses *xiāo huáng cǎo*, effective for bowel disorders and abdominal pain.

Usage

Add 600 mL of water first to decoct *dà huáng* and *gān căo* until 300 mL are left. Remove the dregs and add *máng xiāo* to decoct under mild fire. Take the decoction in a draft while it is warm.

Analysis

As pathogenic heat is bound with dry stool in the intestines, *dà huáng* as the chief ingredient is applied to expel the interior heat by purging and promoting defecation. *Máng xiāo* is used in combination to soften the stool and relieve constipation. *Gān căo* harmonizes the actions of all medicinals in the formula and protects stomach qi from damage by purgation. Altogether, the main aim of the medicinals is to promote defecation, but more importantly, their purpose lies in dispelling pathogenic internal heat.

Tiáo Wèi Chéng Qì Tāng can strengthen gastrointestinal peristalsis, increase intestinal volume, improve intestinal blood circulation, boost immunity, promote gallbladder functions, promote urination, and has antibacterial effects. *Dà huáng* inhibits various bacteria effectively and can resist viruses, fungi, and protozoa, strengthen the stomach, purge gradually, regulate potassium levels, decrease ureic nitrogen, promote gallbladder functions, astringe, diminish inflammation, relieve spasms, lower blood pressure and blood cholesterol, promote urination, increase platelets to arrest bleeding, etc. Therefore, the curative effect of this formula is not only limited in promoting defecation.

Treatment reference

Tiáo Wèi Chéng Qì Tāng has widespread clinical applications. If this formula is applied to treat acute infectious diseases with heat exuberance and the bowel excess pattern, defecation is promoted via bowel relaxation, in which heat is purged quickly followed by the remittance of the disease. It is commonly used to treat acute hepatitis, fulminant hepatitis, intestinal typhoid, epidemic encephalitis B, pneumonia, bacillary dysentery, epidemic hemorrhagic fever, septicemia, acute appendicitis, biliary infection, peritonitis, conjunctivitis, pharyngitis, periodontitis, suppurative tonsillitis, and many more. This formula is also applied as a remedy for diseases of internal damage. For example, in the treatment of acute or chronic nephritis, urination will be promoted by relaxing bowels, thus significantly relieving symptoms. It is also applicable to diabetes, stroke, and hypercortisolism with signs of internal bind of the excess–heat pattern. For gallbladder stones, this formula can also be applied to promote defecation and gallbladder functions.

Tiáo Wèi Chéng Qì Tāng has many variants in practice that have further collaborative uses, such as clearing heat, strengthening healthy qi, rectifying qi, and dissolving stasis. If *gān cǎo* is removed from this formula and *hòu pò* and *zhǐ shí* are added, it becomes *Dà Chéng Qì Tāng* (Major Purgative Decoction), which is indicated for heat bind in the intestine pattern with obvious qi constraint and obstruction. If *gān cǎo* and *máng xiāo* are removed while *hòu pò* and *zhǐ shí* are added, it becomes *Xiǎo Chéng Qì Tāng* (Minor Purgative Decoction), which is mild in purging heat downward, but is strong in diffusing and unblocking qi movement. If *gān cǎo* is removed and *shēng dì*, *xuán shēn*, and *mài dōng* are added, it becomes *Zēng Yè Chéng Qì Tāng* (Humor-Increasing and Qi-Guiding Decoction), which treats heat bind in the intestines with severely impaired body fluids, especially intestinal fluid insufficiency. If *rén shēn*, *dāng guī*, *mài dōng*, *shēng dì*, *xuán shēn*, *hǎi shēn*, and *jiāng zhī* are added, it becomes *Xīn Jiā Huáng Lóng Tāng* (Newly Supplemented Yellow Dragon Decoction), which is used for febrile diseases with heat bind in the intestines and severely impaired healthy qi and body fluids.

Cautions

Though *Tiáo Wèi Chéng Qì Tāng* can be widely applied and can be used for certain diseases without constipation or fever, it does not indicate that it can simply be prescribed at random. Improper application of this formula will damage spleen and stomach yang qi, or even consume healthy qi and body fluids. Therefore, it is crucial to keep its indications in mind, namely pathological changes of heat bind in the intestines. In addition, this formula should not be taken repeatedly after it has exerted its effect of relaxing bowels. As for the decoction method, *máng xiāo* needs to be dissolved. In addition, the decoction of *dà huáng* is fairly complicated. If it is decocted for a long period of time, its purgative effect will be reduced. Therefore, decoct the *dà huáng* for a short while to achieve a strong purgative effect and a long duration to achieve a mild purgative effect. Raw *dà huáng* has a strong purgative effect, while its prepared counterpart is mild. Moreover, purgative formulae should never be applied for externally contracted febrile diseases at the late stage with the absence of pathogenic heat, when the fluids in the intestines are impaired, or for relatively serious interior heat with intestinal fluids insufficiency.

Daily Exercises

1. What are the diagnostic criteria of the *yangming* bowel excess pattern?
2. What are the ingredients of *Tiáo Wèi Chéng Qì Tāng*? Please list three similar/modified formulae.
3. Mr. Luo is a 42-year-old male. He has been complaining of abdominal distention and fullness, being in pain when pressure is applied, and a lack of defecation for 8 days. Other symptoms and signs are low fever in the afternoon, distending pain in the head, a dry mouth and lips, vexation, nausea, a reddish tongue with a grey and dry coating, and a wiry and slippery pulse. Please prescribe a Chinese medicinal formula for this case.

Additional Formulae

Dà Chéng Qì Tāng (Major Purgative Decoction)

Wine-prepared *dà huáng* (Radix et Rhizoma Rhei) 12 g; *hòu pò* (Cortex Magnoliae Officinalis) 6 g; liquid-fried *zhǐ shí* (Fructus Aurantii Immaturus) 12 g; *máng xiāo* (Natrii Sulfas) 9 g. Add water to decoct. *Dà huáng* should be added later and *máng xiāo* needs to be dissolved.

Actions

Drastic purgation of heat binds.

Indications

Yangming bowel pattern presenting abdominal distention, fullness, and hardness with pain felt upon applying pressure, blurred vision, a deep and excessive pulse, cold limbs, cramps, and mania.

Xiǎo Chéng Qì Tāng (Minor Purgative Decoction)

Wine-prepared *dà huáng* (Radix et Rhizoma Rhei) 12 g; liquid-fried *hòu pò* (Cortex Magnoliae Officinalis) 6 g; *zhǐ shí* (Fructus Aurantii Immaturus) 12 g. Add water to decoct.

Actions

Mild purgation of heat bind.

Indications

Yangming bowel pattern presenting tidal fever, delirious speech, chest and abdominal stuffiness and fullness, a dry and yellow tongue coating, a slippery and rapid pulse, or dysentery at the early stage with abdominal pain and tenesmus.

Zēng Yè Chéng Qì Tāng (Humor-Increasing and Qi-Guiding Decoction)

Xuán shēn (Radix Scrophulariae) 30 g; *mài dōng* (Radix Ophiopogonis) with pith 25 g; thin *shēng dì* (Radix Rehmanniae) 25 g; *dà huáng* (Radix et Rhizoma Rhei) 9 g; *máng xiāo* (Natrii Sulfas) 5 g. Add water to decoct; *máng xiāo* needs to be dissolved.

Actions

Nourishing yin and increasing body fluids; purging heat and relaxing bowels.

Indications

Yangming bowel pattern with insufficiency of body fluids, presenting dry stool blockage in the intestines.

Xīn Jiā Huáng Lóng Tāng (Newly Supplemented Yellow Dragon Decoction)

Thin *shēng dì* (Radix Rehmanniae) 15 g; raw *gān cǎo* (Radix et Rhizoma Glycyrrhizae) 6 g; *rén shēn* (Radix et Rhizoma Ginseng) 4.5 g decocted separately; raw *dà huáng* (Radix et Rhizoma Rhei) 9 g; *máng xiāo* (Natrii Sulfas) 3 g; *xuán shēn* (Radix Scrophulariae) 15 g; *mài dōng* (Radix Ophiopogonis) with pith 15 g; *dāng guī* (Radix Angelicae Sinensis) 4.5 g; washed *hǎi shēn* (Stichopus) 2 pieces; ginger juice 6 scoops.

Usage

Add 1.6 L of water to decoct until 600 mL are left. Mix 200 mL of the decoction with a separately decocted *rén shēn* decoction and 2 scoops of ginger juice. Take it orally as a draft. After that, if there are gurgling sounds in the abdomen or if the anus begins to expel gas, defecation will follow shortly. If there is still no defecation for 2–4 h, take the decoction again according to the above method. If no defecation occurs in 6 h, take the decoction for the third time.

DAY SIX

The Fire Toxin Exuberance Pattern

The fire toxin exuberance pattern refers to the accumulation of fire and heat toxins, presenting signs of toxicity such as reddish swellings, pyosis, macules, mania, and bleeding. Fire toxins are similar to pathogenic fire and heat, but are more severe and characterized by accumulation. Thus, "toxin" is used to differentiate from general fire and heat pathogens. Fire toxins are also called heat toxins or fire–heat toxins. It is commonly seen in septicemia, spticopyemia, pneumonia, serious hepatitis, epidemic cerebrospinal meningitis, leptospirosis, acute bacillary dysentery, carbuncles, and sores.

Diagnosis

The main symptoms and signs are fever, restlessness, a bitter taste in the mouth, local reddish swellings or macules, bleeding, mania, and a reddish tongue with a yellow coating. Other indications include a dry mouth and throat, pounding headaches, severe body pains, sores and swellings or a purulent throat, jaundice, unconsciousness, delirium, yellow and scant urine, and carbuncles and sores.

This pattern is largely triggered by local fire toxin accumulation or fire toxins all over the body, thus fever and a dry mouth and throat are definite manifestations. As the accumulation of fire toxins obstructs qi movement, reddish swellings and pain will occur, or even pyosis and carbuncles. Internal exuberance of fire–heat drives blood frenetic, which spills out of vessels and causes skin macules or bleeding (including hematemesis, epistaxis, bloody stool, and hematuria). If the fire disrupts the heart spirit, there will be signs of mania or unconsciousness with ravings. If the fire consumes body fluids, urine will be yellow in color and scant in amount. A bitter taste in the mouth is an important symptom of the internal accumulation of fire toxins; this is one of the key manifestations of this pattern. Headaches and body pain here can be very serious, which are different from those caused by external pathogens invading the body surface and blocking channel qi of the exterior. In this pattern, the headaches are acute and the body pain are agonizing because they result from pathogenic fire and heat burning and impairing body channels. A reddish tongue with a yellow coating is a sign of internal exuberance of fire heat.

Both this pattern and the *yangming* qi heat pattern are caused by invisible pathogenic heat, but that of the latter is exuberant at the body surface, hence resulting in high fever, profuse sweating, extreme thirst, and a surging and large pulse, while that of the former tends to accumulate, inducing reddish swellings, carbuncles, macules, and bleeding without profuse sweating and extreme thirst. It is not difficult to distinguish these two patterns according to their clinical manifestations. However, they sometimes occur simultaneously, leading to the presence of heat toxins throughout the entire body.

Treatment method

Draining fire and resolving toxins.

Formula and ingredients: *Huáng Lián Jiě Dú Tāng* (*Coptis Toxin-Resolving Decoction*)

Huáng lián (Rhizoma Coptidis) 9 g; *huáng qín* (Radix Scutellariae) 6 g; *huáng bǎi* (Cortex Phellodendri Chinensis) 6 g; *zhī zǐ* (Fructus Gardeniae) 9 g.

Formula verse

Huáng Lián Jiě Dú uses *bǎi zhī* qín, with fire exuberance through *sanjiao* as the disease cause; effective for vexation, mania, fever, and sores; also for bloody expectoration and macules.

Usage

Add 1.2 L of water to decoct until 400 mL are left. Remove the dregs and consume it warm 3 times. This formula can also be synthesized as water pills or honey pills for oral intake.

Analysis

In this formula, all four ingredients are bitter and cold, which can clear heat and eliminate toxins. The dose of *huáng lián* is the largest; it is the chief ingredient. The functions of these four ingredients are a little different. *Huáng lián* is used to purge heart fire and assist in purging stomach fire; *huáng qín* is to purge lung fire; *huáng bǎi* is to purge fire in the lower *jiao*; and *zhī zǐ* purges fire all through *sanjiao* and can guide heat downward so that it can be expelled by urination. Although the composition of this formula is relatively simple, it is a classic formula applied for purging fire, resolving toxins, and treating the fire toxin pattern.

According to medicinal natures, the method of clearing invisible heat in Chinese medicine involves three categories: by acrid–cold, bitter–cold, or sweet–cold. Clearing heat with acrid–cold medicinals is indicated for the floating exuberance of pathogenic heat at the *yangming* qi level, such as *Bái Hǔ Tāng*, which can diffuse heat outward. Clearing heat with bitter–cold medicinals is indicated for the internal accumulation of pathogenic fire as fire toxins, such as *Huáng Lián Jiě Dú Tāng*, which can directly diminish fire and clear heat to eliminate toxins. Clearing heat with sweet–cold medicinals is indicated for the deficiency–heat pattern with fever and fluidal insufficiency, which will be discussed later in Chapter 13.

Huáng Lián Jiě Dú Tāng has strong antibacterial and antiviral effects, and can promote phagocytosis and regulate the immune system. *Huáng lián*, *huáng qín*, *huáng bǎi*, and *zhī zǐ* have antibacterial, gallbladder function-promoting, blood pressure-lowering, and immunity-regulating functions, respectively. A combination of these medicinals can exert synergic effects.

Treatment reference

Huáng Lián Jiě Dú Tāng is especially effective for many infectious diseases, and thus many use it as a broad-spectrum antibiotic in Chinese medicine. Its role is not only limited to inhibiting or killing pathogenic microorganisms; it has multiple functions. This formula is indicated for bacillary dysentery, acute enteritis, acute hepatitis, epidemic meningococcal meningitis, leptospirosis, pneumonia, septicemia, burning, carbuncles, and sores presenting the fire toxin pattern. In addition, it is also applicable to some non-infectious diseases with fire toxin symptoms, such as trigeminal neuralgia and allergic purpura.

In practice, proper modification is required. For the internal accumulation of fire toxins with jaundice, add *yīn chén* and *dà huáng*. For heat exuberance, add *shēng dì*, *mài dōng*, and *xuán shēn* to nourish body fluids. There are also several similar formulae that can purge fire and eliminate toxins, which are composed mainly of bitter–cold ingredients for clearing heat and removing toxins. For example, *Xiè Xīn Tāng* (Heart-Draining Decoction) is a formula for exuberant fire toxins driving the frenetic flow of blood, presenting hematemesis and epistaxis. This formula is also called *Dà Huáng Huáng Lián Xiè Xīn Tāng* (Rhubarb and Coptis Heart-Draining Decoction). *Dà huáng* used in the formula is not purely for promoting defecation, but more importantly, to purge fire and eliminate toxins; purging fire is to purge the heart as the heart is attributed to fire.

Cautions

The ingredients of this formula are bitter and cold, which can diminish fire directly, but bitter medicinals are dry and tend to impair body fluids. Moreover, the internal exuberance of fire toxins usually consumes these fluids, so it is important to note the state of body fluids at the time of applying this formula. Do not prescribe it for cases with a severe impairment of fluids and a crimson tongue. When necessary, add yin-nourishing medicinals. In addition, since it is an extremely cold-natured formula, do not prescribe too large a dose or apply it for too long a time in case of impairing yang qi if the patient suffers from the fire toxin pattern with a deficiency–cold physique. This formula is extreme in clearing heat and purging fire toxins, so if it is erroneously applied to treat fever of the exterior pattern or the *yangming* qi heat pattern, it will cause pathogen obstruction without recovery, leading to cold obstruction and latent icy pathogens. It is also not appropriate to apply this formula to treat fevers of visible heat bind in the interior.

Daily Exercises

1. What are fire toxins? What are the main symptoms and signs of the fire toxin exuberance pattern?
2. What are the ingredients of *Huáng Lián Jiě Dú Tāng*? What are its indications?
3. Mr. Chen is a 15-year-old male. He has had fever for 2 days, with other clinical manifestations including severe headaches and body pains, a bitter taste in the mouth, nausea at times, restlessness, brown and scant urine, a wiry and rapid pulse, and a reddish tongue with a dry and yellow coating. Please prescribe a Chinese medicinal formula for this case.

Additional Formulae

Xiè Xīn Tāng (Heart-Draining Decoction)

Dà huáng (Radix et Rhizoma Rhei) 9 g; *huáng lián* (Rhizoma Coptidis) 3 g; *huáng qín* (Radix Scutellariae) 9 g. Soak the above ingredients with boiling water and remove the dregs. Take the decoction warm.

Actions

Draining fire and resolving toxins; drying dampness and dispersing masses.

Indications

Gastric stuffiness and fullness, a "soft" feeling when pressure is applied, fever, vexation and agitation or even mania, constipation, brown and scant urine, hematemesis, epitaxis, red eyes with painful swelling, sores on the mouth and tongue, painful swellings in the gums or jaundice, a red tongue with a yellow coating, and a slippery and rapid pulse.

THE 5TH WEEK

DAY ONE

The Blood Level Heat Exuberance Pattern

This pattern is attributable to the invasion of pathogenic heat into the blood level, causing heat exuberance in the blood and its subsequent frenetic flow. Blood level has two meanings: (1) the four levels of pathological changes of externally contracted febrile diseases, namely the *wei*, qi, *ying*, and blood levels and (2) the pathological changes of blood in diseases of internal damage. This pattern commonly occurs in various infectious diseases at the extreme stage, especially in disseminated intravascular coagulation (DIC). It also occurs in allergic purpura, thrombopenic purpura, other hemorrhagic diseases, acute leukemia, uremia, hepatic comas, presenting blood heat signs.

Diagnosis

The main symptoms and signs are fever, bright red or dark purple macules and papules, or hematemesis, epitaxis, hematuria, bloody stool, a crimson or deep red tongue, and a rapid pulse. Other indications include unconsciousness, delirium, a dry mouth, gargling without a desire to gulp, a false feeling of fullness in the lower abdomen, and dark stool with easy defecation.

An essential pathological feature of the blood level heat exuberance pattern is the presence of heat in blood which drives a frenetic blood flow. This is also known as "heat exuberance driving blood," hence aside from the usual heat signs of fever and a crimson tongue, there are manifestations of blood seeping out of vessels. If the blood leaks from under the skin, it will become macules, which are usually bright red at the beginning and then turn dark purple. If the blood leaks from the collaterals of the lung and stomach, hematemesis and epitaxis will be manifested. If it is from the intestines, bladder, and uterine system, bloody stool, hematuria, and vaginal bleeding will be observed. If the pathogenic heat disrupts the heart spirit, unconsciousness and delirium may occur. As the leaked blood can become static and blood heat can boil blood into static blood, another important pathological change of this pattern is the internal production of static blood binding pathogenic heat and becoming static heat. The internal obstruction of static blood prevents body fluids from being distributed upward, which explains the symptom of a dry mouth. However, as the body fluids have not been too greatly impaired, the patient still tends to consume water, but gargles without any compulsion to gulp.

Although fever is a main symptom of this pattern, high fever is not definite in diseases of internal damage. In this case, the patient experiences a feverish sensation, especially in the soles and palms, and has a flushed face or red lips, which are indications of heat in the blood level.

As the pattern of heat exuberance in the blood level results in macules and bleeding, it is also called the pattern of heat toxins in the blood level, which is classified under the fire toxin exuberance pattern. However, since the pathological changes are mainly limited in the blood level, there are specific symptoms for this particular pattern.

Treatment method

Clearing heat, cooling blood, and dissolving stasis.

Formula and ingredients: Xī Jiǎo Dì Huáng Tāng (Rhinoceros Horn and Rehmannia Decoction)

Xī jiǎo (Cornu Rhinocerotis) 3 g; shēng dì (Radix Rehmanniae) 30 g; sháo yào (Radix Paeoniae) 12 g; mǔ dān pí (Cortex Moutan) 9 g.

Formula verse

Xī jiǎo dì huáng sháo yào dān calm signs of heat exuberance in the blood level.

Usage

Grind xī jiǎo into juice and decoct the other ingredients in water. Remove the dregs and mix the decoction with xī jiǎo juice for oral intake. Alternatively, slice xī jiǎo and decoct it with other ingredients in water.

Analysis

In this formula, *xī jiǎo*, the main ingredient, is salty and cold, which can clear heat, cool blood, and remove toxins. Currently, *xī jiǎo* is forbidden in practice for making medicinals, so *shuǐ niú jiǎo*, a similar medicinal, can be used in its place, but its dose should be increased to more than 30 g and it can be sliced for decocting. *Shēng dì*, sweet and cold, clears heat in the blood level and nourishes blood, being an important ingredient for cooling blood and arresting bleeding. Both *chì sháo* and *mǔ dān pí* can clear heat and cool blood, invigorate blood, and dissipate stasis, which not only strengthens the blood-cooling effect of *xī jiǎo and shēng dì*, but also dispels the static blood produced by heat exuberance in the blood level and avoid the negative consequence of cold medicinals inhibiting blood flow. Though there are only four ingredients in this formula, its combination is carefully designed to exert curative effects of clearing heat, removing toxins, cooling blood, nourishing yin, dispelling stasis, and arresting bleeding.

Xī jiǎo can strengthen the heart and calm the mind. *Shēng dì* not only fortifies the heart, but also stops bleeding by promoting blood coagulation and increasing blood viscosity. *Chì sháo* inhibits various bacteria, quickens blood flow, and dilates blood vessels. *Mǔ dān pí* calms the mind, arrests pain, and has anti-inflammatory and antipyretic effects. It also has certain excitation properties. Overall, this formula not only relieves fever, but also exhibits applications to resolve different aspects of heat exuberance in the blood level.

Treatment reference

Xī Jiǎo Dì Huáng Tāng is extensively applied to critical cases of externally contracted febrile diseases, diseases of internal damage, and surgical and gynecological diseases. In practice, blood heat and bleeding are two major pathological changes. The pattern of heat exuberance in the blood level in externally contracted febrile diseases comprises a definite high fever or a universal scorching sensation over the body and a frenetic blood flow. This manifests as macules and papules or cavity bleeding, often belonging to acute infectious diseases at the DIC level, or other causes, such as epidemic encephalitis B, epidemic meningococal meningitis, epidemic hemorrhagic fever, leptospirosis of lung hemorrhages, intestinal bleeding of intestinal typhoid, fulminant hepatitis, septicemia, measles, or scarlet fever. As for diseases of internal damage, this pattern usually occurs in those with bleeding as the main symptom, such as allergic or thrombopenic purpura, acute leukemia, and so on. Moreover, blood heat and bleeding are both common pathological changes of irregular menstruation, pregnancy, and postpartum diseases. For the treatment of the above cases, *Xī Jiǎo Dì Huáng Tāng* can generally be taken as the primary formula.

In practice, proper modification is required. If the heat toxin is potent, add *huáng lián*, *jīn yín huā*, *lián qiào*, *bǎn lán gēn*, *dà qīng yè*, and other heat-clearing medicinals. If vexation and agitation are resulted from heart fire exuberance, add *huáng lián* and *zhī zǐ* to clear. If there is unconsciousness due to pathogenic heat clouding the pericardium, add *Ān Gōng Niú Huáng Wán* (Peaceful Palace Bovine Bezoar Pill). For severe hematemesis and epitaxis, add *bái máo gēn*, *cè bǎi yè*, and *hàn lián cǎo*. If there is bloody stool, add charred *dì yú* and *huái huā*. If there is hematuria, add *bái máo gēn* and *xiǎo jì*. If the fire toxin exists not only in the blood level, but also all over the body, this formula can be combined with *Huáng Lián Jiě Dú Tāng* (Coptis Toxin-Resolving Decoction), becoming *Qīng Wēn Bài Dú Yǐn* (Epidemic-Clearing Toxin-Resolving Beverage), which is more effective in clearing heat toxins.

Cautions

Most cases treated by this formula are critical, so the accurate application of medicinals is essential. This formula cannot be applied to cases of bleeding caused by yang qi deficiency, the failure of the heart and spleen to control blood, or the insufficiency of body fluids and deficiency–heat, driving frenetic blood flow. It is a cold and cool formula; hence, application should be stopped immediately after curative effects have been achieved in patients with yang deficiency and a weak spleen and stomach. Excluding certain chronic diseases, patients treated by this formula should be nursed with close attention so that once critical symptoms surface, first aid can be performed in time.

Daily Exercises

1. What are the main symptoms and signs of the blood level heat exuberance pattern?
2. What are the ingredients of *Xī Jiǎo Dì Huáng Tāng*? What is/are the function(s) of each ingredient?
3. Mr. Gu is a 19-year-old man. He has been experiencing recurring abdominal pain, hematuria, and skin macules for more than a year. Other clinical manifestations are a lusterless complexion, approximately 7 patches of dark red and purple macules in the lower limbs, a reddish tongue with a thin and white coating, and a wiry and rapid pulse. A physical examination shows a body temperature of 37.4°C, normal heart and lungs, and a flat and soft abdomen without tenderness. Please prescribe a Chinese medicinal formula for this case.

Additional Formulae

Qīng Wēn Bài Dú Yǐn (Epidemic-Clearing Toxin-Resolving Beverage)

Raw *shí gāo* (Gypsum Fibrosum) 180 g; *shēng dì* (Radix Rehmanniae) 18 g; *xī jiǎo* (Cornu Rhinocerotis) 18 g; *huáng lián* (Rhizoma Coptidis) 12 g; *zhī zǐ* (Fructus Gardeniae) 6 g; *jié gěng* (Radix Platycodonis) 3 g; *huáng qín* (Radix Scutellariae) 6 g; *zhī mǔ* (Rhizoma Anemarrhenae) 6 g; *chì sháo* (Radix Paeoniae Rubra) 6 g; *xuán shēn* (Radix Scrophulariae) 6 g; *lián qiào* (Fructus Forsythiae) 6 g; *gān cǎo* (Radix et Rhizoma Glycyrrhizae) 3 g; fresh *zhú yè* (Radix et Rhizoma Glycyrrhizae) 3 g.

Add raw *shí gāo* to decoct with water first and after boiling for 10 min, add the remaining ingredients. For *xī jiǎo*, grind it with water or into powder or add it first to decoct. Take the decoction warm 2 times. If there is no *xī jiǎo* at hand, use *shuǐ niú jiǎo* 120 g instead.

Actions

Clearing heat and resolving toxins; cooling blood and rescuing yin.

Indications

Pathogenic heat exuberance in the qi and blood levels presenting high fever, extreme thirst with a desire to drink, acute headaches, vexation and agitation, loss of consciousness, hematemesis and epitaxis, macules, a crimson tongue with a dry coating, and a rapid pulse.

DAY TWO

The Pathogenic Heat Obstructing Lung Pattern

In this pattern, pathogenic heat obstructs the lung, causing it to function abnormally. This is generally triggered by infection, so it is commonly seen in lobar pneumonia, bronchopneumonia (especially pneumonia complicated by measles), pertussis, diphtheria, scarlet fever, several kinds of acute bronchitis, chronic bronchitis at the acute occurrence stage, and so on.

Diagnosis

The main symptoms and signs of this pattern are fever, coughing, panting, and rapid pulse. Other indications include thirst, chest oppression, chest pain, spitting of thick and yellow sputum, shortness of breath or flaring nasal wings, a red tongue with a thin yellow and dry coating.

Among externally contracted febrile diseases, this pattern can be either caused by exterior wind–cold transforming into heat and entering the interior, or by wind–heat and dry–heat entering the interior to invade the lung, or by pathogenic heat invading the lung directly. As the lung governs respiration and its qi must be able to ascend, diffuse, and descend, heat exuberance in the lung inevitably leads to lung qi obstruction and failure of the lung to ascend and descend. Therefore, aside from some common interior heat manifestations of fever, thirst, a rapid pulse, and a red tongue with a yellow coating, there are symptoms of coughing, panting, and even flaring nasal wings (often among young children). The severity of panting usually reflects the degree of lung qi obstruction and failure of ascension and descension of the lung. The fever, thirst, and a red tongue with a rapid pulse are indicators of the severity of pathogenic fever. In this pattern, the severity of pathogenic heat is sometimes similar to the degree of lung qi obstruction, and at other times, the priority is different. As for chest oppression, chest pain, and thick yellow sputum, they are the results of lung heat burning the lung collaterals and boiling lung fluids. The sputum can be rust-like at times.

Sweating can either be present or absent in this pattern, which is correlated to the state of lung qi obstruction. If it is severe, the sweat pores will also be obstructed, and sweating will not occur. In contrast, if lung qi can still able to diffuse and descend, sweat pores will not be blocked, so sweating is usually observed. In this case, panting is often mild and the pathogenic heat in the lung is able to diffuse outward easily.

Treatment method

Clearing heat and diffusing the lung.

Formula and ingredients: Má Xìng Shí Gān Tāng (Ephedra, Apricot Kernel, Gypsum, and Licorice Decoction)

Má huáng (Herba Ephedrae) 9 g; crushed *xìng rén* (Semen Armeniacae Amarum) without tips 9 g; *zhì gān cǎo* (Radix et Rhizoma Glycyrrhizae Praeparata cum Melle) 9 g; *shí gāo* (Gypsum Fibrosum) 20 g.

Formula verse

Má Xìng Shí Gān has four ingredients, applicable to lung heat exuberance.

Usage

Add 1.4 L of water first to decoct *má huáng* and remove the foam after boiling. Add the remaining ingredients when 1 L is left. Remove the dregs after 400 mL are left. Take the decoction warm 200 mL at a time, 2 times a day.

Analysis

In this formula, *má huáng* and *shí gāo* is a typical combination for treating lung heat. *Má huáng* is acrid–warm, which is generally not applicable to the heat pattern, but as lung qi obstruction cannot be diffused by acrid–warm medicinals, cold-natured *shí gāo* is combined to restrict *má huáng*'s hot nature, thus diffusing lung qi without boosting heat. *Shí gāo* is cold and can stagnate the flow of qi movement, hence it is usually not applicable to lung qi obstruction, but when it is combined with *má huáng*, it is effective in clearing lung heat. These two ingredients complement each other to exert pronounced curative effects. *Xìng rén* lowers lung qi to remove phlegm and assist *má huáng* to relieve coughing and reduce panting. *Gān cǎo* boosts qi, harmonizes the middle and the actions of all medicinals in the formula, and prevents cold *shí gāo* from impairing stomach qi.

It has been shown that each ingredient in the decoction of *Má Xìng Shí Gān Tāng* has certain antibacterial and antiviral effects. *Má huáng* dilates bronchial smooth muscles to calm panting and *xìng rén* relieves coughing and dispels phlegm, and both of them can promote urination and are effective in eliminating cellular edema of the lung. *Shí gāo* relieves fever, quenches thirst, and promotes urination. *Gān cǎo* dispels phlegm, relieves pain, and acts like an adrenocortical hormone. Therefore, the pharmacological function of this formula is fairly complicated. From its clinical applications, its excellent curative efficacy indicates that this formula harbors more portential pharmacological effects that warrant further exploration.

Treatment reference

Má Xìng Shí Gān Tāng is clinically applied to various infectious diseases, and it is especially effective for pneumonia of lung qi obstruction accompanied with panting. Moreover, it can also be applied to allergic asthma of young children that is classified as heat blockage in the lung. It is also used to treat diseases of wind–heat attacking the head and skin, such as rashes, acute occurrence of rhinitis, epidemic pinkeye, corneal ulcers, acute iridocyclitis, stye, and even enuresis and edema due to nephritis. In application, the key to pattern differentiation lies in lung heat, of which the typical signs are fever and coughing. However, wind–heat signs of the nasal cavity, throat, and even head can be used as a reference for lung heat, such as yellow and turbid nasal discharge, yellow and sticky sputum, sticky, yellow, and dry eye discharge, and a sore throat. Thus, the scope of application of this formula is significantly broadened.

In practice, proper modification is required. If this pattern is accompanied by the absence of sweating and aversion to cold, which is usually due to lingering exterior pathogens, thus exterior-releasing medicinals such as *jīng jiè*, *dòu chǐ*, *zǐ sū yè*, and *niú bàng zǐ* should be added. If the patient has a yin-deficient physique or the pathogenic heat has impaired his body fluids, lung yin-nourishing medicinals such as *běi shā shēn*, *mài dōng*, and *lú gēn* should be added. If there is exuberant lung heat resulting in high fever, spitting of rusty or fishy and purulent sputum, add *jīn qiáo mài*, *yú xīng cǎo*, *hǔ zhàng*, *bèi mǔ*, and *yì yǐ rén* to clear lung heat and dissolve phlegm. For pertussis complicated with pneumonia, add *bǎi bù*, *chuān bèi mǔ*, *qián hú*, and *tiān zhú huáng* to dissolve phlegm and relieve coughing. For diphtheria complicated with pneumonia, add *jīn yín huā*, *lián qiào*, *shēng dì*, *xuán shēn*, *huáng lián*, and *bǎn lán gēn* to clear heat, resolve toxins, and nourish yin to moisten the lung. If this formula is used with *guì zhī*, *shēng jiāng*, and *dà zǎo*, it becomes *Dà Qīng Lóng Tāng* (Major Green Dragon Decoction), which is more potent in releasing the exterior and indicated for exterior wind excess–cold pattern accompanied by interior heat. If *xìng rén* is removed and *dà zǎo* and *shēng jiāng* are added to harmonize *ying* and *wei* levels, it becomes *Yuè Bì Tāng* (Maidservant from Yue Decoction), which is indicated for nephritic edema with lung heat.

Cautions

As the causes of coughing and panting are various, this formula is not applicable to wind–cold obstructing the lung, lung qi deficiency, and phlegm–damp obstructing the lung.

In application, the dose ratio of the *má huáng* and *shí gāo* is important. Generally, the proper ratio of *má huáng*:*shí gāo* is 1:5 (traditional ratio 1:2), i.e., more *shí gāo* than *má huáng*. For diphtheria and scarlet fever, the dose of *má huáng* is adjusted to 3 g and *shí gāo* 60 g, the purpose of which is to enhance the lung-clearing effect. If lung qi constraint and obstruction are serious, the dose of *má huáng* can be increased (its acrid–warm and dispersing characteristics should not be taken so much into account).

When this formula is administered to treat bronchopneumonia in young children, it usually works quickly to relieve high fever and panting. However, this disease has a pattern of fast transmission, so close observation is required. If symptoms of a pale complexion, profuse sweating, and dispiritedness occur, apply heart- and kidney-warming and boosting medicinals or send the patient to hospital for appropriate treatment immediately.

Daily Exercises

1. What is the definition of the pattern of pathogenic heat obstructing the lung? Is sweating a definite symptom of the lung heat pattern?
2. In the formula of *Má Xìng Shí Gān Tāng*, what are the functions of the combination of *má huáng* and *shí gāo*? What are the key points with regards to its ratio?
3. Shan is a 4-year-old boy. He caught a cold 3 days ago and had mild fever, an aversion to cold, watery nasal discharge, and paroxysmal cough. He was given antipyretic tablets and there was a little sweating after taking the medicine. However, his body temperature rose quickly yesterday evening. A physical examination showed a temperature of 39.8°C, no aversion to cold, absence of sweating, a dry nose without watery nasal discharge, aggravated coughing, panting, restlessness, a red tongue with a thin yellow and dry coating, and a slippery and rapid pulse. Please prescribe a Chinese medicinal formula for this case.

Additional Formulae

Dà Qīng Lóng Tāng (Major Green Dragon Decoction)

Má huáng (Herba Ephedrae) 10 g; *guì zhī* (Ramulus Cinnamomi) 6 g; *zhì gān cǎo* (Radix et Rhizoma Glycyrrhizae Praeparata cum Melle) 6 g; *xìng rén* (Semen Armeniacae Amarum) without skin and tips 6 g; crushed *shí gāo* (Gypsum Fibrosum) 12 g; *shēng jiāng* (Rhizoma Zingiberis Recens) 9 g, crushed *dà zǎo* (Fructus Jujubae) 5 pieces.

Add water to decoct and take warm to induce mild sweating. If sweating occurs and the disease is cured, stop treatment immediately.

Actions

Inducing sweating to relieve the exterior and clearing interior heat.

Indications

Externally contracted wind–cold with the interior heat pattern, an aversion to cold with fever, cold and heat signs with equal severity, body aches, an absence of sweating, vexation and agitation, and a floating and tight pulse.

Yuè Bì Tāng (Maidservant from Yue Decoction)

Má huáng (Herba Ephedrae) 9 g; *shí gāo* (Gypsum Fibrosum) 30 g; *shēng jiāng* (Rhizoma Zingiberis Recens) 9 g; *gān cǎo* (Radix et Rhizoma Glycyrrhizae) 6 g; *dà zǎo* (Fructus Jujubae) 5 pieces. Add water to decoct.

Actions

Inducing sweating and promoting urination.

Indications

Fever, an aversion to wind, body edema, sweating, a lack of thirst, and a floating pulse.

DAY THREE

The Intestinal Damp–Heat Pattern

The obstruction of the intestines by damp–heat leads to abnormal function and results in diarrhea. This pattern occurs in the course of externally contracted febrile diseases, such as when an exterior pathogen enters the large intestine and when an external damp–heat pathogen attacks the intestine directly. It is commonly seen in acute enteritis, dysentery, intestinal typhoid, epidemic diarrhea in children, and various infectious diseases complicated with enteritis.

Diagnosis

The main symptoms and signs of this pattern are fever, diarrhea with pungent contents, and a burning sensation around the anus. Other indications include a mild aversion to cold, vexing chest and epigastric heat, a dry mouth, thirst, shortness of breath, a yellow and greasy tongue coating, and a rapid pulse.

As damp–heat obstructs the the small and large intestines, they fail to raise the clear, direct the turbid downward, and conduct and transmit intestinal contents. Therefore, the clear and turbid contents will mix together and flow downward and turn into diarrhea. This pattern is caused by a damp–heat pathogen, hence resulting in fever, yellow and pungent stool or urgent watery diarrhea, or diarrhea following abdominal pain. If this pattern is transmitted from the exterior pattern that has not been relieved, there will be a mild aversion to cold. If the damp–heat pathogen disrupts the interior, there will be vexing chest and epigastric heat. If the heat pathogen impairs yin, there will be a dry mouth and thirst. When the interior heat travels outward, sweating will be induced. If the intestinal heat attacks the lung, panting will be observed. An aversion to cold, sweating, and panting are not definite symptoms of this pattern. A yellow and greasy tongue coating and a rapid pulse are signs of damp–heat exuberance in the interior.

Although intestinal damp–heat accumulation in the interior is seen in dysentery that is characterized by tenesmus and purulent hemafecia, it is generally deemed as a bind of food stagnation and a damp–heat pathogen in the intestines in the pattern differentiation of Chinese medicine. Therefore, the diagnosis and treatment of dysentery are not completely similar to this pattern, which will be discussed later.

Treatment method

Clearing and dissolving intestinal damp–heat.

Formula and ingredients: Gé Gēn Huáng Qín Huáng Lián Tāng (Pueraria, Scutellaria, and Coptis Decoction)

Gé gēn (Radix Puerariae Lobatae) 15 g; zhì gān cǎo (Radix et Rhizoma Glycyrrhizae Praeparata cum Melle) 3 g; huáng lián (Rhizoma Coptidis) 6 g; huáng qín (Radix Scutellariae) 9 g.

Formula verse

Gé Gēn Huáng Qín Huáng Lián Tāng, decocted with *gān cǎo* for oral intake; applicable to pathogens in *yangming* and heat dysentery, ensuring health by clearing and dissolving intestinal heat.

Usage

Add 1.6 L of water first to decoct *gé gēn* until 1.2 L are left. Add the remaning ingredients to decoct until 400 mL are left. Remove the dregs and take the decoction twice while warm.

Analysis

In this formula, *gé gēn* is the chief ingredient, which can boost the clear yang qi of the stomach and intestines to ascend and is effective in halting diarrhea as well as relieving the flesh and dispelling the external pathogen by its acrid–cool nature. *Huáng qín* and *huáng lián*, bitter and cold, are combined to clear heat and dry dampness, and dispel damp–heat in the intestines to relieve diarrhea. *Gān cǎo* revives the middle and harmonizes the actions of all medicinals.

This formula is also applicable to the intestinal damp–heat pattern without exterior signs and can be used as a treatment for both the exterior and interior, but its effect of relieving the exterior is weak.

Gé gēn relieves fever, relaxes spasms of smooth muscles, increases the secretion of gastric juices and bile, and improves gastrointestinal functions. *Huáng qín* and *huáng lián* have broad-spectrum antibacterial properties, and are especially effective in combating certain intestinal bacteria. The pharmacological functions of *gān cǎo* have been introduced in previous sections. In conclusion, this formula has seen reliable pharmacological evidence for its good efficacy in treating intestinal inflammation.

Treatment reference

Gé Gēn Huáng Qín Huáng Lián Tāng is applicable to diarrhea due to damp–heat in the intestine regardless of the presence of the exterior pattern. Besides various acute enteritis and bacillary dysentery at the initial stage, it is also indicated for measles, epidemic encephalitis B, viral pneumonia, and other diseases complicated with interior heat diarrhea caused by enteritis or intestinal disorders. In addition, *wú gōng*, *quán xiē*, and *sháo yào* can be added to treat infantile paralysis. For pneumonia presenting an aversion to cold with fever, coughing, panting, abdominal pain, and diarrhea, this formula is potent as it can clear heat, relieve the exterior, alleviate panting, and arrest diarrhea.

If *gé gēn* is removed from this formula, and *sháo yào*, *dà huáng*, *bīng láng*, *dāng guī*, *mù xiāng*, and *ròu guì* are added, it becomes *Sháo Yào Tāng* (Peony Decoction), which can clear damp–heat, move qi and blood, and promote digestion, and is indicated for dysentery caused by damp–heat and food stagnation in the intestines. If *huáng lián* and *gé gēn* are removed from this formula and *sháo yào* and *dà zǎo* are added, it becomes *Huáng Qín Tāng* (Scutellaria Decoction), which can clear heat and treat dysentery. If this pattern is accompanied by vomiting, *jiāng bàn xià* should be added to direct counterflow downward and arrest vomiting. If it is accompanied by food stagnation, add *shān zhā* and *shén qū* to promote digestion. If abdominal pain is severe, add *mù xiāng* and *sháo yào* to move qi, reduce urgency, and relieve pain. If coughing and panting occurs with lung heat, add *sāng bái pí*, *xìng rén*, *bèi mǔ*, and *pí pá yè*, or combine with *Má Xìng Shí Gān Tāng* to clear the lung and dissolve phlegm.

Cautions

The causes and manifestations of diarrhea are numerous. If it is not caused by damp–heat in the intestines, this formula should not be applied. If there are signs of qi stagnation, blood stasis, and food stagnation, the curative effect of this formula is not ideal even for diarrhea due to intestinal damp–heat. Instead, this formula should be combined with other medicinals or formulae to rectify qi, dissolve stasis, and promote food stagnation.

Daily Exercises

1. What are the main symptoms and signs of the intestinal damp–heat pattern?
2. What are the indications of *Gé Gēn Huáng Qín Huáng Lián Tāng*?

3. Ms. Song is an 8-year-old girl. During late summer, she suddenly suffered from diarrhea with yellow, loose, and pungent stool 4 times in half a day, accompanied by thirst with little desire for drinking, nausea, fever (38.1°C), a red tongue with a thin yellow, and mildly greasy coating, and a rapid pulse. Please prescribe a Chinese medicinal formula for this case.

Additional Formulae

Sháo Yào Tāng (Peony Decoction)

Sháo yào (Radix Paeoniae) 15 g; *dāng guī* (Radix Angelicae Sinensis) 9 g; *huáng lián* (Rhizoma Coptidis) 9 g; *bīng láng* (Semen Arecae) 5 g; *mù xiāng* (Radix Aucklandiae) 5 g; *gān cǎo* (Radix et Rhizoma Glycyrrhizae) 5 g; *dà huáng* (Radix et Rhizoma Rhei) 9 g; *huáng qín* (Radix Scutellariae) 9 g; *ròu guì* (Cortex Cinnamomi) 2 g.

Grind the ingredients into a fine powder and take 15 g each time to decoct with 500 mL of water until 250 mL are left. Remove the dregs and take it warm.

Actions

Clearing heat and resolving toxins; rectifying qi and harmonizing blood.

Indications

Damp–heat dysentery presenting abdominal pain, purulent hemafecia, tenesmus, a burning sensation around the anus, scant and brown urine, and a tongue with a greasy and slightly yellow coating.

Huáng Qín Tāng (Scutellaria Decoction)

Huáng qín (Radix Scutellariae) 9 g; *sháo yào* (Radix Paeoniae) 6 g; *zhì gān cǎo* (Radix et Rhizoma Glycyrrhizae Praeparata cum Melle) 3 g; *dà zǎo* (Fructus Jujubae) 4 pieces. Add water to decoct.

Actions

Clearing heat and treating dysentery; harmonizing the middle and arresting pain.

Indications

Dysentery with abdominal pain, fever, a bitter taste in the mouth, a red tongue, and a wiry and rapid pulse.

DAY FOUR

The Damp–Heat Accumulation in the Middle Pattern

The accumulation of damp–heat in the middle is triggered by damp–heat pathogen accumulation in the spleen and stomach of the middle *jiao*, which causes disorder of the spleen and stomach in their ascending and descending actions. This pattern often occurs in externally contracted febrile diseases and is primarily induced by the invasion of an external damp–heat pathogen. In some cases, the damp–heat pathogen attacks the body surface first and then enters the spleen and stomach, gradually transforming into heat and causing exuberance of both dampness and heat in the middle *jiao*. In other patients, the damp–heat pathogen mounts a direct invasion of the spleen and stomach of the middle *jiao*. This pattern is commonly seen in intestinal typhoid, acute gastroenteritis, cholera, leptospirosis, etc.

Diagnosis

The main symptoms and signs are chest and epigastric stuffiness and fullness, vomiting, diarrhea, and a tongue with a yellow and greasy coating. Other indications include fever, lingering sweat, thirst without any compulsion for heavy drinking, scant and brown urine, and a rapid pulse.

The damp–heat pathogen tends to invade the spleen and stomach and is especially common in the later period of summer, thus this pattern usually occurs in summer and autumn. It is often caused by a contaminated diet. The invasion of the damp–heat pathogen inevitably stagnates the qi movement of the middle *jiao*, so there are sensations of chest and epigastric stuffiness and fullness, and perhaps abdominal distention and fullness. The obstruction of the middle by damp–heat also influences spleen–stomach functions, particularly in raising the clear and directing the turbid downward. Failure of stomach qi to descend manifests as nausea and vomiting, while failure of spleen qi to ascend clear qi results in diarrhea. If the accumulation of damp–heat in the middle consumes body fluids, it will result in fever, thirst, scant and brown urine, a red tongue with a yellow and greasy coating, and a rapid pulse. As the pathogen is damp and turbid, thirst is present without any desire for substantial drinking.

During diagnosis, the dominance of dampness or heat should be determined. If there are severe epigastric fullness and abdominal distention, with no obvious thirst or a desire for drinking warm water, whitish and turbid urine, and a white and greasy tongue coating, it can be classified as severe dampness and mild heat. If high fever, persistent sweating, significant thirst, scant, brown, and inhibited urination, a yellow and greasy tongue coating, and a slippery and rapid pulse are observed, it pertains to severe heat and mild dampness. In addition, the degree of fever in this pattern is related to the disease. For example, intestinal typhoid with this pattern usually triggers a high fever of above 39°C, but when it occurs in acute gastroenteritis, dysentery, and cholera, the body temperature may not necessarily be that high.

Treatment method

Clearing heat and removing dampness; rectifying qi and harmonizing the middle.

Formula and ingredients: Lián Pò Yǐn (Coptis and Officinal Magnolia Bark Beverage)

Prepared *hòu pò* (Cortex Magnoliae Officinalis) 6 g; ginger juice-fried *huáng lián* (Rhizoma Coptidis) 3 g; *shí chāng pú* (Rhizoma Acori Tatarinowii) 3 g; prepared *bàn xià* (Rhizoma Pinelliae) 3 g; dry-fried *xiāng dòu chǐ* (Semen Sojae Praeparatum) 9 g; *jiāo zhī zǐ* (Fructus Gardeniae Praeparatus) 9 g; *lú gēn* (Rhizoma Phragmitis) 60 g.

Formula verse

Lián Pò Yǐn uses *dòu chǐ, chāng pú bàn xià lú gēn zhī*; applicable to chest and epigastric oppression with vomiting and diarrhea, indicating for damp–heat accumulation in the middle.

Usage

Add water to decoct.

Analysis

In this formula, *huáng lián* dries dampness and clears heat, while *hòu pò* moves qi and dissolves dampness. These two ingredients are the chief medicinals, which move qi to dissolve dampness and dissolves dampness to clear heat. *Zhī zǐ* is used to assist *huáng lián* in clearing heat and drying dampness. *Xiāng dòu chǐ* diffuses qi to disperse heat outward. *Shí chāng pú* is aromatic, which resolves damp–turbidity to harmonize the spleen and stomach. *Bàn xià* dries dampness to check counterflow and arrest vomiting. *Lú gēn* clears heat, removes dampness, harmonizes the stomach, and relieves vomiting. The key feature of this formula is the combination of bitter–cold (e.g., *huáng lián* and *zhī zǐ*) and acrid–warm medicinals (e.g., *hòu pò* and *bàn xià*). This type of combination is called the "opening of acrid medicinals and bitter medicinals promoting descent," or "unblocking and purging with bitter–acrid medicinals." The bitter–cold nature is applied to clear heat and dry dampness, and the acrid–warm nature to dissolve dampness and diffuse qi movement. Therefore, this formula can clear damp–heat, harmonize the spleen and stomach, raise the clear and direct the turbid downward, and stop vomiting and diarrhea.

  Huáng lián, hòu pò, and *zhī zǐ* have positive effects on inhibiting bacteria. *Bàn xià, hòu pò*, and *shí chāng pú* can rectify gastrointestinal functions. As a result, *Lián Pò Yǐn* is favorable for treating various infectious diseases.

Treatment reference

Clinically, this formula is applied to cure acute diseases of digestive infection, such as acute gastroenteritis, intestinal typhoid, paratyphoid, and
bacillary dysentery presenting internal damp–heat accumulation. If vomiting is severe, add dry-fried *zhú rú* and ginger juice, or add *Yù Shū Dān*
(Jade Pivot Elixir). For cholera and systremma, it is better to use *Cán Shǐ
Tāng* (Silkworm Droppings Decoction). If the dampness of this pattern is
severe, add *huò xiāng*, *pèi lán*, and fresh lotus leaves; if heat is severe, add
huáng qín and *shí gāo*.

Cautions

In application, the ingredients and dosages should be adapted according
to the dominance of dampness or heat. If this pattern is accompanied by
severe vomiting and diarrhea, or even with obvious dehydration, fluid
infusion should be secondary. If the appearances of the vomit and diarrhea
contents are similar to that of rice-washed water, laboratory tests should
be carried out immediately to diagnose whether it is the fulminating contagious disease cholera, so that timely quarantine and other measures can
be appropriated.

Daily Exercises

1. List the diagnostic criteria of the damp–heat accumulation in the
   middle pattern. How do you identify if dampness or heat holds
   priority?
2. What are the ingredients of *Lián Pò Yǐn*?
3. Ms. Zhang is a 24-year-old female. She has been ill for 10 days.
   Initially, she experienced an aversion to cold and had a fever. During
   this week, the aversion to cold has been relieved, but her body
   temperature has gradually risen, especially in the afternoon, and
   peaked at 40.3°C. Her other symptoms and signs are chest oppression,
   a lack of hunger pangs, seldomly sweating, thirst without any desire
   for much drinking, occasional nausea, head heaviness, fatigue, a red
   tongue with a thin, yellow, and greasy coating, a slippery and rapid

pulse, scant and brown urine, and loose stool 2 times a day. Please prescribe a Chinese medicinal formula for this case.

Additional Formulae

Yù Shū Dān (Jade Pivot Elixir)

Shān cí gū (Pseudobulbus Cremastrae seu Pleiones) 90 g; hóng dà jǐ (Radix Knoxiae) 45 g; qiān jīn zǐ shuāng (Semen Euphorbiae Pulveratum) 30 g; wǔ bèi zǐ (Galla Chinensis) 90 g; shè xiāng (Moschus) 9 g; xióng huáng (Realgar) 30 g; zhū shā (Cinnabaris) 30 g.

Grind the ingredients into a fine powder, mix them with cooked glutinous rice flour evenly to make into lozenges, and dry them in the shade. Take orally 0.6–1.5 g at a time, 2 times day. It is also sold as a powder in the market, usually 6 g a bottle; 1.5 g to be consumed orally each time, 2 times a day.

Actions

Dispelling filth and resolving toxins; dissolving phlegm and arresting vomiting; and relieving swelling and pain.

Indications

Contraction of summer heat and dampness filth presenting abdominal distention, oppression, pain, nausea, vomiting, diarrhea, and external diseases with red swellings, hot pain, or animal bites.

Cán Shǐ Tāng (Silkworm Droppings Decoction)

Cán shā (Faeces Bombycis) 15 g; yì yǐ rén (Semen Coicis) 12 g; dà dòu juǎn (Semen Sojae Germinatum) 12 g; mù guā (Fructus Chaenomelis) 9 g; ginger juice-fried huáng lián (Rhizoma Coptidis) 9 g; prepared bàn xià (Rhizoma Pinelliae) 3 g; wine-fried huáng qín (Radix Scutellariae) 3 g; tōng cǎo (Medulla Tetrapanacis) 3 g; jiāo zhī zǐ (Fructus Gardeniae Praeparatus) 5 g; wú zhū yú (Fructus Evodiae) 1 g. Add water to decoct and take the decoction cool.

Actions

Clearing heat and draining dampness; raising the clear and directing the turbid downward.

Indications

Damp–heat accumulation and obstruction or cholera presenting vomiting, diarrhea, abdominal pain, cramps, thirst, vexation and agitation, a tongue with a yellow, thick, and greasy coating, and a rapid pulse.

DAY FIVE

The Liver–Gallbladder Damp–Heat Pattern

The liver–gallbladder damp–heat pattern is caused by the obstruction of the liver, gallbladder, and their channels by damp–heat. The liver and gallbladder are attached to each other and their functions are hence closely related. Dysfunction of one organ influences the other, and thus there exist many instances of the simultaneous disorder of both the liver and gallbladder. For this pattern, the location of the disease may be in the liver, the gallbladder, the liver channel, the gallbladder channel, both the liver and gallbladder, or in both channels. The damp–heat pathogen travels downward, so consequently, there are manifestations of damp–heat pouring downward. However, if the heat is strong enough, it may also manifest as up-flaming of liver fire or gallbladder fire. This pattern is often seen in various hepatitic diseases, cholecystitis, herpes zoster, and inflammation of the ear, breast, and genitals. It also occurs in diseases of internal damage, such as hypertesion and schizophrenia.

Diagnosis

For damp–heat pouring downward, the main symptoms and signs are inhibited urination, pungent vaginal discharge in women, and swellings and pain in the genitals; for up-flaming of liver-gallbladder fire, there may be vertigo, headaches, a bitter taste in the mouth, red eyes, and tinnitus. Other indications include distending chest and rib-side pain, jaundice, nausea, epigastric stuffiness, swelling and itching or rashes with exudates in the genitals, deafness, ear swellings, red eyes, tearing, a red tongue with a yellow and greasy coating.

The clinical manifestations of this pattern are extremely complicated. In diagnosis, aside from the main symptoms of damp–heat pouring downward and up-flaming of liver–gallbladder fire, the following two aspects should be noted in pattern differentiation: (1) the disease location and (2) the disease nature. The site of the disease, for some cases, are in the liver and gallbladder, particularly in the rib-side regions. In Chinese medicine, these regions are dominated by the liver and gallbladder, which is different from modern anatomical classification; hence, distending rib-side pain and fullness are attributed to the liver and gallbladder. Others may be apparent in the regions of distribution of the liver and gallbladder channels, mainly in the head (especially both sides and the ear regions), chest, rib-sides, breasts, genitals, and toes. Yet, more are present in the openings of the liver and gallbladder. Since the liver opens into the eye, many such diseases are ophthalmologically related. As for the nature of the disease, it can be due to either damp–heat or fire–heat. Indeed, the disease nature is judged from the specific symptoms and signs. In this pattern, if the up-flaming of liver and gallbladder fire upsets the head, there will be vertigo and headaches that are usually more serious at the sides, with head distention. If the fire–heat attacks the eyes, there will be red eyes, tearing, and photophobia. If it attacks the ear, there will be tinnitus, deafness, and ear swelling. A bitter taste in the mouth is often an indication of heat in the liver and gallbladder. For liver–gallbladder damp–heat, apart from symptoms involving the urinary and reproductive systems, such as inhibited and urgent urination, turbid urine, increased leukorrhea with a pungent odor or is yellowish-green, painful swelling in the genitals, itching, and exudates, there may also be leg swelling and masses. In addition, the obstruction of the liver and gallbladder channels by damp–heat or fire–heat may present distending chest and rib-side pain, distending lower abdominal pain, etc. The pathogen in the liver and gallbladder can also affect the normal functions of the spleen and stomach, manifesting as nausea, epigastric stuffiness and fullness, a lack of appetite, and an absence of taste for greasy foods. If the pathogenic heat in the liver and gallbladder disrupts the interior, there will be vexation and insomnia, even mania and restlessness, or fever and feverish sensations in the chest, palms, and soles.

Treatment method

Clearing and resolving liver–gallbladder damp–heat.

Formula and ingredients: *Lóng Dǎn Xiè Gān Tāng* (*Gentian Liver-Draining Decoction*)

Wine-fried *lóng dǎn cǎo* (Radix et Rhizoma Gentianae) 6 g; dry-fried *huáng qín* (Radix Scutellariae) 9 g; wine-fried *zhī zǐ* (Fructus Gardeniae) 9 g; *zé xiè* (Rhizoma Alismatis) 12 g; *chuān mù tōng* (Caulis Clematidis Armandii) 6 g; dry-fried *chē qián zǐ* (Semen Plantaginis) wrapped 9 g; wine-washed *dāng guī* (Radix Angelicae Sinensis) 3 g; wine-fried *shēng dì* (Radix Rehmanniae) 6 g; *chái hú* (Radix Bupleuri) 6 g; *gān cǎo* (Radix et Rhizoma Glycyrrhizae) 3 g.

Formula verse

Lóng Dǎn Xiè Gān uses *zhī qín chái*, together with *chē qián shēng dì* and *zé xiè*; also *mù tōng gān cǎo* and *dāng guī*, effective for clearing liver–gallbladder damp–heat.

Usage

Add water to decoct or prepare into pills, termed *Lóng Dǎn Xiè Gān Wán* (Gentian Liver-Draining Pill) for oral intake 3–6 g each time, 2–3 times a day.

Analysis

This formula not only clears and reduces liver–gallbladder damp–heat, but also clears fire–heat pathogens. *Lóng dǎn cǎo* is bitter and cold and can purge fire and dry dampness, being the chief ingredient. *Zhī zǐ* and *huáng qín*, which are also cold and bitter, are added to assist *lóng dǎn cǎo* to clear heat and dry dampness. As these ingredients are all bitter and cold, this formula has the effect of clearing heat and removing toxins. *Chē qián zǐ*, *zé xiè*, and *chuān mù tōng* are bland and can percolate and drain dampness through urination and pave a way for the external drainage of the fire–heat pathogen. They can also be added for treating the up-flaming of liver–gallbladder fire. Extremely bitter and cold medicinals easily induce dryness and impair yin, and those that are dampness-percolating and urination-promoting also can impair yin, thus *shēng dì* and *dāng guī* are used to nourish yin and ensure that this formula dispel pathogens without impairing healthy qi. The damp–heat pathogen in the liver and gallbladder channels inevitably influences qi movement and in turn, qi stagnation makes it more difficult to expel the damp–heat pathogen. Therefore, *chái hú* is added to soothe liver and gallbladder qi. *Gān cǎo* harmonizes the actions of all medicinals and also clears heat and removes toxins. Many ingredients of this formula are prepared by wine, the purpose of which is to avoid extreme coldness that checks spleen and stomach qi, and to guide its medicinal efficacy upward. In summary, this formula is mainly used to clear heat by dispelling pathogens with the supplementary boosting of healthy qi, and promoting urination with the nourishment of yin.

This formula has many antibacterial and anti-inflammatory properties, especially in treating acute inflammation. It also can induce urination, promote gallbladder functions, and arrest pain. *Lóng dǎn cǎo* calms the mind and has anti-inflammatory effects. It can also relieve fever. *Zhī zǐ* inhibits bacteria, calms the mind, relieves pain, relax spasms, promotes gallbladder functions, and lowers blood pressure. The effects of *huáng qín*, *chái hú*, and *dāng guī* have been introduced in previous sections. Thus, the efficacy of this formula not only lies in inhibiting bacteria and relieving inflammation, but also in regulating immunity.

Treatment reference

The manifestations of the pattern of damp–heat in the liver and gallbladder are very complex, and the indications of *Lóng Dǎn Xiè Gān Tāng* are fairly broad. It is estimated that there are more than 60 of them, including externally contracted febrile diseases, diseases of internal damage, external medicine, gynecology, pediatrics, ENT, dermatology, etc. This formula is applicable to the following diseases presenting damp–heat and fire–heat in the liver and gallbladder: acute and chronic hepatitis, acute and chronic cholecystitis, pneumonia, pleuritis, cystitis, acute pyelonephritis, acute and chronic testitis, adnexitis, vaginitis, perineum abscess, acute tympanitis, acute conjunctivitis, ear furuncle, leg erysipelas, herpes zoster, acute appendicitis, hypertension, acute nephritis, schizophrenia, nervous prostration, prosopalgia, nervous headaches, Cushing syndrome, eczema, allergic dermatitis, and functional uterine bleeding.

In practice, proper modification is required. For headaches and dizziness due to the up-flaming of liver fire, add *jú huā*, *shí jué míng*, and *líng yáng jiǎo*. For hematemesis and hemoptysis due to liver–gallbladder heat invading the stomach or lung, add *cè bǎi yè*, *ǒu jié*, and *bái jí*. For numerous exudates at lesions due to damp–heat pouring downward with excessive dampness, add *cāng zhú* and *kǔ shēn*. For diseases caused by damp–heat pouring downward presenting flaccid legs, red ankle and knee swelling and pain, leg erythema nodosum, red genital or anal swelling and pain, or itching with exudates, *Sān Miào Sǎn* (Wonderfully Effective Three Powder) is also an option. If constipation occurs due to the liver fire flaming upward which prevents the purgation of fire–heat outward, use *Dāng Guī Lóng Huì Wán* (Chinese Angelica, Gentian, and Aloe Pill), which has a more potent effect in purging fire.

Cautions

Although *Lóng Dǎn Xiè Gān Tāng* has healthy qi-boosting ingredients, it is an extremely bitter and cold formula, which tends to impair the spleen and stomach. Therefore, patients of spleen–stomach weakness should take it with caution with reduced dosages. *Mù tōng* used in the formula is faced with controversy in the market, so it is sometimes replaced by *mǎ dōu líng* (Fructus Aristolochiae); the same also applies to *guān mù tōng* (Caulis Aristolochiae Manshuriensis), which can cause poisoning. This formula is not intended to be taken for a long period of time or in large doses, lest the spleen and stomach be impaired. Do not consume greasy, raw, and cold food in the duration of taking this decoction.

Daily Exercises

1. What are the clinical features of the liver–gallbladder damp–heat pattern?
2. What are the ingredients of *Lóng Dǎn Xiè Gān Tāng*?

3. Ms. Su is a 23-year-old woman. She often experiences hemilateral headaches, vexation, agitation, a bitter taste in the mouth, and chest and rib-side fullness and oppression. This morning, she suddenly had blurred vision, an aggravated headache which is especially acute in the upper left region of her head, brown, inhibited, and painful urination, a red tongue with a thin yellow and greasy coating, and a wiry, slippery, and rapid pulse. Her blood pressure is recorded as 190/120 mmHg. Please prescribe a Chinese medicinal formula for this case.

Additional Formulae

Sān Miào Săn (Wonderfully Effective Three Powder)

Wine-fried *huáng băi* (Cortex Phellodendri Chinensis) 120 g; *cāng zhú* (Rhizoma Atractylodis) soaked in rice-washed water and then dried 180 g; *chuān niú xī* (Radix Cyathulae) 60 g. Grind into a fine powder and mix with flour and water to make into pills. It is indicated for oral intake with ginger and salty soup, 6–9 g each time.

Actions

Clearing heat and drying dampness.

Indications

Damp–heat pouring downward presenting leg numbness or with a burning sensation, red ankle and knee swellings and burning pain, leg weakness, eczema, scant and brown urine, and a yellow and greasy tongue coating.

Dāng Guī Lóng Huì Wán (Chinese Angelica, Gentian, and Aloe Pill)

Dāng guī (Radix Angelicae Sinensis) 30 g; *lóng dăn căo* (Radix et Rhizoma Gentianae) 15 g; *zhī zǐ* (Fructus Gardeniae) 30 g; *huáng lián* (Rhizoma Coptidis) 30 g; *huáng băi* (Cortex Phellodendri Chinensis) 30 g; *huáng qín* (Radix Scutellariae) 30 g; *dà huáng* (Radix et Rhizoma Rhei) 15 g; *lú huì* (Aloe) 15 g; *qīng dài* (Indigo Naturalis) 15 g; *mù xiāng*

(Radix Aucklandiae) 5 g; *shè xiāng* (Moschus) 1.5 g. The ingredients are ground into powder and made into water pills. Take 6 g orally each time with warm water, 2 times a day.

Actions

Clearing heat and purging the liver; relaxing bowels and dispelling stagnation.

Indications

Excess fire in the liver and gallbladder pattern presenting headaches, dizziness, vexation, restlessness, mania or delirium, constipation, inhibited urination, and brown urine.

CHAPTER 7

The Phlegm–Rheum
and Water–Dampness Pattern

DAY SIX

This is a disease pattern displaying various manifestations caused by pathological products such as phlegm–rheum and water–dampness in the body. This pattern can be seen either in externally contracted diseases or in diseases of internal damage. Patterns of exterior dampness, phlegm–heat in the *shaoyang*, *shaoyang* water retention, intestinal damp–heat, middle *jiao* damp–heat, and damp–heat in the liver and gallbladder (Chapter 6) are all in relation to phlegm–rheum and water pathogens. In this section, it mainly discusses phlegm–rheum and water–dampness patterns due to functional disorder of water transportation and transformation.

Features of the Phlegm–Rheum and Water–Dampness Pattern

The diagnosis is mainly based on its clinical manifestations. However, these manifestations are so complicated and various that it is challenging to outline common features. Some diseases have evident characteristics, such as spitting of sputum, vomiting of loose drool, a water-shaking sensation in the stomach, the gurgling sound of water in the intestines, pleural effusion, ascites, and edema, which are all visible indications of phlegm–rheum and water–dampness. In such a case, diagnosis is not difficult. On the other hand, there are other diseases that do not present the above manifestations, but they are still diagnosed as a type of phlegm–rheum and water–dampness pattern. For example, headaches, dizziness, palpitations, and vomiting are common symptoms in the phlegm–rheum pattern; dizziness, head heaviness, chest oppression, coughing, and panting often reflect the accumulation of damp–turbidity in the upper body; stomach distention and fullness, nausea, vomiting, and a sticky feeling or a sweet taste in the mouth indicate damp–turbidity buildup in the middle part of the body; loose stool, turbid urine, leg edema, and profuse leukorrhea in women show damp–turbidity accumulating in the lower body. It is a quite difficult to diagnose the existence of phlegm–rheum and water–dampness solely by the above symptoms, thus the tongue and pulse conditions should be combined in analysis. The patient of the phlegm–rheum and water–dampness pattern usually shows a greasy and turbid or slippery tongue coating with lots of fluids, and a slippery or wiry or soggy and soft pulse.

Therefore, the phlegm–rheum and water–dampness pattern involves many diseases, such as chronic gastritis, gastroptosis, chronic enteritis, chronic hepatitis, hypertension, hyperlipemia, vertigo, neurosis, neurosis, pleuritis, chronic peritonitis, chirrhosis ascites, chronic nephritis, heart disease, chronic adnexitis, and chronic bronchitis.

Formation and Manifestations of the Phlegm–Rheum and Water–Dampness Pattern

Phlegm–rheum

Phlegm–rheum is a product of disorders of fluid metabolism and once it is synthesized, it inevitably adopts the role of a novel pathological factor. In Chinese medicine, the distribution of phlegm–rheum is widespread and can occur at various *zang–fu* organs and tissues. Phlegm and rheum are similar, but the latter, which is also called water retention, is loose and accumulates in the stomach, intestines, chest, rib sides, and abdomen to become stagnated stomach fluids, pleural effusion, and ascites. Phlegm is sticky and usually exists in a fixed form and manifestation, and apart from the sputum expectorated from the lung, it can remain in the *zang–fu* organs, tendons, bones, and skin, e.g., clouding the heart (which causes coma), disrupting the liver with wind (which causes dizziness, numbness, and cramps), obstructing the channels and collaterals (which causes spasms and paralysis), accumulating in the skin (which causes masses), and stagnating in the joints (which causes joint swelling, ankylosis, or deformation). Phlegm–rheum is commonly regarded as a tangible pathogen, although it is not in some cases, such as dizziness and limb numbness.

Water–dampness

Dampness is one of the six pathogenic factors that pertain to external dampness. If disorders of the spleen and stomach result in the failure of food transportation and conversion, it will also lead to water–dampness retention, which is a type of internal dampness. The pathological features of internal dampness are similar those of external dampness, which include heaviness, stickiness, difficulty in relief, or swollen limbs and exudates. Internal dampness can be caused either by abnormal functions in the transportation and transformation by the spleen and stomach after the invasion of external dampness, or by spleen–stomach weakness and hypofunction of the distribution of water affected by other *zang–fu* disorders. Moreover, when there is the presence of internal dampness, the patient will be more vulnerable to external dampness. It demonstrates the close relationship between the pathomechanism and pathological changes of internal dampness and external dampness.

Categories of the Phlegm–Rheum and Water–Dampness Pattern

The phlegm–rheum and water–dampness pattern is further categorized according to different natures and locations, such as phlegm–dampness clouding the heart, phlegm–heat obstructing the pericardium, phlegm–dampness obstructing the lung, phlegm–heat accumulation in the lung, dampness encumbering the spleen and stomach, heat–dampness accumulation in the middle, dysfunction of the kidney with excessive water, phlegm–rheum obstructing the stomach, water accumulation in the bladder, wind–phlegm entering the collaterals, water retention in the ribsides, water retention in the abdomen, excessive water in the skin, and phlegm accumulation under the skin.

In this chapter, the diagnosis and treatment of the following patterns will be discussed: water amassment syndrome, the phlegm–rheum pattern, yang deficiency and water diffusion, dampness encumbering the spleen and stomach, the phlegm–damp pattern, phlegm–heat affecting the interior, wind–phlegm affecting the upper body, and water (fluid) retention.

Treatment Methods of the Phlegm–Rheum and Water–Dampness Pattern

The key methods for treating the phlegm–rheum and water–dampness pattern are dispelling phlegm, expelling water retention, promoting urination, and resolving dampness, which pertain to the methods of dispersion and purgation. The goal is to clear pathogens of phlegm and water retention. Only when the pathological products have been eliminated, the diseases can then be rectified. Medicinals whose functions encompass removing phlegm–rheum and water–dampness by promoting urination, relaxing bowels, or restoring normal transportation and conversion functions of the spleen and stomach are frequently applied. In addition to dispelling pathogens, it is also important to correct and restore *zang–fu* functions affected by phlegm–rheum and water–dampness.

As there are many sub-types of the phlegm–rheum and water–dampness pattern, the specific treatment methods are different. In this section, we will review the methods of unblocking yang to promote urination, warming and removing phlegm–rheum, warming yang to transform water, fortifying the spleen to resolving dampness, drying dampness to dispel phlegm, clearing and dissolving phlegm–heat, dispelling wind and dissolving phlegm, and expelling water by purgation. It should be noted that the induction of urination by percolating bland herbs is usually effected in each method; it can be said that "the only correct treatment for dampness is to promote urination."

For the treatment of the phlegm–rheum and water retention pattern, qi must be regulated in a healthy state to avoid impairment in the course of expelling pathogens. Meanwhile, it is also beneficial to restore the normal functions of the spleen and stomach to boost yang qi. Focus should also be given to the existence of other pathological products, such as qi stagnation, blood stasis, and pathogenic heat. Therefore, the management of this pattern is also combined with methods of boosting the spleen, benefiting qi, warming yang, rectifying qi, dissolving stasis, and clearing heat. As the medicinals and formulae for treating phlegm–rheum and water retention are often acrid, aromatic, warm, dry, sweet, or bland, which tend to consume yin and fluids, they should be applied with caution to patients with yin deficiency and a weak physique, and also pregnant women.

Daily Exercises

1. Where do the phlegm–rheum and water–dampness originate from?
2. What are the diagnostic criteria of the phlegm–rheum and water–dampness pattern?
3. What are the treatment principles for phlegm–rheum and water retention pattern? What aspects should be noted?

THE 6TH WEEK

DAY ONE

Water Amassment Syndrome

This syndrome is caused by pathogenic factors entering the bladder, resulting in the failure of the bladder to transform qi, leading to water retention in the interior. As water is usually accumulated in the bladder, it is also called bladder water amassment syndrome. However, the disease location can also involve other regions in the body. It is commonly seen in edema, urine retention, and acute gastroenteritis caused by acute and chronic nephritis.

Diagnosis

The main symptoms and signs are thirst with a compulsion for drinking or vomiting immediately after drinking water, inhibited urination, and edema. Other indications include fever, an aversion to wind and cold, headaches, vertigo, distention and fullness in the lower abdomen, diarrhea, a white tongue coating, and a floating pulse.

Since the bladder's function on qi transformation is affected by pathogenic factors, water distribution and discharge becomes erratic and a series of symptoms is resulted. If water retention prevents fluids from reaching the mouth, it will lead to thirst. However, as the body does not actually lack fluids, water taken in is usually regurgitated. Internal water retention in the bladder causes inhibited urination and abdominal distention and fullness. Excessive water in the body surface leads to edema. The "flooding" of water in the large intestine contributes to diarrhea. If water retention flows upward (which is in a reverse direction) or blocks clear yang qi, headaches and vertigo are resulted. If the exterior pattern still exists, it will be accompanied by fever and an aversion to wind and cold. If the exterior pattern has been relieved but pathogens are transmitted internally with exuberant heat as well as water, fever or high fever may also be present. Hence, the sub-patterns described in this chapter can either be of the interior pattern, or patterns involving both the exterior and interior.

Treatment method

Draining dampness and dispelling dampness; warming and blocking yang qi.

Formula and ingredients: Wŭ Líng Săn (Five Substances Powder with Poria)

Skinless *zhū líng* (Polyporus) 9 g; *zé xiè* (Rhizoma Alismatis) 12 g; *fú líng* (Poria) 9 g; *bái zhú* (Rhizoma Atractylodis Macrocephalae) 9 g; skinless *guì zhī* (Ramulus Cinnamomi) 5 g.

Formula verse

Wŭ Líng Săn uses *guì zhī*, together with *zé xiè, zhū ling, and bái zhú.* Originally for water amassment in the bladder, it also treats spleen impairment and dampness retention.

Usage

The above five ingredients are to be pounded into powder and taken orally 3 g each time with water, 3 times a day. Also drink sufficient hot water to induce sweating. Alternatively, decoct the above ingredients in water. They can also be made into pills for oral intake with water, 4–6 g each time. The ingredients can also be wrapped in gauze, 9–15 g for decoction in water.

Analysis

In this formula, the dose of the chief medicinal, *zé xiè*, is the highest, as its sweet and bland nature with its urine-promoting function can reduce internal water amassment. *Zhū líng* and *fú líng*, which are both sweet, bland, and dampness-percolating, are combined to strengthen the potency of eliminating water–dampness. *Bái zhú* is bitter, warm, and dry, and can either dry dampness or strengthen the spleen's functions so as to expel water–dampness. *Guì zhī* works in two aspects: its acrid and warm natures are beneficial in warming and unblocking yang qi, hence when yang qi is distributed normally, water–dampness can be easily transformed; and its exterior-relieving function can be helpful in dispersing retained external pathogens on the body surface. Therefore, regardless of the existence of the exterior pattern, *guì zhī* should be added. As for effectiveness, this formula mainly promotes urination through its bland nature and concurrently, it also focuses on strengthening the spleen to convert dampness and warming and unblocking yang qi, so internal water amassment can be eliminated.

Wǔ Líng Sǎn, to a certain extent, can regulate the metabolism of water, electrolytes, fats, sugar, and proteins, and is particularly significant in promoting urination. It has preventive and curative properties on acute or chronic alcoholism. Each ingredient in this formula can stimulate urination. Furthermore, *zhū líng*, *bái zhú*, and *fú líng* can fortify immunity, protect the liver, relax smooth muscles, and bring down blood cholesterol levels. *Guì zhī* and *zhū líng* can also inhibit bacteria. *Guì zhī* dilates blood vessels, improves blood circulation of organs, and disperses heat by promoting sweating. This formula thus has multiple complex pharmacological functions aside from promoting urination.

Treatment reference

Wǔ Líng Sǎn is a classic formula for treating internal water retention and enjoys a broad spectrum of application. It can be used for diseases of many systems, such as the urinary, digestive, nervous, and endocrine systems. Specifically, these include acute nephritis, chronic nephritis, urinary stones, pyelonephritis, cystitis, urethritis, urine retention after an operation or during pregnancy, acute gastroenteritis, acute infectious hepatitis, ascites due to cirrhosis, nervous headaches, Meniere's syndrome, prosopalgia, encephaledema, hydrocephalus, and so on. Moreover, it is applicable to skin diseases like eczema and herpes zoster. Generally, referential symptoms of this formula are inhibited urination, edema, vomiting, diarrhea, dizziness, and skin exudates. With respect to application, it demonstrates some form of regulation of body functions. For instance, it can treat diarrhea and is also able to relieve severe constipation. It cures thirst and inhibited urination, and also diabetic insipidus with profuse urine. These indicate *Wǔ Líng Sǎn* can restore the normal state of the body by rectifying disorders of the body.

In practice, proper modification is required. If edema is serious, add *chē qián zǐ*, *dōng guā pí*, *dà fù pí*, *shēng jiāng pí*, and so on. If water amassment syndrome is complicated by yin deficiency and heat, remove *guì zhī* and *bái zhú* from this formula, and add *huá shí* and *ē jiāo*, becoming *Zhū*

Líng Tāng (Polyporus Decoction). If dizziness and vomiting are present, add *yù jīn*, *gōu téng*, and *shí jué míng*. If difficult and painful urination, thirst, vexation, back soreness, a red tongue, and a rapid pulse, which indicates the internal accumulation of damp–heat in both the affected spleen and kidney, are observed, add *shēng dì*, *shú dì huáng, zhī mǔ*, and *huáng bǎi*. If it is accompanied by inhibited urination and qi deficiency, add *rén shēn*, becoming *Chūn Zé Tāng* (Spring Lustrous Decoction).

Cautions

Wǔ Líng Sǎn is applied to promote urination and expel dampness. Improper use may impair fluids of the human body. Due to this reason, it should not be taken for a long period of time, especially for patients with yin deficiency. In addition, water amassment syndrome treated by this formula should not display any signs of attacks by heat pathogens; otherwise, it should be treated by clearing damp–heat instead of prescribing acrid and warm ingredients such as *guì zhī*.

Daily Exercises

1. What are the key points of pattern differentiation of water amassment syndrome?
2. What are the ingredients of *Wǔ Líng Sǎn*?
3. Ms. Chen is a 7-year-old girl. She suffered from facial and lower limb edema 2 years ago. The edema remitted for some time after treatment, but has since relapsed. In the recent weeks, the edema has been aggravated, accompanied by an aversion to cold, low fever in the afternoon, thirst without any desire to drink, dark and scant urine, abdominal fullness, a white and slightly greasy tongue coating, and a floating and rapid pulse. Please prescribe a Chinese medicinal formula for this case.

Additional Formulae

Zhū Líng Tāng (*Polyporus Decoction*)

Skinless *zhū líng* (Polyporus); *zé xiè* (Rhizoma Alismatis); *fú líng* (Poria); crushed *huá shí* (Talcum); *ē jiāo* (Colla Corii Asini); 9 g each. Decoct the above ingredients in water. For *ē jiāo*, melt it in the decoction for oral consumption.

Actions

Promoting urination and percolating dampness; clearing heat and nourishing yin.

Indications

Inhibited urination, fever, thirst with a desire to drink, nausea, vomiting, dysentery, bloody urine, heat strangury, and difficult and painful urination.

Chūn Zé Tāng (Spring Lustrous Decoction)

Ingredients of *Wǔ Líng Sǎn* together with *rén shēn* (Radix et Rhizoma Ginseng). Decoct in water for oral consumption.

Actions

Boosting qi and promoting urination.

Indications

Internal retention of qi deficiency and water–dampness presenting fatigue, thirst, and inhibited urination.

DAY TWO

The Phlegm–Rheum Pattern

The phlegm–rheum pattern is indicated by the internal retention of phlegm–rheum due to yang qi deficiency in the middle *jiao* and the spleen failing to convert and transport fluids. The site of retention of phlegm–rheum for this pattern is mainly in the middle *jiao*, and naturally, phlegm–rheum that particular region will influence the functions of other organs as well. This pattern is commonly seen in bronchitis, vertigo syndrome, chronic gastritis, and some cardiovascular and related diseases.

Diagnosis

The main symptoms and signs of this pattern are distention in the chest, rib sides, and stomach, dizziness, vomiting of lucid fluids and phlegm–drool, and a white and slippery tongue coating. Other indications include adverse qi rising from the stomach to the chest, dizziness after standing up, palpitations, coughing, panting, a fear of cold in the back, a wiry and slippery or deep and tight pulse.

As the phlegm–rheum resides in the middle *jiao*, qi movement will definitely be affected. Together with phlegm–rheum as a substantial pathogen, distention and fullness may be observed in the chest, rib sides, and stomach, and also a barrel chest caused by emphysema. Phlegm–rheum in the middle *jiao* can prevent clear yang from ascending and results in vertigo and blurred vision. It also causes antagonistic rising of stomach qi, so lucid fluids and phlegm–drool may be vomited. Phlegm–rheum attacking the heart in an upward direction causes the heart spirit to be disrupted, thus resulting in palpitations. If the lung's function on diffusing and descending is influenced, coughing and panting will occur. Phlegm–rheum in the middle *jiao* also affects the distribution of yang qi, which leads to a fear of feeling cold in the back. A tongue with a white and slippery coating and a wiry and slippery or deep and tight pulse are signs of latent phlegm–rheum.

Dizziness occurring in this pattern is different from common vertigo and head heaviness, which is usually manifested as swirling vision, and difficulty in opening the eyes, with obvious nausea or vomiting (commonly seen in hypertension), edema in the inner ear, and even brain concussions. Coughing and panting are often accompanied by the massive production of white, foamy, and sticky sputum, which is prevalent in chronic bronchitis. Vomiting of lucid fluids and phlegm–drool may be accompanied by a sensation of water wobbling in the stomach, which may be audible.

As there are various reasons accounting for distention in the chest, rib-sides, and stomach, dizziness, vomiting, and coughing and panting, other causes must be excluded for the diagnosis of phlegm–rheum retention in the middle *jiao*. For diagnosis, pay attention to the condition of the tongue coating, the symptoms of middle yang deficiency, the abnormal functions of the spleen, and the features of the phlegm–rheum.

Treatment method

Boosting the spleen to percolate dampness and transforming phlegm–rheum by warming.

Formula and ingredients: Líng Guì Zhú Gān Tāng (Poria, Cinnamon Twig, Atractylodes Macrocephala, and Licorice Decoction)

Fú líng (Poria) 12 g; *bái zhú* (Rhizoma Atractylodis Macrocephalae) 6 g; skinless *guì zhī* (Ramulus Cinnamomi) 9 g, dry-fried *gān cǎo* (Radix et Rhizoma Glycyrrhizae) 6 g.

Formula verse

Líng Guì Zhú Gān treats fluid retention, especially for transforming phlegm–rheum by warming.

Usage

Add 1.2 L of water to decoct until 600 mL are left. Remove the dregs and take the decoction warm, 200 mL each time, 3 times a day.

Analysis

Líng Guì Zhú Gān Tāng is an important formula for transforming phlegm–rheum in the middle *jiao* by warming. In this formula, *fú líng* fortifies the spleen to assist transportation, percolates dampness, and promotes urination, being the chief ingredient. *Guì zhī* is added to unblock yang qi by warming, and thus aid the transportation and transformation of water–dampness. *Bái zhú* strengthens the spleen and dries dampness. *Zhì gān cǎo* is applied to fortify the spleen and boost qi for the restoration of spleen's transportation function, and it also harmonizes the actions of all medicinals. In terms of formula composition, it is similar to that of *Wǔ Líng Sǎn* (Five Substances Powder with Poria), but *Wǔ Líng Sǎn* is used for water retention in the lower *jiao* with bland ingredients percolating dampness and promoting urination in large doses, i.e., a large dose of *zé xiè* together with *zhū líng* to discharge fluids in the lower *jiao* through urination, while this formula is for middle yang deficiency and water retention in the middle *jiao* with spleen-fortifying and qi-boosting *zhì gān cǎo* instead of *zé xiè* and *zhū líng*.

In summary, *Líng Guì Zhú Gān Tāng* boosts the stomach, promotes urination, calms the mind, relieves pain, and strengthens the heart. The pharmacological functions of main ingredients have been discussed in previous sections.

Treatment reference

Líng Guì Zhú Gān Tāng is widely prescribed in the clinic, for example for illnesses such as dizziness due to Meniere's syndrome, hypertension and cerebral concussion, edema and hydropericardium caused by chronic bronchitis, asthma, heart failure, and nephritis. This formula is also applicable to arthritis due to the contraction of wind–dampness with yang qi deficiency, low fever and sweating due to yang deficiency, insipidus, and neurogenic thirst. Clinically, as long as the states of yang qi deficiency, the abnormal transportation function of the spleen, and internal retention of phlegm–rheum are thoroughly defined, this formula can be used accordingly.

If the vomited lucid fluids and phlegm–drool are in massive amounts, add *fǎ bàn xià* and *chén pí*. If dizziness is serious, add *tiān má*, *fǎ bàn xià*, and *zé xiè*. If coughing and panting are severe, add dry-fried *má huáng*, *fǎ bàn xià*, *chén pí*, and *bái guǒ*. If spleen function is highly irregular, add *dǎng shēn*. If cutaneous edema is present, add *chē qián zǐ*, *zé xiè*, and *dōng guā pí*. If arthralgia is observed, add *wū shāo shé*, *wēi líng xiān*, and *qiāng huó*. If *guì zhī* is removed from this formula and *gān jiāng* is added, it is termed *Shèn Zhuó Tāng* (Kidney Fixity Decoction), which is strong in warming the spleen and transforming dampness.

Cautions

This formula is warm in nature, so it is not suitable for patients affected by heat pathogens or having a physique of yin deficiency. Although this formula is spleen-boosting, it is primary indicated for eliminating water retention. Therefore, it is not prescribed for dizziness and edema caused by dysfunction of the liver and kidney and qi and blood deficiencies, as well as coughing and panting due to wind–cold, phlegm–heat, and lung dysfunction.

Daily Exercises

1. What are the definitions of phlegm–rheum and the phlegm–rheum pattern? What are the clinical features of the phlegm–rheum pattern?
2. What are the actions and indications of *Líng Guì Zhú Gān Tāng*?
3. Mr. Huang is a 67-year-old male. He is afflicted with hypertension and in recent years, he has been suffering from palpitations and shortness of breath, especially after exertion. He often coughs up white and foamy sputum, with edema in the lower limbs, occasional dizziness, chest and stomach stuffiness, an absence of thirst, a white and slippery tongue coating, and a wiry and slippery pulse. Please prescribe a Chinese medicinal formula for this case.

Additional Formulae

*Shèn Zhuó Tāng (**Kidney Fixity Decoction**)*

Fú líng (Poria) 12 g; *bái zhú* (Rhizoma Atractylodis Macrocephalae) 6 g; *gān cǎo* (Radix et Rhizoma Glycyrrhizae) 6 g; *gān jiāng* (Rhizoma Zingiberis) 12 g. Add water to decoct.

Actions

Warming the spleen and overcoming dampness.

Indications

Downward attack of cold dampness, body heaviness, cold pain below the lumbar region, normal appetite, an absence of thirst, and normal urination.

DAY THREE

The Yang Deficiency and Water Diffusion Pattern

The yang deficiency and water diffusion pattern is a syndrome arising from the failure of spleen and kidney yang qi to warm and transform water–dampness or spleen–kidney dysfunction caused by chronic water (fluid) retention. Edema occurring in this pattern may involve all parts of the body, but the key disease locations are the spleen and kidney. It is a pattern encompassing a deficiency–excess complex with yang deficiency and deficiency–cold in the interior, as well as the retention of water–dampness. This pattern is commonly seen in chronic nephritis, nephrotic syndrome, cardiac edema, edema due to chronic hepatitis or ascites, and various endocrine diseases.

Diagnosis

The main symptoms and signs of this pattern are inhibited urination, edema in the limbs, an absence of thirst, a white and slippery tongue coating, and a deep and thin pulse. Other indications include heaviness and aches in the four extremities, abdominal pain, diarrhea, palpitations, dizziness, muscular throbbing or trembling, instability when standing, vomiting, a fear of cold, and cold limbs.

The absorption, distribution, and discharge of body fluids are connected to multiple organs in the body, among which the spleen's transportation function and kidney's opening and closing function are the most vital, especially in the context of the functions of yang qi. Spleen yang and kidney yang supplement each other, so chronic spleen yang deficiency can lead to kidney yang deficiency, while kidney yang insufficiency in turn causes spleen yang deficiency. Hence, it is not particularly difficult to understand the source of the yang deficiency and water diffusion pattern and the etiology of its various symptoms. As the spleen and kidney are both in dysfunction, water is unable to be discharged outward, manifesting as inhibited urination and edema in the limbs. The internal retention of water–dampness contributes to the absence of thirst, a white and slippery tongue coating, and a deep and thin pulse. Water–dampness that overflows in the muscles and skin results in heaviness and aches of the four limbs, or even edema. The ascending counterflow of water triggers dizziness and vomiting, and if it attacks the heart, there will be palpitations. Failure of water transportation due to spleen dysfunction is manifested as abdominal pain and diarrhea.

The essence of this pattern can be regarded as an interior cold pattern, because the main patho-mechanism lies in spleen–kidney yang deficiency, while water–dampness in the interior is only a secondary cause. Fear of cold and cold limbs are manifestations of deficiency–cold. Yang qi failing to warm channels manifests as muscular throbbing or trembling, instability in standing, vomiting, a fear of cold, cold limbs, and so on.

Treatment method

Warming yang and promoting urination.

Formula and ingredients: Zhēn Wǔ Tāng (True Warrior Decoction)

Fú líng (Poria) 9 g; sháo yào (Radix Paeoniae) 9 g; shēng jiāng (Rhizoma Zingiberis Recens) sliced 9 g; bái zhú (Rhizoma Atractylodis Macrocephalae) 6 g; cooked fù zǐ (Radix Aconiti Lateralis Praeparata) crushed and skinless 9 g.

Formula verse

Zhēn Wǔ Tāng strengthens kidney yang, and uses líng sháo zhú fù and shēng jiāng. It is applicable to abdominal pain of shaoyin and accumulation of cold water, and also palpitations, dizziness, vomiting, and diarrhea.

Usage

Add 1.4 L of water to decoct until 600 mL are left. Remove the dregs and take 150 mL warm each time, 3–4 times a day.

Analysis

Fù zǐ is the chief ingredient in Zhēn Wǔ Tāng; it is used to warm and supplement kidney yang and spleen yang and assist in the transportation and transformation of water–dampness. Bái zhú and fú líng are combined to strengthen the spleen, transport dampness, and percolate water. The collective effect of bái zhú and fù zǐ is to boost the spleen and kidney, dispel interior cold, warm channels, remove dampness, and relieve pain. Shēng jiāng aids fù zǐ to warm yang and dispel cold, and supports fú líng and bái zhú to disperse water. Sháo yào is the supplementary ingredient that promotes urination, relieves cramps and pain, harmonizes blood, and supplements yin; it alleviates the acrid and dry natures of *shēng jiāng* and *fù zǐ* without impairing yin. All in all, this formula warms the spleen and kidney, promotes transportation and transformation, and transforms water–dampness.

Fú líng, *bái zhú*, and *fù zǐ* have been proven to induce urination. In addition, *fù zǐ* strengthens the heart, increases blood pressure, and relieves pain. *Sháo yào* calms the mind, relieves pain, alleviates spasms of smooth muscles, promotes urination, inhibits bacteria, and reduces sweating. The combination of *fù zǐ* and *sháo yào* can enhance the effect of relieving pain and calming the mind, so it is often applied to treat pain of the four limbs caused by deficiency–cold abdominal pain and pathogens of wind, cold, and dampness.

Treatment reference

Zhēn Wǔ Tāng is indicated for many diseases in clinical practice. The most common disorders are the various kinds of edema, regardless of source, which can be from the heart, the kidney, the liver, nutrition, endocrine secretion, and pregnancy, but only if there are symptoms of spleen–kidney yang deficiency. However, its action is not only limited to promoting urination, but also has been demonstrated to strengthen the heart, fortify the kidney, protect the liver, and rectify endocrine secretion. It is also applicable to hypertension, in which it can lower blood pressure levels, especially if complicated with heart failure or irregular heartbeats. This formula is also used for treating many digestive diseases, such as gastritis, gastroptosis, gastric or duodenal ulcers, chronic enteritis, and chronic abdominal pain. This formula exerts bidirectional effects on treating gastroenteral diseases, either chronic diarrhea or constipation caused by spleen–kidney yang deficiency. In addition, it is also prescribed for chronic nephritis, chronic bronchitis, emphysema, Meniere's syndrome, functional disorder of autonomic nerves, and various kinds of arthritis. If this formula is applied according to the internal exuberance of deficiency–cold, manifesting as a pale complexion, a fear of cold, cold limbs, severe edema in the lower limbs, diarrhea with undigested food in the stool, and cold abdominal pain, its main difference from the indications of *Lǐ Zhōng Wán* (Center-Regulating Pill) and *Sì Nì Tāng* (Frigid Extremities Decoction) lies in the internal over-flowing of water.

In practice, proper modification is required. If edema is severe and there is inhibited urination, add *chē qián zǐ*, *zé xiè*, and *dōng guā pí*. If it is accompanied with coughing, panting, and spitting and vomiting of lucid and loose phlegm–drool, add *wǔ wèi zǐ*, *xì xīn*, and *gān jiāng*. For serious spleen yang deficiency and diarrhea, remove *sháo yào* and add *gān jiāng*. For serious kidney yang deficiency, add *ròu guì*, *huáng qí*, and *shú dì huáng*. If the doses of *fù zǐ* and *bái zhú* are doubled, while *shēng jiāng* is removed from this formula and *rén shēn* is added, it becomes *Fù Zǐ Tāng* (Aconite Decoction), which can warm yang and expel cold dampness, which is mainly indicated for joint pain due to attacks of wind–cold in the interior.

Cautions

The yang deficiency and water diffusion pattern is usually chronic and cases may be critical, so it is encouraged to be alert when dealing with such a pattern. In addition, although this formula is applicable to feverish conditions, it must be ascertained that the disease is caused by yang qi deficiency or floating of yang qi. If it is an exterior heat pattern or an interior heat pattern, this formula should not be prescribed.

Daily Exercises

1. What are the clinical features of the yang deficiency and water diffusion pattern?
2. What are the ingredients of *Zhēn Wǔ Tāng*?
3. Mr. Yan is a 64-year-old male. He has had chronic bronchitis for more than a decade. In recent years, his coughing and panting are aggravated in winter and edema is seen in his face and four limbs, especially the lower extremities. This winter, the symptoms have worsened; he has developed a fear of cold and experiences a cold sensation and a feeling of heaviness in his four limbs. He is also unable to lie on his back due to coughing and panting and he lacks strength. Other symptoms include loose stool, dark purple lips, a dark red tongue with a greasy

and thin coating, and a deep, thin, and slippery pulse. Please prescribe a Chinese medicinal formula for this case.

Additional Formulae

Fù Zǐ Tāng (*Aconite Decoction*)

Blast-fried *fù zǐ* (Radix Aconiti Lateralis Praeparata) without skin 15 g; *fú líng* (Poria) 9 g; *sháo yào* (Radix Paeoniae) 9 g; *bái zhú* (Rhizoma Atractylodis Macrocephalae) 12 g; *rén shēn* (Radix et Rhizoma Ginseng) 6 g. Add water to decoct.

Actions

Warming channels and boosting yang, dispelling cold, and transforming dampness.

Indications

Yang qi deficiency and attacks of cold–dampness in the interior presenting joint pain, an aversion to cold, cold limbs, a tongue with a white and slippery coating, and a deep and thin pulse.

DAY FOUR

The Dampness Encumbering the Spleen and Stomach Pattern

The pattern of dampness encumbering the spleen and stomach refers to the spleen and stomach affected by the obstruction and attacks of damp–turbidity on the spleen and stomach, or simply, disorders of the spleen and stomach. It has been mentioned in previous chapters that pathogenic dampness can be classified under external dampness and internal dampness. This pattern may either exist in externally contracted diseases due to the attack of exterior dampness, or in diseases of internal damage mainly due to internal dampness. The following digestive diseases often present this pattern: acute and chronic gastroenteritis, intestinal typhoid, acute and chronic hepatitis, dysentery, gastric and duodenal ulcers, and gastric neurosis.

Diagnosis

The main symptoms and signs of this pattern are gastric and abdominal distention and fullness, nausea, loose stool, and a tongue with a greasy coating. Other indications include a lack of appetite, an absence of taste in the mouth, fatigue, lethargy, body heaviness, and a moderate pulse.

As the spleen and stomach are encumbered by damp–turbidity and qi movement is blocked, gastric and abdominal distention and fullness will be triggered. Pathogenic dampness can affect the functions of the spleen and stomach in raising the clear and directing turbidity downward, manifesting as nausea, loose stool, and a lack of appetite. The obstruction of the middle *jiao* by dampness prevents clear yang from being distributed throughout the whole body, leading to fatigue and lethargy, which is different from the fatigue and dispiritedness caused by general yang qi weakness. The greasy coating of the tongue is an important piece of evidence for the existence of internal dampness. The absence of taste in the mouth and a moderate pulse are crucial supplementary proofs in diagnosis.

This pattern is characterized by encumbered yang qi of the spleen and stomach and internal obstruction by damp–turbidity. If it is accompanied by manifestations of pathogenic heat, it pertains to the pattern of damp–heat accumulation in the middle. If there are obvious middle yang deficiency and internal obstruction of cold–dampness, then it belongs to the *taiyin* deficiency–cold pattern. These two other patterns mentioned are similar to this pattern; they must not be confused with one another.

Treatment method

Fortifying the spleen and removing dampness.

Formula and ingredients: Píng Wèi Săn (Stomach-Calming Powder)

Skinless *cāng zhú* (Rhizoma Atractylodis) soaked in rice-washed water for 2 days 250 g; skinless *hòu pò* (Cortex Magnoliae Officinalis) prepared by ginger juice and fried with aroma 156 g; *chén pí* (Pericarpium Citri Reticulatae) 156 g; dry-fried *gān căo* (Radix et Rhizoma Glycyrrhizae).

Formula verse

Píng Wèi Săn is made up of four ingredients, namely *pò chén pí*, *cāng zhú*, and *gān căo*. It functions to dry dampness and fortify the spleen, and also to disperse distention and fullness. It is especially effective for moving qi and harmonizing the stomach.

Usage

Grind ingredients into a fine powder and decoct 6–9 g each time in water with 2 pieces of ginger and 2 pieces of date. Remove the dregs and take the decoction warm. Alternatively, decoct in water with *cāng zhú* (Rhizoma Atractylodis) 10 g; *hòu pò* (Cortex Magnoliae Officinalis) 5 g; *chén pí* (Pericarpium Citri Reticulatae) 5 g; *gān căo* (Radix et Rhizoma Glycyrrhizae) 3 g; 2 pieces of ginger; and 2 pieces of jujubes. The ingredients can also be made into pills, to be taken 6 g each time, 2 times a day.

Analysis

Píng Wèi Săn is a typical formula prescribed for removing dampness from the spleen and kidney by drying, moving qi, and boosting the spleen. The bitter- and warm-natured *cāng zhú*, which is the chief ingredient, is used in a large dose to dry dampness and enhance the spleen in transporting and transforming water–dampness. The similarly bitter and warm *hòu pò* is added to rectify qi and distention, as well as to dry dampness and direct counterflow downward; *chén pí* is used to rectify qi and fortify the spleen; and *gān căo* and *dà zăo* are to restore the functions of transportation and transformation by regulating the spleen and stomach. Qi-moving medicinals are used in this formula because the dampness encumbering the interior inevitably inhibits the movement of qi and in turn, inhibited qi movement further affects the elimination of dampness. Therefore, the most appropriate way to move qi is to remove dampness.

　　Píng Wèi Săn has been shown to work effectively in restoring gastrointestinal functions. *Cāng zhú* fortifies the stomach, promotes urination, induces sweating, calms the mind, decreases blood sugar levels, and has other secondary properties. *Hòu pò* is able to strengthen the stomach, calm the mind, relieve pain, relax muscular stiffness, and also inhibit bacteria.

Chén pí works by fortifying the stomach, relieving vomiting, and expelling phlegm. *Gān cǎo* functions to relieve spasms, protect the stomach mucosal membrane, and regulate adrenocortical hormones. This formula not only boosts the stomach and aids in digestion, but also has wide pharmacological applications.

Treatment reference

Practically, *Píng Wèi Sǎn* can be applied to all the disease patterns caused by pathogenic dampness. Although the main disease location lies in the spleen and stomach, it is not limited to these. For example, many stomach diseases tend to present symptoms of dampness encumbering the middle *jiao*, such as chronic gastritis, gastroptosis, gastric neurosis, and stomach and duodenal ulcers. Hence, this formula is often adopted. In addition, this formula can often be applied to many non-digestive diseases, but only if there is a presence of pathogenic dampness. Such diseases include coronary disease, insomnia, chronic nephritis, scant menses, amenorrhea, infertility, and leukorrhea.

Clinically, *Píng Wèi Sǎn* is usually prescribed as a basic formula for removing dampness, which can be modified in application. For the dampness encumbering the spleen and stomach pattern with severe qi stagnation, add *mù xiāng* and *shā rén* to strengthen the force of moving qi. If it is with food stagnation, add dry-fried *shén qū*, *mài yá*, and scorch-fried *shān zhā*. If abdominal distention and constipation are present, add *bīng láng*, *lái fú zǐ*, and *zhǐ shí*. If fatigue, a lack of strength, a loss of appetite, and loose stool occur due to spleen–stomach weakness, add dry-fried *bái zhú*, *fú líng*, and *dǎng shēn*. If it is accompanied by cold abdominal pain and diarrhea due to cold exuberance in the spleen and stomach, add *gān jiāng* and *ròu guì*. If there is frequent vomiting or hiccups due to severe ascending counterflow of stomach qi, add *jiāng bàn xià* and *zǐ sū gěng*. If dampness is mingled with heat in the spleen and stomach, the diagnosis and treatment of the damp–heat accumulation in the middle *jiao* pattern can serve as a guide. If it is accompanied by exterior dampness yet to be removed and the exterior pattern is apparent, the exterior dampness pattern can be used as a reference for treatment.

If this formula is used with *Wǔ Líng Sǎn* (Five Substances Powder with Poria), it becomes *Wèi Líng Tāng* (Stomach-Calming Poria Decoction), which is indicated for exuberant water–dampness or the presence of edema and inhibited urination. If *xiāng fù* and *shā rén* are added to this formula, it becomes *Xiāng Shā Píng Wèi Wán* (Costusroot and Amomum Stomach-Calming Pill), which is more potent in dispersing distention and rectifying qi.

Cautions

Although *Píng Wèi Sǎn* can be applied to many disease patterns, its nature is relatively warm and dry, which is not suitable for diseases without signs of dampness or even to diseases with dampness accompanied by yin deficiency or pathogenic heat; it should not be applied at random, and proper combinatorial techniques with other medicinals are required.

Daily Exercises

1. What are the clinical features of the dampness encumbering the spleen and stomach pattern? What are the differences of its symptoms compared to the damp–heat accumulation in the middle pattern?
2. What are the ingredients of *Píng Wèi Sǎn*?
3. Ms. Yan is a 43-year-old female. She has suffered from stomach disease for 7–8 years, which was previously diagnosed as superficial gastritis. In the past week, she has been experiencing gastric distention, fullness, and discomfort, especially after having food. She also had occasional mild stomach pain, nausea, loose stool 2 times a day, a lack of appetite, a white, turbid, and greasy tongue coating, and a soggy and thin pulse. Please prescribe a Chinese medicinal formula for this case.

Additional Formulae

Wèi Líng Tāng (Stomach-Calming Poria Decoction)

Wǔ Líng Sǎn (Five Substances Powder with Poria) 3 g and *Píng Wèi Sǎn* (Stomach-Calming Powder) 3 g. Mix the ingredients of both formulae evenly and add 3 pieces of ginger and 2 pieces of jujubes for decocting in water.

Actions

Fortifying the spleen and harmonizing the middle; draining dampness and moving qi.

Indications

Obstruction of the spleen and stomach by dampness or food poisoning presenting gastric and abdominal distention and fullness, diarrhea, scant urine, and a white and greasy tongue coating.

Xiāng Shā Píng Wèi Wán (Costusroot and Amomum Stomach-Calming Pill)

Cāng zhú (Rhizoma Atractylodis) 10 g; *hòu pò* (Cortex Magnoliae Officinalis) 8 g; *chén pí* (Pericarpium Citri Reticulatae) 8 g; *xiāng fù* (Fructus Amomi) 8 g; *shā rén* (Fructus Amomi) 4 g; *gān cǎo* (Radix et Rhizoma Glycyrrhizae) 4 g. The ingredients are made into small pills. Take pills 6 g orally each time, 2 times a day.

Actions

Drying dampness and fortifying the spleen; rectifying qi and loosening the center.

Indications

Obstruction of the spleen and stomach by dampness, presenting gastric and abdominal distention and fullness.

DAY FIVE

The Phlegm–Damp Pattern

The phlegm–damp pattern is caused by the disorder of various *zang–fu* organs in transporting and transforming water–dampness, and thus dysfunctional fluid metabolism and accumulation of water are present. In addition to a direct connection with the spleen and stomach, fluid metabolism is also closely related to the diffusion and descent of lung qi, vaporization of kidney yang, dredging function of the liver and gallbladder, and unblocking of triple *jiao*. Therefore, dysregulation of any one organ may contribute to the formation of phlegm–damp. Phlegm–damp can be distributed to any part of the body. In broad terms, it includes phlegm–rheum, water–dampness, and damp–turbidity mentioned in the previous chapters. Specifically, it refers to phlegm, also called damp–phlegm, which is either visible or simply a presumed pathological product. Its circulation is far wider than the dampness covering the spleen and stomach in the dampness encumbering the spleen and stomach pattern. The phlegm–damp pattern in this section pertains to the latter definition.

This pattern is commonly seen in many respiratory and digestive diseases, such as chronic bronchitis, emphysema, chronic gastritis, gastric or duodenal ulcers, chronic enteritis, chronic hepatitis, and chronic cholecystitis. As phlegm–damp can interact with pathogens of wind, cold, heat, food stagnation, and stasis, and be distributed to various organs, channels, tendons, bones, muscles, and skin, it involves a great number of diseases.

Diagnosis

The main symptoms and signs of this pattern are coughing, usually producing white sputum, a white and greasy tongue coating, and a slippery pulse. Other indications include chest oppression, gastric stuffiness, poor appetite and digestion, nausea, vomiting, fatigue, dizziness, palpitations, panting, mania, insomnia or lethargy, susceptibility to fright, phlegm nodes, scrofula, flowing phlegm, profuse leukorrhea, and obesity.

Chinese medicine believes that the spleen is the source of phlegm production, while the lung is the container that holds the phlegm. It denotes the failure of the spleen in transportation as the cause of phlegm–damp production, which is then usually stored in the lung. Phlegm obstruction in the lung inevitably affects the diffusion and descent of lung qi, which presents coughing with white sputum produced and panting. A tongue with a white greasy coating and a slippery pulse are key indications of the accumulation of phlegm in the body. As phlegm–damp hinders qi movement, there will appear to be chest oppression and gastric stuffiness. Phlegm–damp in the spleen and stomach influences functions of transportation, transformation, raising the clear, and directing the turbid downward, thus a lack of appetite, nausea, and vomiting will occur. Phlegm–damp obstruction in the middle prevents clear yang qi from distributing throughout the whole body and head, triggering fatigue and dizziness. Phlegm–damp clouding clear yang qi can also lead to drowsiness and lethargy. If the phlegm–damp disrupts the heart spirit, it may manifest as palpitations, mania, insomnia, restlessness due to fright, cramps, and even the loss of consciousness. If the phlegm–damp stagnates in the tendons, bones, and channels to become bumps, they are called phlegm nodes as they are movable, painless, and not reddish, which is unlike general inflammation with reddish swellings and hot pain. Phlegm nodes occurring in the neck usually come under scrofula, i.e., lymphatic tuberculosis, while those occurring deep in the muscles or bones are usually flowing phlegm (tuberculosis of the bone and joint). If the phlegm–damp flows downward, women will suffer from profuse leukorrhea and even infertility if the uterus is involved. Unresolved phlegm–damp will be infused throughout the entire body, manifesting as obesity. That is why it is said overweight individuals are usually flooded with phlegm. Certain types of high blood fat levels also pertain to phlegm–damp.

Treatment method

Drying dampness and dissolving phlegm; rectifying qi and harmonizing the middle.

Formula and ingredients: Èr Chén Tāng (Two Matured Substances Decoction)

Fǎ bàn xià (Rhizoma Pinelliae Praeparatum) 15 g; *jú hóng* (Exocarpium Citri Rubrum) 15 g; *fú líng* (Poria) 9 g; *zhì gān cǎo* (Radix et Rhizoma Glycyrrhizae Praeparata cum Melle) 5 g.

Formula verse

Èr Chén Tāng uses *xià* and *chén*, *gān cǎo*, and *fú líng*. It is beneficial to qi, expels phlegm, and dries dampness, making it effective in treating phlegm–damp.

Usage

Grind the above ingredients into a crude powder and administer 12 g each time for decocting with 7 pieces of ginger, 1 piece of smoked plum, and water. Take the decoction warm.

Analysis

Èr Chén Tāng is a basic formula for treating phlegm–damp. Here, *bàn xià*, the main medicinal, dries dampness and removes phlegm, and also serves to harmonize the stomach and relieve vomiting, move qi, and alleviate cough. As qi stagnation is an important factor that causes the internal production of phlegm–damp, *chén pí* is supplemented to dredge qi movement and free qi flow, which is beneficial to the elimination of phlegm–damp. Meanwhile, the internal obstruction phlegm–damp by impedes qi movement and results in chest oppression and gastric and abdominal distention and fullness. The application of *chén pí* can relieve the above symptoms and *chén pí* itself resolves phlegm, so it is a vital ingredient for the treatment of the phlegm–damp pattern. *Fú líng* boosts the spleen and percolates dampness. Dampness can be removed as long as the spleen is efficient in transportation, and so arresting the production of phlegm. *Gān cǎo* harmonizes the middle and boosts qi. If middle qi is sufficient, phlegm–damp will not be generated. *Shēng jiāng* harmonizes the stomach, stops vomiting, and also reduces the toxicity of *bàn xià*. A small amount of *wū méi* can astringe lung qi due to its sour nature, and together with the acrid *bàn xià* that is dispersing, the formula becomes both astringing and dispersing, which makes it able to dry dampness and dissolve phlegm without impairing yin through its original warm and dispersing natures. Since it has long been regarded that the staler *bàn xià* and *chén pí* are, the better the formula works, it is also termed *Èr Chén* (Two Stale Ones).

Through research, *bàn xià* has been shown to relieve coughing and vomiting. *Chén pí* can promote the secretion of digestive juices, drain flatulence, fortify the gallbladder, relieve inflammation, dilate bronchi, and remove phlegm. *Fú líng* promotes urination, protects the liver, and calms the mind. *Gān cǎo* relieves spasms of the smooth muscles and inflammation and allergy, and if combined with *chén pí* and *fú líng*, it can protect the mucosal membrane of the stomach and intestines and also cure ulcers. Undoubtedly, pharmacological studies are still far from revealing the complete pharmacological function of *Èr Chén Tāng*. In clinical application, this formula regulates the digestive, respiratory, nervous, cardiovascular, endocrine, reproductive, and urinary systems.

Treatment reference

Èr Chén Tāng is indicated for a wide range of diseases. Almost all formulae for phlegm–damp are based on this formula. In practice, flexible modification is required according to the different natures and locations of the interacting pathogens of phlegm–damp. If a cold pathogen acts together with phlegm, add *cāng zhú* and s*hēng jiāng zhī*. If the cold is severe, add *wú zhū yú* and *fù zǐ*. If the heat is mixed with fire, add *shí gāo*, *qīng dài*, *huáng lián*, and *zhú lì*. If it is mixed with wind as wind– phlegm, add *tiān má*, *zhì tiān nán xīng*, *bái fù zǐ*, *zào jiǎo*, and *dì lóng*. If it is accompanied by food stagnation, add *shān zhā*, *shén qū*, and *mài yá*. If it is affected by stasis becoming static phlegm, add *táo rén*, *hóng huā*, and *dān shēn*. If it is with heat accumulation in the intestines, add *dà huáng*, *máng xiāo*, and whole *guā lóu*. If it is with qi stagnation, add prepared *xiāng fù*, *zhǐ qiào*, and *chái hú*. If the phlegm–damp remains in the spleen, stomach, or lung, this formula is often combined with *Píng Wèi Sǎn* (Stomach-Calming Powder) to treat the following diseases with obvious symptoms of phlegm–damp: dyspepsia, chronic bronchitis, emphysema, chronic gastritis, gastric neurosis, peptic ulcers, chronic enteritis, chronic hepatitis, and bronchial asthma. For phlegm–damp clouding the heart spirit, add *shí chāng pú*, *yù jīn*, *méng shí*, and *fǎ bàn xià*. If this formula is used together with *dǎn nán xīng*, *zhǐ shí*, *rén shēn*, *shí chāng pú*, and *zhú rú*, it becomes *Dí Tán Tāng* (Phlegm-Flushing Decoction), which is indicated for stroke and unconsciousness as a result of phlegm affecting the heart orifices. If phlegm–damp obstructs the uterus leading to profuse leukorrhea or infertility, add *cāng zhú*, prepared *xiāng fù*, *dāng guī*, and *tiān nán xīng*, becoming *Cāng Fù Dǎo Tán Wán* (Atractylodis and Cyperi Phlegm-Expelling Pill). If phlegm–damp stagnates in the muscles and under the skin, add *bái jiè zǐ* and *zào jiǎo cì*. If phlegm–damp obstructs the middle with spleen and stomach deficiency–cold, it can be combined with *Lǐ Zhōng Wán* (Center-Regulating Pill), becoming *Lǐ Zhōng Huà Tán Wán* (Center-Regulating and Phlegm-Transforming Pill). If there is coughing with yellow phlegm due to the internal combination of lung heat and phlegm–heat, add *guā lóu rén*, *huáng qín*, *zhǐ shí*, and *dǎn nán xīng*, becoming *Qīng Qì Huà Tán Wán* (Qi-Clearing and Phlegm-Transforming Pill).

Cautions

Èr Chén Tāng is a warm- and dry-natured formula. Be cautious in prescribing it to patients with yin deficiency or heat pathogens. In some cases, yin-nourishing and heat-clearing medicinals should be used together. For patients susceptible to hemoptysis, do not administer *bàn xià* because its extreme dryness may lead to massive coughing with the production of blood.

Daily Exercises

1. What are the clinical features of the phlegm–damp pattern? What are the differences compared to the dampness encumbering the spleen and stomach pattern?
2. What are the ingredients of *Èr Chén Tāng*? What are the major modified formulae?
3. Mr. Qian is a 58-year-old male. He has had chronic bronchitis and emphysema for more than a decade, which critically worsens in winter. Several days earlier, he contracted wind–cold which triggered a bad cough with massive amounts of white and foamy sputum, panting, chest oppression, gastric and abdominal distention and fullness, an absence of thirst, a loss of appetite, a tongue with a white,

thick and greasy coating, and a thin and slippery pulse. Please prescribe a Chinese medicinal formula for this case.

Additional Formulae

Dí Tán Tāng (Phlegm-Flushing Decoction)

Jiāng bàn xià (Rhizoma Pinelliae Praeparatum) 8 g; *dǎn nán xīng* (Arisaema cum Bile) 8 g; *jú hóng* (Exocarpium Citri Rubrum) 6 g; *zhǐ shí* (Fructus Aurantii Immaturus) 6 g; *fú líng* (Poria) 6 g; *rén shēn* (Radix et Rhizoma Ginseng) 3 g; *shí chāng pú* (Rhizoma Acori Tatarinowii) 3 g; *zhú rú* (Caulis Bambusae in Taenia) 2 g; *gān cǎo* (Radix et Rhizoma Glycyrrhizae) 1.5 g. Add water, ginger, and jujubes to decoct.

Actions

Clearing up phlegm and opening the orifices.

Indications

Stroke due to phlegm affecting the heart orifices presenting tongue stiffness, inability to speak, a yellow and greasy tongue coating, and a deep and slippery or wiry and tight pulse.

Cāng Fù Dǎo Tán Wán (Atractylodis and Cyperi Phlegm-Expelling Pill)

Cāng zhú (Rhizoma Atractylodis) 8 g; *xiāng fù* (Rhizoma Cyperi) 8 g; *zhǐ qiào* (Fructus Aurantii) 8 g; *chén pí* (Pericarpium Citri Reticulatae) 6 g; *fú líng* (Poria) 6 g; *dǎn nán xīng* (Arisaema cum Bile) 4 g; *gān cǎo* (Radix et Rhizoma Glycyrrhizae) 4 g.

The ingredients are ground into powder and made into pills with ginger juice and *shén qū* (Massa Medicata Fermentata). Take the pills 9 g orally each time along with light ginger soup. Alternatively, similar dosages of the above ingredients can be decocted in water for oral intake.

Actions

Drying dampness and dissolving phlegm; rectifying qi and invigorating blood.

Indications

Obese women or exuberant phlegm–drool presenting amenorrhea, profuse and sticky leukorrhea, and infertility.

Qīng Qì Huà Tán Wán (Qi-Clearing and Phlegm-Transforming Pill)

Guā lóu rén (Semen Trichosanthis) with oil removed 30 g; *chén pí* (Pericarpium Citri Reticulatae) without the white part 30 g; wine-fried *huáng qín* (Radix Scutellariae) 30 g; *xìng rén* (Semen Armeniacae Amarum) 30 g; *zhǐ shí* (Fructus Aurantii Immaturus) 30 g; *fú líng* (Poria) 30 g; *dǎn nán xīng* (Arisaema cum Bile) 45 g; *bàn xià* (Rhizoma Pinelliae) 45 g.

The ingredients are ground into powder and made into pills with ginger juice. Take the pills 6 g orally for each time with warm water, 2–3 times a day.

DAY SIX

The Phlegm–Heat Harassing the Interior Pattern

This a pattern of phlegm–heat in the body affecting *zang–fu* functions. Phlegm–heat refers to phlegm–damp complicated with pathogenic heat, so this pattern actually extends from the phlegm–damp pattern. Many organs can be influenced by phlegm–heat, among which are phlegm–heat accumulation in the lung, phlegm–heat invading the gallbladder and stomach, phlegm–heat blocking the heart orifices, phlegm–heat stagnation in the liver, and phlegm–heat impeding the channels and collaterals. In this section, we will mainly discuss the consequences of internal obstruction by phlegm–heat with disharmony of gallbladder and stomach, which is commonly seen in acute or chronic gastritis, pernicious vomiting during pregnancy, dizziness, epilepsy, mania, palpitations, and stroke.

Diagnosis

The main symptoms and signs of this pattern are insomnia, a bitter taste in the mouth, palpitations, mental disorder, and a tongue with a yellow and greasy coating. Other indications may include vexation, restlessness, fright, occasional mania, unconsciousness, vomiting, hiccups, chest oppression, and a wiry and slippery pulse.

Phlegm–heat of this pattern mainly resides in the gallbladder, hence also often involving the stomach, presenting symptoms such as nausea and vomiting which indicate the failure of the stomach to harmonize and descend. Phlegm–heat of the gallbladder can also disrupt the heart spirit, causing insomnia, palpitations, vexation, restlessness, and susceptibility to fright in mild cases, with mental disorder in severe cases. When this pattern occurs in diseases of internal damage, the manifestations can either be depressive and indifferent insanity, or excited and restless mania. When it occurs in externally contracted febrile diseases, the manifestations can either be unconsciousness or delirious speech. A bitter taste in the mouth, a tongue with a yellow and greasy coating, and a wiry and slippery pulse are signs of phlegm–heat. Furthermore, phlegm–heat blocks qi movement, leading to chest oppression.

Treatment method

Clearing heat and removing dampness; rectifying qi and harmonizing the stomach.

Formula and ingredients: Wēn Dǎn Tāng (Gallbladder-Warming Decoction)

Bàn xià (Rhizoma Pinelliae) 6 g; zhú rú (Caulis Bambusae in Taenia) 6 g; dry-fried zhǐ shí (Fructus Aurantii Immaturus) 6 g; chén pí (Pericarpium Citri Reticulatae) 9 g; zhì gān cǎo (Radix et Rhizoma Glycyrrhizae Praeparata cum Melle) 3 g; fú líng (Poria) 5 g.

Formula verse

Wēn Dǎn Tāng uses líng bàn cǎo and zhǐ zhú chén pí along with ginger and jujubes. It is indicated for deficiency, vexation, insomnia, palpations, and also the gallbladder heat harassing pattern.

Usage

Grind the above ingredients into a crude powder and administer 15 g each time for decocting with 5 pieces of ginger, 2 pieces of jujubes, and water. Take the decoction warm.

Analysis

Wēn Dǎn Tāng is in fact a modified formula of *Èr Chén Tāng* (Two Matured Substances Decoction). In this formula, *bàn xià, chén pí, fú líng, gān cǎo*, and ginger are all key ingredients of *Èr Chén Tāng*, which have functions of drying dampness and dissolving phlegm, and rectifying qi and harmonizing the middle. Due to complications with pathogenic heat, *zhú rú* is added to clear and dissolve hot phlegm. *Zhǐ shí* serves to strengthen the effect of moving qi and resolving phlegm. Overall, this formula is indicated for the phlegm–damp pattern with pathogenic heat or with the tendency of transforming heat. Although the formula is named "Gallbladder-Warming," it actually is "Gallbladder-Clearing."

Aside from some pharmacological functions of the ingredients in *Èr Chén Tāng*, this formula attaches more importance to calming the mind and regulating the central nervous system, so it is a commonly used formula for mental disorders.

Treatment reference

Wēn Dǎn Tāng is widely used in clinical practice. It is indicated for acute and chronic gastritis, peptic ulcers, chronic hepatitis, and chronic cholecystitis presenting pain, distention, and fullness in the stomach, abdomen, chest, and rib sides, a bitter taste in the mouth, nausea, vexing heat, and a tongue with a yellow and greasy coating. It has moderate effects on relieving pain, distention, and vomiting. Moreover, this formula is applicable to diseases of the phlegm–heat nature, such as insomnia, palpitations, dizziness, schizophrenia, neurosis, cerebral concussion sequela, strokes, mania, and mental disorder of acute febrile diseases. As the final target site of phlegm–heat varies from disease to disease, this formula can also be used to treat phlegm–heat caused by coronary diseases, arrhythmia, hyperthyroidism, Meniere's syndrome, pernicious vomiting during pregnancy, chronic bronchitis, pulmonary infection, and so on. In application, tongue coating is an important indicator. A yellow and greasy coating usually denotes phlegm–heat, but it usually fades away after the application of this formula, which indicates the gradual resolution of phelgm–heat.

Clinically, there are many modifications. For severe dizziness, add *tiān má*, *jú huā*, or *cì jí lí*. For severe vomiting, add *zǐ sū yè*, *huáng lián*, or *dài zhě shí*. For severe pathogenic heat, add *huáng lián*, *huáng qín*, or *zhī zǐ*. For exuberant phlegm–heat, add whole *guā lóu*, *xuán míng fěn*, *lái fú zǐ*, or *zhú lì*. For insomnia and palpitations due to phlegm–heat affecting the heart, add *yuǎn zhì*, raw *mǔ lì*, or *suān zǎo rén*. For episodes of mania, add *yù jīn*, *bái fán*, *dǎn nán xīng*, or *shí chāng pú*. If *huáng lián* is added to this formula, it becomes *Huáng Lián Wēn Dǎn Tāng* (Coptis Gallbladder-Warming Decoction), which is for severe pathogenic heat. If qi and blood deficiencies are present, add *shú dì huáng*, *rén shēn*, *suān zǎo rén*, and *yuǎn zhì*, becoming *Shí Wèi Wēn Dǎn Tāng* (Ten-Ingredient Gallbladder-Warming Decoction). If there is stubborn fire–heat phlegm, this formula is too weak; it can be modified into *Gǔn Tán Wán* (Phlegm-Removing Pill).

Cautions

Wēn Dǎn Tāng is used to treat the phlegm–heat harassing the interior pattern. Its heat-clearing function is admittedly not very potent, so for patterns of serious heat signs or the phlegm–fire pattern, other heat-clearing and fire-purging medicinals should be added. If there is constipation with internal exuberance of phlegm–fire, purgation is usually effected, often by applying *dà huáng*. As this formula is warm- and dry-natured, it is not advisable to use it to treat patients with blood deficiencies. Exuberant fire–heat tends to impair fluids, so under such a circumstance, add some *shēng dì*, *shā shēn*, *shí hú*, or an equivalent ingredient to nourish yin.

Daily Exercises

1. What is phlegm–heat? What are the manifestations of phlegm–heat disturbance of the gallbladder?

2. What are the ingredients of *Wēn Dǎn Tāng*? What are its indications?
3. Ms. Shen is a 32-year-old female. She has had insomnia for 5–6 years. On some nights, she is unable to fall asleep. Other manifestations are sores in the tongue and mouth, vexation, a bitter taste in the mouth, amnesia, head dizziness, chest oppression, a red tongue with a thin coating that is yellow and greasy in the center, and a wiry and slippery pulse. Please prescribe a Chinese medicinal formula for this case.

Additional Formulae

Huáng Lián Wēn Dǎn Tāng (*Coptis Gallbladder-Warming Decoction*)

Ingredients of *Wēn Dǎn Tāng* plus *huáng lián* (Rhizoma Coptidis) 3 g. Add water to decoct.

Actions

Clearing and dissolving hot phlegm.

Indications

Insomnia, dizziness, vexation, yellow urine, a bitter taste in the mouth, a red tongue with a yellow and greasy tongue coating, and a slippery and rapid pulse.

Shí Wèi Wēn Dǎn Tāng (*Ten-Ingredient Gallbladder-Warming Decoction*)

Fǎ bàn xià (Rhizoma Pinelliae Praeparatum) 6 g; dry-fried *zhǐ shí* (Fructus Aurantii Immaturus) 6 g; *chén pí* (Pericarpium Citri Reticulatae) 6 g; *fú líng* (Poria) 4.5 g; dry-fried *suān zǎo rén* (Semen Ziziphi Spinosae) 3 g; *yuǎn zhì* (Radix Polygalae) 3 g; *wǔ wèi zǐ* (Fructus Schisandrae Chinensis) 3 g; *shú dì huáng* (Radix Rehmanniae Praeparata) 3 g; *rén shēn* (Radix et Rhizoma Ginseng) 3 g; *zhì gān cǎo* (Radix et Rhizoma Glycyrrhizae Praeparata cum Melle) 1.5 g; ginger 5 pieces; jujube 1 piece. Add water to decoct.

Actions

Dissolving phlegm and boosting qi; calming the mind and the heart.

Indications

Heart dysregulation presenting timidity, edema on the four limbs, an absence of taste for food, palpitations, vexation, poor sleep, and restlessness.

Gǔn Tán Wán (*Phlegm-Removing Pill*)

Wine-steamed *dà huáng* (Radix et Rhizoma Rhei) 24 g; wine-washed *huáng qín* (Radix Scutellariae) 24 g; *méng shí* (Chlorite-schist) 3 g; and *chén xiāng* (Lignum Aquilariae Resinatum) 15 g.

The processing of *méng shí* is as follows: first, crush it and add 3 g of sodium sulfate in a small earthen pot. Cover the pot and use a piece of iron thread to bind it. Use salt of the earth to block the opening of the pot and dry it under the sun. Then, calcine it till it turns red and extract *méng shí* when it is cool. Grind the ingredients into a fine powder and make into water pills. Take the pills 5–9 g each time with light tea or warm water after meals, 1–2 times a day.

Actions

Draining fire and eliminating phlegm.

Indications

Stubborn excess phlegm–heat presenting mania, palpitations due to fright, and coma; coughing producing yellow and sticky sputum, panting, and chest and stomach stuffiness and oppression; dizziness, tinnitus, insomnia, and dreaminess; or neck tuberculosis, constipation, a yellow, thick, and greasy tongue coating, and a slippery, rapid, and forceful pulse.

THE 7TH WEEK

DAY ONE

The Wind–Phlegm Harassing the Upper Body Pattern

This pattern is caused by the internal accumulation of phlegm–damp together with liver wind harassing the upper part of the body. Wind–phlegm refers to phlegm–damp complicated with pathogenic wind, and pathogenic wind can be further classified as external wind and internal wind. The concepts of external wind and internal wind will be discussed in Chapter 8. Regardless of the source of wind, both can be complicated with phlegm–damp and result in diseases. For phlegm complicated with external wind, the disease is usually located at the lung, leading to an aversion to cold with fever, and cough with expectoration. For phlegm with internal wind, the disease is usually located at the liver, leading to dizziness, headaches, and shock. The wind–phlegm harassing the upper body pattern discussed here refers to phlegm with internal wind, which is also within the scope of the phlegm–damp pattern. This pattern is commonly observed in dizziness, hypertension, nervous prostration, stroke, and epilepsy.

Diagnosis

The main symptoms and signs of this pattern are dizziness, head heaviness, pain, nausea, vomiting, and a tongue with a white and greasy coating. Other indications may include chest stuffiness and fullness, nausea, and vomiting of phlegm–drool during episodes of dizziness and headaches, sudden unconsciousness, hemiplegia, epilepsy, and numbness of the four limbs.

As this pattern results from a combination of phlegm–damp and liver wind, its symptoms are exclusively associated with phlegm–damp and liver wind. Internal obstruction by phlegm–damp can cloud the clear yang in the upper body and together with the ascending counterflow of liver wind, the phlegm–damp attacks the head, causing dizziness or headaches. The dizziness is usually characterized by vertigo (the sense that the surroundings are spinning or moving) or by the patient himself unable to open his eyes. Concurrently, as the wind–phlegm attacks the stomach, nausea and vomiting are caused, sometimes very acute. Phlegm–turbidity obstruction in the interior renders inhibited qi movement, so chest or gastric distention and fullness may be observed. Vomiting of phlegm–drool and a white and greasy tongue coating are important indicators of the phlegm–damp pattern. If the phlegm–damp and the ascending counterflow of liver wind are serious, it may lead to wind–phlegm clouding the heart orifice, manifesting as sudden unconsciousness and hemiplegia of stroke or epilepsy. If the wind–phlegm flows along the channels and collaterals, numbness will occur and this symptom may be presented individually or with other symptoms.

Treatment method

Removing dampness and resolving phlegm; extinguishing wind and boosting the spleen.

Formula and ingredients: Bàn Xià Bái Zhú Tiān Má Tāng (Pinellia, Atractylodes Macrocephala, and Gastrodia Decoction)

Bàn xià (Rhizoma Pinelliae) 9 g; *tiān má* (Rhizoma Gastrodiae) 6 g; *fú líng* (Poria) 9 g; *jú hóng* (Exocarpium Citri Rubrum) 6 g; *bái zhú* (Rhizoma Atractylodis Macrocephalae) 9 g; *gān cǎo* (Radix et Rhizoma Glycyrrhizae) 3 g; *shēng jiāng* (Rhizoma Zingiberis Recens) 2 pieces; *dà zǎo* (Fructus Jujubae) 3 pieces.

Formula verse

Bàn Xià Bái Zhú Tiān Má Tāng, with *líng, cǎo, jú hóng, zǎ*, and *shēng jiāng*, treats dizziness and headaches due to wind–phlegm exuberance, and restores health by resolving phlegm and extinguishing wind.

Usage

Add 800 mL of water to decoct until 250 mL are left. Remove the dregs and take the decoction warm. Add another 400 mL of water to decoct with the dregs until there 250 mL are left and take the decoction warm. Take the decoction 2 times a day.

Analysis

Bàn Xià Bái Zhú Tiān Má Tāng is formulated on the basis of *Èr Chén Tāng* (Two Matured Substances Decoction) together with *tiān má* and *bái zhú*. *Èr Chén Tāng* can dry dampness and resolve phlegm, and rectify qi and harmonize the middle, but this pattern pertains to phlegm–damp complicated with the ascending counterflow of liver wind, so *tiān má* is added to calm the liver and extinguish wind. This formula consists of *bàn xià* for removing phlegm and *tiān má* for extinguishing wind, both of which are chief ingredients. *Bái zhú* is added to fortify the spleen and remove dampness, targeting the source of phlegm production. Therefore, this formula functions to calm liver wind, boost the spleen, and remove phlegm–damp.

According to modern pharmacological researches, *tiān má* can calm the mind, relieve spasms, and prevent epilepsy. It also decreases the resistance of coronary arteries, cerebral vessels, and peripheral vessels, improves blood circulation, and nourishes nerves, so it is beneficial in the treatment of dizziness from nervous, vascular, and anemic sources. *Bái zhú* has multiple functions, some of which include boosting the stomach, promoting urination, calming the mind, supplementing and protecting the liver, and exerting synergic pharmacological effects with *tiān má*.

Treatment reference

Bàn Xià Bái Zhú Tiān Má Tāng is a commonly used formula for dizziness and headaches. These are usually caused by hypertension, nervous prostration, and vestibular edema. It is clinically characterized by whirling dizziness not unlike motion sickness and seasickness, nausea, vomiting, a white and greasy tongue coating, and a slippery pulse. For severe dizziness, add *jiāng cán*, *gōu téng*, *dǎn nán xīng*, or *shí jué míng*. For severe headaches, add *quán xiē*, *dì lóng*, *wú gong*, or *màn jīng zǐ*. For a spleen with weak food transportation and conversion functions, add *dǎng shēn* and *huáng qí*.

Cautions

In clinical practice, there are various disease causes of dizziness and headaches, such as exuberant liver yang, kidney deficiency, qi deficiency, blood deficiency, and static blood in diseases of internal damage. This formula is only indicated for phlegm–damp complicated with liver wind. If the ascending counterflow of liver wind is so strong that it causes unconsciousness, medicinals that can suppress fright, open the orifices, and extinguish wind should be added because this formula is too weak for the above-mentioned applications.

Daily Exercises

1. What is wind–phlegm? What are the main symptoms and signs of the wind–phlegm harassing the upper body pattern?
2. What are the ingredients of *Bàn Xià Bái Zhú Tiān Má Tāng*?
3. Ms. He is a 36-year-old female. For 3 years, she has been experiencing dizziness, where the last occurrence was only yesterday as she felt her surroundings swirling even in bed with her eyes closed. Vomiting of phlegm–drool was also triggered, with food dregs followed by clear fluid. Other symptoms and signs were chest and stomach stuffiness and fullness, an absence of thirst, tinnitus, hearing loss, a white and greasy tongue coating, and a thin and slippery pulse. Please prescribe a Chinese medicinal formula for this case.

DAY TWO

The Fluid Retention Pattern

The fluid retention pattern is triggered by disorder of water metabolism, bringing about fluid stagnation and accumulation, and resulting in water retention, which is a type of loose substantial pathogen. The pattern reviewed here usually presents exudates and edema, which are commonly seen in exudative pleuritis, ascites of cirrhosis, and edema of nephritis.

Diagnosis

The main symptoms and signs of this pattern are chest and rib-side pain, shortness of breath, an enlarged abdomen, or cutaneous edema. Other indications may include gastric stuffiness and fullness or hardness, occasional dry vomiting, coughing, headaches, dizziness, delocalized edema (greater severity in the lower body), abdominal distention, scant urine, constipation, a slippery and moist tongue coating, and a deep and wiry pulse.

Water retention in different sites in the body may present different corresponding symptoms. If water is retained in the chest and rib sides, it is called pleural effusion, which will impede the diffusion and descending functions of the lung, so there will be shortness of breath and even panting. It may also affect the chest and rib sides, featuring pain aggravated during coughing and deep breaths, which spread to the back. If the lung is involved, coughing is triggered, while dry vomiting occurs if the stomach is affected. If water is retained in the abdomen, it gives rise to ascites, manifesting as abdominal distention and enlargement not unlike a drum. Water retention blocks qi movement, causing gastric stuffiness, fullness, distention, and even hardness. If water retention diffuses in the skin, it becomes edema, which is characterized by serious and lingering swellings much more severe in the lower body. Due to water retention, fluids cannot be discharged normally, thus urine is scant. Some patients may experience constipation, which is in relation to the dysfunction of intestinal conduction and transmission resulting from water retention and qi stagnation. A slippery and moist tongue coating and a deep and wiry pulse are signs of internal water retention.

The symptoms of water retention are hence caused by substantial pathogens and for diagnosis, aside from referring to the clinical manifestations, modern examinations on pleural effusion and ascites, including auscultation, percussion, X-ray, ultrasound, and punctures can be performed. Water retention usually follows disorders of the spleen, lung, heart, kidney, liver, *sanjiao*, and other organs that have dysfunctional water metabolism.

After the detection of water retention, further examinations should be carried out to identify further causes instead of remaining at the present stage of diagnosis.

Treatment method

Expelling water by purgation.

Formula and ingredients: Shí Zǎo Tāng (Ten Jujubes Decoction)

Equal doses of dry-fried *yuán huā* (Flos Genkwa); *gān suì* (Radix Kansui); *jīng dà jǐ* (Radix Euphorbiae Pekinensis).

Formula verse

Shí Zǎo uses *suì*, *jǐ* and *yuán huā*, excellent at expelling water by purgation.

Usage

Grind the above ingredients into a fine powder and mix them evenly. Decoct with 300 mL of water with 10 pieces of jujubes until 160 mL are left. Then, remove the jujubes. For patients with a strong physique, add 1–1.5 g of medicinal powder to the decoction each time, while for patients with a weak physique, add 0.6–1 g. Take the decoction warm in the morning, once a day. After oral intake of the decoction, if water retention still exists even though there has been watery stool, take the decoction at the same dosage again the next day. If the watery stool is severe, consume some thin porridge while suspending this medicinal powder therapy.

Today, the above ingredients are made into powder and filled into capsules for oral intake, 0.6–1.5 g each time, once a day. Before taking the capsules, decoct 10–15 pieces of jujubes with water and use the decoction to swallow the capsules in the morning on an empty stomach.

Analysis

Water retention that is treated by *Shí Zǎo Tāng* is a type of massive accumulation of fluid, which is beyond the indication of general dampness-resolving and urination-promoting methods. The ingredients of this formula are all potent water-expelling medicinals. Traditionally, *yuán huā* is good at removing recurrent rheum in the chest and rib-sides, *gān suì* at moving water–dampness in the channels and collaterals, and *dà jǐ* at draining water pathogens in the intestines and stomach. The combination of these ingredients exerts synergic effects on expelling water–rheum, relieving swellings and fullness. However, due to their strength at expelling, damage to the body will occur easily. In addition, before the accumulation and retention of water, the *zang–fu* organs will have been in deficiency for some time. The application of these potent medicinals will further weaken healthy qi. Therefore, the ingredients are required to be decocted with jujubes, which can mitigate the extreme nature of the medicinals on one hand, and boost the spleen and stomach and protect healthy qi on the other hand by eliminating pathogens without impairing qi. Because jujubes (*dà zǎo* in Chinese) are a vital ingredient in the formula, it is named *Shí Zǎo* (Ten Jujubes).

It has been shown that *gān suì*, *yuán huā*, and *dà jǐ* can stimulate intestinal walls, increase intestinal peristalsis, and cause diarrhea, especially watery diarrhea. All of them can also promote urination, among which the effect of *dà jǐ* is relatively mild with its lower toxicity. Aside from inducing bowel movements and urination, these ingredients have certain effects on regulating internal organs, blood circulation, and the nervous and immune systems.

Treatment reference

Shí Zǎo Tāng is the classic formula for expelling water by purgation. It is clinically applied to treat chest or abdominal effusions due to tuberculous pleuritis, ascites of hepatitis, ascites of advanced schistosomiasis, and tuberculous peritonitis. It also treats general edema caused by chronic nephritis. After taking this formula, the patient will experience watery diarrhea and increased urine discharge, and water retained in the body will be gradually drained. Since this formula has certain regulating effects on the internal organs, blood circulation, and the nervous and immune systems, it is also administered to treat excessive secretion of gastric acids, schizophrenia, neuralgia, and other disorders presenting similar symptoms as those of water retention. This formula is especially applicable to persistent water retention.

The preparation of the medicinals into powder and decoction with jujubes are said to possess greater efficacy. Other forms of preparation are pills and capsules. If *yuán huā* is replaced with *bái jiè zǐ* and the ingredients are made into water pills, it becomes *Kòng Xián Dān* (Drool-Controlling Pellet), whose efficacy is similar to that of *Shí Zǎo Tāng*, but is comparatively milder and much better at draining phlegm–rheum in the channels, collaterals, tendons, and bones.

Cautions

Shí Zǎo Tāng is a formula for expelling pathogens to treat the branch. Although jujubes can protect stomach qi, they may impair it instead if diagnosis is erroneous. Therefore, if this formula is prescribed, the pattern differentiation of water retention must be accurate and the patient's physique and reaction after taking the medicine should be noted. If the patient has a very weak physique, it is a must to first boost healthy qi or apply treatment with both attack and supplementation. If water retention still persists after undergoing this therapy and the patient is not weak, continue with this formula, or suspend it until the patient's healthy qi restores. As for the dosage, it is advised to administer an initial small dose and then increase the dose gradually. If diarrhea persists for a long time, consume some cold porridge. After excessive water has been expelled, attention should be given to treat its root cause.

Daily Exercises

1. What are the clinical features of the water retention pattern?
2. What are the ingredients of *Shí Zǎo Tāng*? What are the cautions when applying this formula?
3. Ms. Jin is an 18-year-old female. She has had fever for 5 days. She complains of chest pain (greater severity on the right), which is aggravated during deep breaths and coughing. She experiences head heaviness, shallow respiration, right chest cavity and rib-side fullness, decreased respiratory movement, and trachea deviation to the left. An examination shows chest dullness on the right, a solid sound in the lower region on percussion, decreased breathing sounds and disappearing vocal fremitus on auscultation, a reddish tongue with a white and slippery coating, and a deep and wiry pulse on inspection. Please prescribe a Chinese medicinal formula for this case.

Additional Formulae

Kòng Xián Dān (Drool-Controlling Pellet)

Even doses of *gān suì* (Radix Kansui) without cores; skinless *jīng dà jǐ* (Radix Euphorbiae Pekinensis); *bái jiè zǐ* (Semen Sinapis). All the ingredients are ground into a fine powder and made into water pills the size of mung beans. Take the pills 1–3 g each time with warm water or mild ginger soup after meals or before sleep.

Actions

Expelling phlegm–rheum.

Indications

Stagnation of phlegm–drool in and around the chest presenting sudden unbearable dull pain in the chest and back, nape, or hip; radiating pain in the tendons and bones; restlessness; cold pain in the four limbs; intolerable headaches; lethargy; a lack of appetite; thick and sticky sputum; phlegm rales in the evening; and massive secretion of drool and saliva.

CHAPTER 8

The Wind Pattern

DAY THREE

Wind is one of the six pathogenic factors, and it is commonly referred to as pathogenic wind. There are two types of wind: external wind and internal wind. The former is the cause of many diseases, and exuberant fire–heat or deficiencies of the blood may present similar symptoms to external wind. Internal wind, on the other hand, is triggered from the interior. Both internal wind and external wind can result in disease patterns characterized by inconsistent disease sites, rapid disease changes, and shaking limbs or cramps.

Features of the Wind Pattern

The wind pattern is determined by the features of its main symptoms. It encompasses a wide range of manifestations, but all of them have characteristics of pathogenic wind-engendering diseases. Some are manifested as shifting disease locations, such as delocalized pain of the joints or muscles, delocalized pain in the head, and itching skin or relapsing of macules and remission at different locations. Others are manifested as an acute onset or quick changes in the disease course, such as sudden fainting and unconsciousness due to stroke. The rest are manifested as uncontrollable shaking, including signs of cramps of the four limbs, trembling, stiffness, hemiplegia, and facial palsy, as well as symptoms of vertigo, "flowery" vision, and numbness. The diagnosis of the wind pattern can usually be performed according to one set of the above-mentioned manifestations rather than all of them.

215

Thus, the wind pattern is not only closely related to diseases of the nervous system, such as stroke, epilepsy, convulsions due to high fever, tetanus, tremor, numbness, and various neuritis, but also to many other diseases, such as hypertension, rheumatoid arthritis, systemic lupus erythematosus (SLE), skin pruritus, urticaria, and eczema.

Categories of the Wind Pattern

The wind pattern has many sub-patterns. Clinically, the most commonly used classification is based on the source of pathogenic wind, namely the external wind pattern and internal wind pattern. The external wind pattern is a type of exterior pattern (Chapter 3), usually accompanied by an aversion to cold and fever without any disorder of the internal organs. Delving deeper, the external wind pattern includes the external wind engendering itching pattern, the external wind attacking the upper body pattern, the external wind obstructing the facial collaterals pattern, the external wind causing spasms pattern (e.g., tetanus), and the wind–cold or wind–damp stagnating the muscles or joints pattern. The internal wind pattern occurs either in the heat exuberance stage or impaired yin stage of externally contracted diseases, or in miscellaneous diseases of internal damage, which are caused by disorders of internal organs, with an especially close relationship with the liver. It includes the liver yang transforming into wind pattern, the liver heat engendering wind pattern, the yin deficiency stirring the wind pattern, and the blood dryness producing wind pattern.

Another system of classification is based on deficiency and excess, namely the excess–wind pattern and the deficiency–wind pattern. The excess–wind pattern results from pathogenic wind and heat, while the deficiency–wind pattern is caused by yin deficiency and blood deficiency.

Treatment Methods of the Wind Pattern

The treatment for the wind pattern should be based on the root cause of the disease. If it is an external wind pattern, the basic form of treatment is to expel the exogenous wind pathogen by a wind-scattering method.

According to the various accompanying pathogens, combinatorial methods of dispelling cold, clearing heat, removing dampness, eliminating phlegm, invigorating blood, and unblocking collaterals can be used. If it is an internal wind pattern, the disease is cured mainly by calming liver wind. In order to do so, the methods of calming the liver and subduing yang, clearing heat and cooling the liver, nourishing yin and fluids, and nourishing blood and moistening dryness can be carried out according to the cause of wind-stirring.

Naturally, the treatment methods for the external wind pattern and internal wind pattern are completely different. If the scattering method is erroneously applied to treat the internal wind pattern, it will boost fire–heat or further consume yin and blood, worsening the disease. Similarly, if the heat-clearing or nourishing method is mistakenly prescribed to treat the external wind pattern, it will further complicate the condition of the patient, aggravating the disease and prolonging the disease course. However, in clinical practice, it is common to observe internal wind triggered by external wind or stirring of internal wind accompanied by external wind. In such cases, internal wind and external wind interact with each other, so in treatment, a comprehensive therapy is required by targeting the major and minor aspects.

Daily Exercises

1. What are the external wind pattern and internal wind pattern?
2. What are the clinical features of the wind pattern?
3. What is the main treatment principle for the wind pattern? What aspects should be paid attention to?

DAY FOUR

The External Wind Engendering Itching Pattern

This pattern is indicated by itching of the skin caused by exogenous wind pathogens. It is commonly seen in urticaria, eczema, skin pruritus, and various kinds of allergic dermatitis. Though its main pathogen is external wind, it is often accompanied by pathogens of cold, heat, and dampness in attacking the body surface. If it is complicated by pathogenic cold, the swellings on skin are often light in color, with manifestations of an aversion to cold, absence of sweating, and aggravation following contact with coldness. If it is complicated by pathogenic heat, the swellings on the skin are usually red and painful with a burning sensation, and dysphoria, a bitter taste in the mouth, and aggravation after contact with heat may occur. If it is complicated by pathogenic dampness, there are always exudates on the skin. The external wind engendering itching pattern discussed in this section pertains to pathogenic wind complicated by damp and heat pathogens.

Diagnosis

The main symptom of this pattern is itching of the skin, lumps of rash, or exudates. Other indications can be relapsing and remitting or lasting cutaneous lamps of rash, dysphoria, a bitter taste in the mouth, a white or yellow tongue coating, and a floating, rapid, and powerful pulse.

Itching of skin in this pattern is not confined to a fixed location, which can be explained by the attack of flowing wind pathogens, being a characteristic of external wind engendering diseases and also the main indicator for the diagnosis of this pattern. As the wind pathogen is mingled with the damp pathogen, wind–damp accumulates in the muscles, skin, and blood vessels, causing skin erosion and persistent excretion of exudates. As this pattern is often accompanied by the heat pathogen, there are often also symptoms of heat, such as dysphoria and a bitter taste in the mouth. If this pattern lasts for a long period of time, an external pathogen stagnating in the muscle and skin may also be contracted, causing inhibited blood flow, lack of blood nourishment in the skin, and aggravated skin itching and lesions. In addition, if the patient is elderly or has a physique of blood deficiency, he will be more susceptible to the contraction of external wind and recovery will be more difficult. Note that itching of the skin purely caused by the lack of blood nourishment, namely blood dryness producing wind, is beyond the scope of the external wind pattern.

Treatment method

Scattering wind and harmonizing blood; clearing heat and removing dampness.

Formula and ingredients: Xiāo Fēng Sǎn (Wind-Dispersing Powder)

Dāng guī (Radix Angelicae Sinensis) 3 g; *shēng dì* (Radix Rehmanniae) 3 g; *fáng fēng* (Radix Saposhnikoviae) 3 g; *chán tuì* (Periostracum Cicadae) 3 g; *zhī mǔ* (Rhizoma Anemarrhenae) 3 g; *kǔ shēn* (Radix Sophorae Flavescentis) 3 g; *hú má* (Semen Sesami Nigrum) 3 g; *jīng jiè* (Herba Schizonepetae) 3 g; *cāng zhú* (Rhizoma Atractylodis) 3 g; *niú bàng zǐ* (Fructus Arctii) 3 g; *shí gāo* (Gypsum Fibrosum) 3 g; *gān cǎo* (Radix et Rhizoma Glycyrrhizae) 1.5 g; *chuān mù tōng* (Caulis Clematidis Armandii) 1.5 g.

Formula verse

Xiāo Fēng Sǎn has jīng fáng, chán tuì hú má kǔ shēn cāng; zhī gāo bàng tōng guī dì cǎo, beneficial to the skin itching pattern.

Usage

Grind ingredients into a crude powder and add 600 mL of water to decoct until 400 mL are left. Take the decoction orally on an empty stomach, 2 times a day.

Analysis

Xiāo Fēng Sǎn applies acrid-natured, wind-scattering, and exterior-releasing medicinals (*jīng jiè, fáng fēng, niú bàng zǐ*, and *chán tuì*) as chief ingredients to remove external wind in the muscles and skin. *Cāng zhú* and *chuān mù tōng* are added to remove dampness and promote urination. *Shí gāo, zhī mǔ*, and *kǔ shēn* help to clear heat. *Dāng guī, shēng dì*, and *hú má* nourish blood and harmonize fluids, serving to moisten dryness and remove wind. They can also prevent the dryness triggered by other wind-dispelling ingredients from impairing blood. Raw *gān cǎo* clears heat and resolves toxins, and harmonizes the actions of all medicinals. In summary, this formula has functions of dispelling wind, removing dampness, clearing heat, and nourishing blood.

Research has shown that *fáng fēng* and *gān cǎo* can relieve allergy, and *jīng jiè, cāng zhú*, and *dāng guī* can dilate blood vessels in the skin to improve blood circulation, and also have effects on relieving inflammation and inhibiting bacteria. *Chán tuì* can calm the mind. *Kŭ shēn* is potent in relieving itching and inhibiting bacteria, and like *dāng guī* and *shēng dì*, it can restrain the production of antibodies. Thus, this formula has comprehensive effects on regulating immunity, relieving allergy and inflammation, improving blood circulation, and inhibiting bacteria.

Treatment reference

Xiāo Fēng Sǎn is a common formula for treating various skin-itching diseases, such as skin urticaria, acute and chronic eczema, and senile skin itch. It is also applicable to allergic dermatitis, drug eruptions, neurodermatitis, and paddy-field dermatitis. It is also sometimes used to treat acute nephritis. Clinically, many patients with persistent dermatopathy fail to respond favorably to various allergy-relieving modern drugs, such as antihistamines and hormone therapies, but the application of this formula can often achieve a good result.

In practice, proper modification is required. If it is accompanied by constipation, add 3–6 g of raw *dà huáng*. If there are massive skin exudates, which indicate severe dampness, add *dì fū zĭ*, *bì xiè*, *chē qián zĭ*, or *bái xiān pí*. If there are reddish and extremely itchy lumps of rash, which indicate severe heat, add *jīn yín huā*, *lián qiào*, *chì sháo*, or *mŭ dān pí*, and increase the dose of *kŭ shēn* by a little. If the disease lingers with serious skin lesions, add *shé tuì*, *wū shāo shé*, or *băi bù shé*.

For external wind engendering itching presenting wind–cold signs, such as fever, a mild aversion to cold about 2–3 times of onset each day, an absence of sweating, itching of body, pale white or pale red lumps of rash that are aggravated by contact with cold, a tongue with a white and moist coating, and a floating pulse, *Guì Zhī Má Huáng Gè Bà Tāng* (Half-Cinnamon Twig and Half-Ephedra Decoction) should be applied. This formula features acrid and warm ingredients that can treat the itching pattern by dispelling exterior wind–cold to restore normal qi and blood flows in the muscles and skin. Moreover, a medicinal washing therapy can be combined to treat the external wind engendering itching pattern. For example, washing of lesions by the decoction of *jīng jiè* (Herba Schizonepetae) 10 g; *fáng fēng* (Radix Saposhnikoviae) 10 g; *kŭ shēn*

(Radix Sophorae Flavescentis) 15 g; *bái xiān pí* (Cortex Dictamni) 10 g; *dì fū zǐ* (Fructus Kochiae) 10 g; and *bái fán* (Alumen) 15 g, can also achieve favorable effects.

Cautions

During the treatment course, avoid catching wind and cold, and it is not recommended to consume fatty fish foods and dairy products. Maintain a light diet and a decent mood.

Daily Exercises

1. What are the main symptoms and signs of the external wind engendering itching pattern?
2. What are the ingredients of *Xiāo Fēng Sǎn*? How can it be modified according to different situations?
3. Ms. Zheng is a 14-year-old female. In the past 3 days, she has been suffering from general lumps of rubella that relapses and remits, and itching is quite severe till a point where she cannot fall asleep at night. The situation worsens if she catches wind outside. Other manifestations are vexation and agitation, a bitter taste in the mouth, dark urine, a tongue with a thin and white coating, a slightly reddish tongue tip, and a wiry and slippery pulse. Please prescribe a Chinese medicinal formula for this case.

Additional Formulae

Guì Zhī Má Huáng Gè Bà Tāng (Half-Cinnamon Twig and Half-Ephedra Decoction)

Guì zhī (Ramulus Cinnamomi) 5 g; *sháo yào* (Radix Paeoniae) 3 g; sliced *shēng jiāng* (Rhizoma Zingiberis Recens) 3 g; dry-fried *gān cǎo* (Radix et Rhizoma Glycyrrhizae) 3 g; *má huáng* (Herba Ephedrae) without knots 3 g; crushed *dà zǎo* (Fructus Jujubae) 4 pieces; soaked *xìng rén* (Semen Armeniacae Amarum) without skin and tip 6 g.

Add 1 L of water first to decoct *má huáng*. After boiling for 1–2 times, remove the foam and add the other ingredients to decoct until 360 mL are left. Remove the dregs and take the decoction warm, 120 mL each dose.

Actions

Dispelling wind and dispersing cold; harmonizing *ying* and *wei* levels.

Indications

Wind–cold stagnating the exterior presenting fever and an aversion to cold not unlike malaria, with fever more severe than the cold and occurring 2–3 times a day, a flushed face, itching of body, an absence of sweating, or general lumps of rubella.

DAY FIVE

The Wind Obstructing Facial Collaterals Pattern

This pattern is manifested as facial palsy after contracting external wind, which obstructs the facial channels and collaterals. It generally involves facial nervous paralysis, and is also called simple facial paralysis. Modern medicine believes that the onset of this disease is connected to a disorder of facial nerves instead of having a direct relation to external wind. However, Chinese medicine considers this disease to be induced by the sudden contraction of external wind, especially wind–cold, and after its onset, it is accompanied by a mild aversion to cold and facial cramps, which are symptoms in accordance with the features of pathogenic wind causing diseases. More importantly, favorable clinical effects can be achieved by applying medicinals that can dispel external wind, which hence indicates that the pathogen is in fact external wind. In addition, the idea that external wind can attack the facial channels and collaterals and cause diseases is to some extent related to the internal factor of deficiency of body qi and failure of blood to nourish the channels and collaterals.

Diagnosis

The main symptoms and signs mainly affect one side of the face, such as drooping of the mouth, inability to purse the lips, leakage of water or soup during drinking, and inability to close an eye. Other indications include a mild aversion to cold, twitches or cramps of facial muscles, or pain located at the back of the ear.

Facial palsy is the main symptom of this pattern. It is caused by an attack of external wind at one side of the facial channels and collaterals, leading to local disorder of qi and blood flow, with tendons and muscles lacking nourishment. To be specific, facial muscles of one side become slack and loose, while the muscles of the normal opposite side are relatively more tense, causing a deviated mouth and eye. Therefore, distorted facial expressions, an absence of wrinkles in the forehead of the affected side, an inability to frown and close the eyes, occasional tearing, a flat nasal groove, an upturned mouth on one side, and involuntary leakage of saliva are several manifestations of this pattern. As external wind attacks the body and clashes with defensive qi, some patients experience mild fever and an aversion to cold. Local pain is related to the blockage of the channels and collaterals and stagnation of qi and blood.

Facial palsy not only appears in simple facial paralysis, but also in other diseases, such as swelling of parotid glands, mastoiditis, syphilis, nasopharyngeal cancer, fibroma of the auditory nerve, and so on, although they may not be very common. Patients with hemiplegia due to stroke may also present a drooping mouth and eyes, but its manifestation is different from that of external wind obstructing the collaterals. For the latter, stroke not only results in limb paralysis of one side, but also a drooping mouth, leakage during drinking, and a flat labial groove, but the presence of wrinkles in the forehead distinguishes it from the external wind obstructing facial collaterals pattern.

Treatment method

Dispelling wind and unblocking the collaterals.

Formula and ingredients: Qiān Zhèng Săn (Symmetry-Correcting Powder)

Equal doses of *bái fù zǐ* (Rhizoma Typhonii); *jiāng cán* (Bombyx Batryticatus); *quán xiē* (Scorpion) with toxin removed.

Formula verse

Qiān Zhèng Sǎn treats facial palsy, by using *bái fù*, *jiāng cán*, and *quán xiē*. Take the ingredients with wine after being finely grounded, and efficacy is evident for wind striking the collaterals.

Usage

Grind the above ingredients into a fine powder and take 3 g each time orally with warm water or wine. It can also be modified into a decoction and in such a case, decoct 5 g of each ingredient in water. Take the decoction 2 times a day.

Analysis

Qiān Zhèng Sǎn takes advantage of *jiāng cán* and *quán xiē*, which are arthropod-based medicinals, to dispel external wind and dredge channels and collaterals, exerting stronger effects than general herbs. *Bái fù zǐ* is acrid and hot and its acrid-dispersing nature can be used to dispel wind and unblock collaterals. This pattern results from pathogenic wind obstructing the channels and collaterals that stagnates fluids into phlegm. Therefore, the phlegm and pathogenic wind mix together and become wind–phlegm, which is a substantial pathogen that blocks qi and blood flow and causes prolonged illness. The three ingredients are all excellent in expelling wind–phlegm. Although there are few ingredients in the formula, they exert significant effects. Ingredients are taken with warm wine to smooth blood vessels by the wine's diffusing and unblocking natures and to direct the effects of the medicinals to the face.

    Bái fù zǐ can calm the mind and relieve pain, while *quán xiē* and *jiāng cán* can relieve convulsions and calm the mind. This formula has effects on treating disorders of the nervous system.

Treatment reference

Qiān Zhèng Sǎn is specific in treating facial palsy, but it has also been applied to treat many diseases of the nervous system in modern practice, such as facial spasms, hemiplegia due to stroke, trigeminal neuralgia, migraines, and peripheral polyneuritis, achieiving favorable effects.

If wind obstructing the facial collaterals is accompanied by symptoms of heat, add *shēng dì*, *huáng qín*, or *shí gāo* to clear heat. If external wind is complicated by cold presenting an aversion to cold, an absence of sweating, and facial pain and cramps, add *fáng fēng*, *qiāng huó*, or *qín jiāo* to dispel wind. If external wind attacks the body with cold–damp presenting facial palsy and cramps, heaviness, cold pain, and numbness in the limbs, add *má huáng*, *fù zǐ*, or *guì zhī* to unblock channels, disperse cold, and remove dampness by warming. If the disease persists due to internal obstruction of phlegm stasis, add *chuān xiōng*, *dāng guī*, and *sháo yào* to harmonize blood and unblock collaterals. In order to strengthen this formula's effect on dispelling wind, unblocking collaterals, and relieving spasms, some wind-dispelling and spasm-relieving medicinals, such as *wú gōng*, *tiān má* and *dì long*, may also be added.

Cautions

Qiān Zhèng Sǎn is relatively warm-natured and is more applicable to the wind obstructing facial collaterals pattern with a cold nature. If there are signs of heat, e.g., red swellings behind the ear, a bitter taste in the mouth and a presence of thirst, it is inappropriate to prescribe this formula singly. This formula tends to impair body fluids due to its dry nature, so oral intake for a long period of time is strongly discouraged, especially for patients with yin deficiency and internal heat, and in this case, heat-clearing and blood-nourishing medicinals should be considered.

Daily Exercises

1. What are the main symptoms and signs of the wind obstructing facial collaterals pattern?
2. What are the ingredients of *Qiān Zhèng Sǎn*? How can it be modified according to different situations?
3. Mr. Shen is a 62-year-old male. Three days ago in the morning, he felt facial cramps and discomfort when he was outdoors but did not pay much attention. One hour later, he returned home and his family members found the corner of his mouth deviated to the right. He looked at himself in the mirror and also noticed a distortion in his labial groove and he could not close his left eye. His other symptoms and signs are

a mild aversion to wind, mild pain behind his left ear, leakage of soup from the mouth from one side when drinking, tears in the left eye, drooling, a thin and greasy tongue coating, and a thin and wiry pulse. Please prescribe a Chinese medicinal formula for this case.

DAY SIX

The Wind Attacking the Upper Body Pattern

Wind attacking the upper body refers to the attack of external wind on the head and causes disharmony of channels and inhibited clear yang. This pattern is commonly seen in headaches due to the common cold, migraines, and other kinds of headaches.

Pathogenic wind is characterized by a tendency in attacking the upper part of the body and mixing with other pathogens such as cold, heat, and dampness. Therefore, to be more specific, headaches triggered by wind attacking the upper body should be classified into patterns of wind–cold, wind–heat, and wind–damp. This section mainly focuses on the wind–cold pattern.

Diagnosis

The main symptoms and signs are headaches (at one side or at the top). Other indications include fever, an aversion to cold, a stuffy nose, loose nasal discharge, aching limbs, a thin and white tongue coating, and a floating pulse.

This pattern is resulted from exogenous wind–cold that attacks the head and obstructs the channels and collaterals, rendering inhibited qi and blood flow. The degree and location of each headache can be different, examples of which are dull pain, acute pain, continuous pain, relapsing and remitting pain, pain at one side, pain at the top of the head, non-fixed pain, or pain affecting the whole head. This type of headache usually aggravates after catching wind–cold. If wind–cold attacks the fleshy exterior, it will inhibit *wei* qi and show symptoms of the exterior pattern, such as fever, an aversion to cold, a stuffy nose, loose nasal discharge, or aching limbs.

As the wind pathogen often mix with other external pathogens, varying clinical pictures thus emerge. If it is complicated by a cold pathogen, the headache is acute and worsens when encountered with wind and cold, and there are accompanying symptoms of an aversion to cold and absence of sweating. If it is complicated by heat, the headache is distending and there are symptoms of thirst, a red tongue, and yellowish urine. If it is complicated by dampness, the headache comes with a heavy sensation and there are symptoms of chest and stomach stuffiness and oppression, nausea, and a greasy tongue coating.

Headaches are foremost a symptom of the exterior pattern, so the wind attacking the upper body pattern is closely related to the exterior pattern. However, the former considers headaches as a main symptom and discounts other exterior symptoms, while the exterior pattern takes an aversion to cold with fever as the main symptom with the symptom of headache demoted as a secondary indicator (i.e., it can be present or absent, and serious or mild).

Treatment method

Dispelling wind and unblocking the collaterals to relieve pain.

Formula and ingredients: Chuān Xiōng Chá Tiáo Sǎn (Tea-Mix and Chuanxiong Powder)

Chuān xiōng (Rhizoma Chuanxiong) 12 g; *jīng jiè* (Herba Schizonepetae) without stem 12 g; *bái zhǐ* (Radix Angelicae Dahuricae) 6 g; *qiāng huó* (Rhizoma et Radix Notopterygii) 6 g; *gān cǎo* (Radix et Rhizoma Glycyrrhizae) 6 g; *xì xīn* (Radix et Rhizoma Asari) without top 3 g; *fáng fēng* (Radix Saposhnikoviae) without top 4.5 g; *bò he* (Herba Menthae) 24 g.

Formula verse

Chuān Xiōng Chá Tiáo Sǎn applies *jīng fáng* and *xīn zhǐ bò he gān cǎo qiāng*. It frees the body from a stuffy nose, dizziness, wind attacking the upper body, and migraines.

Usage

Grind the ingredients into a fine powder, take 6 g orally each time, and follow up by drinking tea. Alternatively, add water to decoct, 2 times a day. If the headache is accompanied by an aversion to cold with fever and an absence of sweating, it is advisable to cover the body with sheets after taking the medicine to induce mild sweating.

Analysis

Chuān xiōng has a strong acrid taste and due to its potent aromatic piercing effect, it is excellent at unblocking collaterals and relieving pain, and is especially applicable to headaches at the top and the sides. *Qiāng huó*, greatly acrid-natured and wind-dispelling, is good at treating headaches at the back radiating to the neck, while *bái zhǐ*, acrid–warm and aromatic, is good for headaches at the forehead. A combination of the above three ingredients can be applied to different areas of the headache. *Xì xīn* also has a strong acrid taste and is penetrating, which is good for dispelling wind and unblocking collaterals, and is combined with *jīng jiè* and *fáng fēng* to dispel the wind pathogen in the head. *Bò he* is applied in large doses due to its acrid nature and wind-dispelling and head-resuscitating effects. Drinking of tea following the intake of medicinals can be explained by taking advantage of its bitter and cold natures for awakening the head and regulating channels, and preventing the warmth and dryness of other medicinals from consuming and impairing fluids.

Chuān xiōng has been demonstrated to be efficacious in dilating blood vessels, relieving spasms, calming the mind, and lowering blood pressure. *Fáng fēng*, *xì xīn*, *qiāng huó*, and *bái zhǐ* can relieve pain and fever to a certain extent, hence this formula is effective for headaches caused by fever or other factors.

Treatment reference

Chuān Xiōng Chá Tiáo Sǎn is mainly indicated for headaches of externally contracted diseases, but it is also applicable to headaches of internal damage with characteristics of pathogenic wind attacking the upper body.

Therefore, it is widely administered to treat headaches due to various infections or from angioneurotic sources. The headaches could have occurred recently or are chronic.

In practice, proper modification is required according to the pathogens complicated by external wind. In general, this formula is suitable to headaches with the wind–cold nature. If the symptoms of cold are significant, or there are cold limbs and a fear of cold, add some *má huáng* or cooked *fù zǐ*, and more *chuān xiōng*. If there are (heat) signs of thirst, red eyes, yellowish urine, and a red tongue, remove or reduce the dose of acrid–warm ingredients and add some *huáng qín, zhī zǐ, jú huā, màn jīng zǐ, bái jiāng cán*, and *sāng yè*, or use *Jú Huā Chá Tiáo Sǎn* (Tea-Mix and Chrysanthemum Powder). If it is accompanied by symptoms of dampness such as headaches with heaviness, chest and stomach stuffiness and fullness, fatigue, body heaviness, and a white and greasy tongue coating, add *dú huó, cāng zhú*, or *hòu pò*. If the headache lingers for a long time and is fixed at one point and stabbing, it is complicated by internal obstruction of phlegm stasis, so add *táo rén, hóng huā, chì sháo, quán xiē*, and *dì lóng* to dispel phlegm and stasis. The dosages of the chief ingredients can be modified according to the different areas of the headaches. For example, if the headache is mainly limited at the top of the head or at both sides, the dose of *chuān xiōng* can be increased and *chái hú* can be added. Clinical practice shows the importance of the use of *chuān xiōng*, especially for treating migraines. Regardless of external contraction or internal damage, this ingredient is often considered the key component in the formula. For instance, the dose of *chuān xiōng* in *Sàn Piān Tāng* (Migraine-Dispersing Decoction) is as large as 30 g. If the headache radiating to the neck is severe, add more *qiāng huó*. If the headache in the forehead is severe, add more *bái zhǐ*.

Cautions

Many factors can cause headaches, including those of internal damage, such as ascendant hyperactivity of liver yang, up-flaming of gallbladder fire, kidney water deficiency, deficiency of qi and blood, internal obstruction by phlegm–damp, and blockage of blood stasis, all of which are *not* indications of this formula. Most critically, if this formula is incorrectly applied to treat headaches due to internal exuberance of fire or deficiency, it will boost fire pathogens, stir wind, and impair yin. As a result, pattern differentiation must be precise and this formula should not be prescribed simply as a unique recipe for headaches without pattern differentiation.

Daily Exercises

1. What are the main symptoms and signs of the wind attacking the upper body pattern?
2. What are the ingredients of *Chuān Xiōng Chá Tiáo Sǎn*? How can medicinals be applied according to different areas of headaches?
3. Ms. Tan is a 36-year-old female. She has been suffering from migraines for about a decade which tend to occur in the winter or after catching wind and cold. During her episodes, there is no obvious point of tenderness, but she feels cold pain within the brain. It is accompanied by cold limbs, chest oppression, and nausea. Her tongue is pale with a thin and white coating, and she has a pulse that is thin and deep. Please prescribe a Chinese medicinal formula for this case.

Additional Formulae

Jú Huā Chá Tiáo Sǎn (Tea-Mix and Chrysanthemum Powder)

Chuān Xiōng Chá Tiáo Sǎn together with *jú huā* (Flos Chrysanthemi) 6 g; *jiāng cán* (Bombyx Batryticatus) 3 g. Decoct with water. Alternatively, make into a powder with proportional dosages; take 6 g each time, and then drink light tea.

Actions

Scattering wind and relieving pain; clearing heat from head and eyes.

Indications

Wind–heat affecting the head and eyes presenting migraines, dizziness, thirst, red eyes, and a red tongue tip.

Sàn Piān Tāng (Migraine-Dispersing Decoction)

Chuān xiōng (Rhizoma Chuanxiong) 30 g; *sháo yào* (Radix Paeoniae) 15 g; *yù lǐ rén* (Semen Pruni) 3 g; *chái hú* (Radix Bupleuri) 3 g; *gān cǎo* (Radix et Rhizoma Glycyrrhizae) 3 g; *bái jiè zǐ* (Semen Sinapis) 9 g; *xiāng fù* (Rhizoma Cyperi) 6 g; *bái zhǐ* (Radix Angelicae Dahuricae) 1.5 g. Add water to decoct.

Actions

Invigorating blood and unblocking collaterals; dispersing wind and relieving pain.

Indications

Migraines.

THE 8TH WEEK

DAY ONE

The Liver Yang Transforming into Wind Pattern

This pattern is characterized by the rising counterflow of hyperactive liver yang and internal stirring of liver wind due to the liver and kidney's failure to nourish the liver following yin and fluid insufficiencies and disharmony of yin and yang. This pattern pertains to an internal wind pattern. Internal stirring of liver wind is manifested as dizziness, headaches, numbness of limbs, even sudden unconsciousness, hemiplegia, convulsions, etc. Its symptoms are similar to those of an excess pattern, but since it is essentially caused by liver and kidney yin deficiency, this pattern is regarded as an excess–root and deficiency–branch pattern. This pattern is commonly seen in hypertension, hypertensive encephalopathy, cerebrovascular accidents, and certain types of epilepsy, mental disorders, neurosis, and so on.

Diagnosis

The main symptoms and signs of this pattern are dizziness or headaches, numbness or trembling of limbs, even sudden unconsciousness, twitches of limbs, or hemiplegia. Other indications may include difficulty in speech, blurred vision, unsteady walking, vexation, insomnia, and a wiry and thin pulse.

This pattern usually develops from the ascendant hyperactivity of liver yang, characteristics of which include dizziness, tinnitus, distending or throbbing pain in the head, which are aggravated after labor work or feeling angry, an occasional flushed face or a red face and eyes the whole day, impatience, irascibility, a bitter taste in the mouth, poor-quality sleep, dreaminess, and a red tongue with a yellow coating. This pattern is formed by the rising counterflow of liver wind, so when it affects the head, dizziness, headaches, and blurred vision are induced. The liver and kidney fail to moisten and nourish tendons, and together with liver wind disrupting the channels and collaterals, numbness or tremor of the limbs are resulted. The rising counterflow of liver wind can affect qi and blood flow, and hyperactive liver yang can concentrate fluids into phlegm. The liver wind together with phlegm may cloud the heart and cause sudden unconsciousness. Such a case is within the scope of wind–phlegm, which is similar to the wind–phlegm disturbing the upper body pattern (7th week, Day 1). However, in this pattern, the liver wind is severe and there are manifestations of liver yang exuberance and symptoms of affected tendons, channels, and collaterals, so it is not difficult to differentiate them. If wind–phlegm blocks the tongue root or one side of the channels and collaterals, there will be difficulty in speech or movement of one side of the body.

In diagnosis, clinical manifestations of liver yang transforming into wind should be noted. Some patients only present numbness of the fingers or tongue tip, or involuntary wriggling of fingers, while others can suffer from comas, spasms, and paralysis. All in all, this pattern generally signifies that the patient is in a critical condition, hence even if the initial state is mild and seemingly temporary, it should not be treated lightly. If ascendant hyperactivity of liver yang, numbness of fingers or the tongue tip, wriggling of fingers, and transient unconsciousness are observed, it is often a precursor of the stirring of wind, in which the patient must receive timely treatment. Contemporary tests of blood pressure, viscosity of blood, elasticity of blood vessels, and hemodynamics can be combined to diagnose stroke (wind stirring) as early as possible.

Treatment method

Calming and extinguishing liver wind, and boosting the liver and kidney.

Formula and ingredients: Tiān Má Gōu Téng Tāng (Gastrodia and Uncaria Decoction)

Tiān má (Rhizoma Gastrodiae) 9 g; *gōu téng* (Ramulus Uncariae Cum Uncis) 12 g added later; *shí jué míng* (Concha Haliotidis) 18 g decocted first; *zhī zǐ* (Fructus Gardeniae) 9 g; *huáng qín* (Radix Scutellariae) 9 g; *chuān niú xī* (Radix Cyathulae) 12 g; *dù zhòng* (Cortex Eucommiae) 9 g; *yì mǔ cǎo* (Herba Leonuri) 9 g; *sāng jì shēng* (Herba Taxilli) 9 g; *yè jiāo téng* (Caulis Polygoni Multiflori) 9 g; *fú shén* (Sclerotium Poriae Pararadicis) 9 g.

Formula verse

Tiān Má Gōu Téng Tāng uses *jué míng, zhī dù jì shēng xī huáng qín; yè téng fú shén yì mǔ cǎo*, and treats symptoms of internal stirring of liver wind.

Usage

Add 1.5 L of water to decoct until 300 mL are left. Take the decoction orally and add 1 L of water to decoct the dregs until 300 mL are left. Take the decoction warm, 2 times a day.

Analysis

Tiān má, gōu téng, and *shí jué míng*, the chief ingredients of this formula, extinguish liver wind. As the production of liver wind is related to hyperactive yang heat in the liver channel, this formula is combined with *zhī zǐ* and *huáng qín* to clear liver heat. Liver yang hyperactivity and the rising counterflow of liver wind in this pattern are both caused by liver and kidney deficiency, so *dù zhòng* and *sāng jì shēng* are used to boost the liver and kidney. This formula focuses on three aspects of treating liver yang transforming into wind: boosting the liver and kidney, clearing heat, and extinguishing wind. In addition, due to the existence of the ascendant hyperactivity of liver yang and the rising counterflow of wind–fire, *niú xī* is added to direct the counterflow of qi and blood downward. *Yè jiāo téng* and *fú shén* are applied to calm the mind. *Yì mǔ cǎo* also dredges blood vessels and can direct blood flow downward to strengthen the efficacy of *niú xī*.

Studies have shown that the decoction of this formula bears no effect on bringing down the blood pressure of a normal animal, but has a blood pressure-lowering effect on animals with hypertension. It indicates that this formula is effective for treating hypertension and furthermore, its efficacy is not only limited to reducing blood pressure.

Treatment reference

Tiān Má Gōu Téng Tāng is indicated for hypertension of liver yang hyperactivity and liver wind affecting the upper body. The effect of this formula is in accordance with the treatment principle for liver yang transforming into wind. However, its strength on extinguishing liver wind, pacifying liver yang, and supplementing the liver and kidney are generally weak, so it is in fact more applicable to mild cases of the liver yang transforming into wind pattern, consisting of symptoms such as dizziness, insomnia, vexation, and numbness of limbs. If the disease belongs to a serious case of liver yang transforming into wind, presenting unconsciousness, hemiplegia, cramps of four limbs, and tremors, using only this formula is not sufficient. It requires reinforcement for extinguishing liver wind. Hence, *dài zhě shí*, *líng yáng jiǎo*, *lóng gǔ*, or *mǔ lì* is added. If the effect of boosting the liver and kidney needs to be strengthened, *shēng dì*, *bái sháo*, *xuán shēn*, *tiān dōng*, *guī bǎn*, or *biē jiǎ* should be added. If internal heat is severe presenting thirst with massive consumption of fluids, and a red face and eyes, *shí gāo*, *lóng dǎn cǎo*, and so on should be added. If it belongs to a critical pattern of liver yang transforming into wind presenting unconsciousness and hemiplegia, prescribe *Zhèn Gān Xī Fēng Tāng* (Liver-Sedating and Wind-Extinguishing Decoction), which is indicated for the early stage of stroke with hot pain in the head, a red face and eyes, and vexing heat in the heart.

Cautions

Aside from liver yang transforming into wind and wind–phlegm affecting the upper body, many factors may contribute to symptoms of dizziness, headaches, and numbness of limbs, such as blood deficiency, phlegm–damp, and static blood. Thus, the formula must be applied according to accurate pattern differentiation. For the treatment of this pattern, dietary regulation must also be considered. The patient should consume light and bland foods, and avoid having acrid, sweet, and fatty foods, smoking cigarettes, and drinking alcohol. Always maintain a good mood, lead a healthy lifestyle, keep your temper under control, and do not overstrain.

Daily Exercises

1. What are the similarities and differences between the liver yang transforming into wind pattern and the ascendant hyperactivity of liver yang pattern in their pathologies and clinical manifestations?

2. What are the ingredients of *Tiān Má Gōu Téng Tāng*? What are its indications?
3. Mr. Zhao is a 58-year-old male. For 6 months, he often experiences vertigo, throbbing pain in the temporal region of both sides of the head, chest oppression, vexation, irascibility, and an occasional numbness of his fingers. He also dreams a lot in the sleep, has a red tongue edge and tip with a thin and white coating, and a wiry and slippery pulse. His blood pressure is recorded as 170/110 mmHg. Please prescribe a Chinese medicinal formula for this case.

Additional Formulae

Zhèn Gān Xī Fēng Tāng (Liver-Sedating and Wind-Extinguishing Decoction)

Niú xī (Radix Achyranthis Bidentatae) 30 g; raw *zhě shí* (Haematitum) 30 g; crushed *lóng gǔ* (Os Draconis) 15 g; raw *mǔ lì* (Concha Ostreae) 15 g; raw *guī bǎn* (Plastrum Testudinis) 15 g; raw *bái sháo* (Radix Paeoniae Alba) 15 g; *tiān dōng* (Radix Asparagi) 15 g; *xuán shēn* (Radix Scrophulariae) 15 g; *chuān liàn zǐ* (Fructus Toosendan) 6 g; raw *mài yá* (Fructus Hordei Germinatus) 6 g; *yīn chén* (Herba Artemisiae Scopariae) 6 g; *gān cǎo* (Radix et Rhizoma Glycyrrhizae) 4.5 g. Add water to decoct.

Actions

Calming the liver and extinguishing wind; nourishing yin and subduing yang.

Indications

Stroke presenting dizziness, a distending feeling in the eyes, tinnitus, hot pain in the head, vexing heat in the heart, a flushed facial complexion not unlike after drinking alcohol, belching, limbs with a gradual loss of control, a distorted mouth, consciousness restored soon after shock, sequelae after resuming consciousness, dispiritedness, and a wiry, long, and forceful pulse.

DAY TWO

The Liver Heat Stirring Wind Pattern

The liver heat stirring wind pattern results from exuberant fire–heat entering the liver channel and causing internal stirring of liver wind that is manifested as spasms of limbs. This pattern also belongs to the internal wind pattern. As pathogenic heat enters the liver channel, exuberant liver heat will inevitably influence the tendons controlled by the liver, causing cramps of tendons and convulsions and stiffness of limbs. Although body fluids in this pattern can be impaired by the exuberant fire–heat, the underlying cause of the disorder lies in pathogenic heat. Therefore, it is an excess pattern, or more specifically, an excess–wind pattern. This pattern is commonly seen at the peak stage of externally contracted febrile diseases, including epidemic encephalitis B, meningococal meningitis, cerebral malaria, various toxic encephalopathies, febrile convulsions, and so on.

Diagnosis

The main symptoms and signs of this pattern are high fever, trembling or continuous spasms, and stiffness. Other indications may include vexation, thirst, unconsciousness, lockjaw, upturned eyes, a deep red and dry tongue with a yellow/dark greyish or scorched/prickling coating, and a wiry and rapid pulse.

This pattern results from exuberant heat, so there must be high fever accompanied by vexation and thirst. The heat pathogen will burn the tendons and vessels, causing spasms or stiffness of limbs. Cases with relapsing and remitting periods are mild, while those occurring continuously without remission are critical ones with unfavorable prognosis. In episodes of spasms, it may be accompanied by unconsciousness, lockjaw, upturned eyes, and even opisthotonos (stiffness of the nape and back) with the body bending backward like a bow. High fever and cramps are the main symptoms of this pattern, by which the diagnosis of liver heat stirring wind can be made. A dry and red tongue with a yellow/dark greyish or scorched/prickling coating, and a wiry and rapid pulse are all signs of liver heat stirring wind.

The diagnosis of the liver heat stirring wind pattern should be distinguished from the deficiency–wind pattern at the late stage of externally contracted febrile diseases or from certain chronic diseases with blood deficiency or liver–kidney yin deficiency. The deficiency–wind pattern is characterized by low or no fever, dispiritedness, wriggling or slow twitches of the extremities, a dry and crimson or pale red tongue, and a weak and thin pulse, all of which are manifestations that can be easily differentiated from the internal stirring of liver wind pattern.

Treatment method

Cooling the liver and extinguishing wind.

Formula and ingredients: Líng Jiǎo Gōu Téng Tāng (Antelope Horn and Uncaria Decoction)

Líng yáng jiǎo (Cornu Saigae Tataricae) 4.5 g decocted first; *sāng yè* (Folium Mori) after frosty days 6 g; *chuān bèi mǔ* (Bulbus Fritillariae Cirrhosae) without the core 12 g; *shēng dì* (Radix Rehmanniae) 15 g; *gōu téng* (Ramulus Uncariae Cum Uncis) 9 g added later; *jú huā* (Flos Chrysanthemi) 9 g; *fú shén* (Sclerotium Poriae Pararadicis) 9 g; *bái sháo* (Radix Paeoniae Alba) 9 g; *gān cǎo* (Radix et Rhizoma Glycyrrhizae) 2.4 g; fresh *zhú rú* (Caulis Bambusae in Taenia) 15 g.

Formula verse

Líng Jiǎo Gōu Téng fú jú sāng, bèi cǎo zhú rú sháo dì huáng; for fire–heat exuberance triggering spasms, take immediately to treat internal stirring of liver wind.

Usage

Add 1.2 L of water to decoct *líng yáng jiǎo* and *zhú rú* first for 30 min. Remove the dregs and add the other ingredients to decoct until 400 mL are left. Take the decoction warm 2 times, 2–4 times a day. Alternatively, decoct *líng yáng jiǎo* slices and 300 mL of water with slow fire until 50 mL are left and then mix this decoction with the decoction of other medicinals. If the patient is unconscious, nasal feeding through a stomach tube can be used, but the insertion should be gentle lest spasms are induced.

Analysis

As exuberant heat is the main cause of internal stirring of liver wind, *líng yáng jiǎo* and *gōu téng* that can clear heat and cool the liver are incorporated as chief ingredients. *Sāng yè*, *jú huā*, *zhú rú*, and *shēng dì* are added to clear interior heat. Since the heat pathogen impairs fluids and fluid deficiency will deprive tendons and vessels of nourishment and worsen cramps, *bái sháo* is combined with *shēng dì* to nourish fluids and moisten tendons and vessels. The heat pathogen can also boil and concentrate fluids into phlegm and phlegm obstruction in the tendons makes the heat much more difficult to be removed, so *chuān bèi mǔ* is mixed with *zhú rú* to clear heat and dissolve phlegm. As the heat pathogen affects the mind, *fú shén* is used to calm the heart and mind.

In pharmalogical terms, *líng yáng jiǎo* and *gōu téng* can calm the mind, and relieve spasms and fever. *Shēng dì* can strengthen the heart, promote urination, and stop bleeding, while *bái sháo* has functions of relieving spasms, calming the mind, inhibiting bacteria, and promoting urination. Through a comprehensive effect on relieving spasms, fever, and decreasing intracranial pressure, this formula achieves the purpose of treating spasms due to exuberant heat.

Treatment reference

The liver heat stirring wind pattern is a critical pattern of febrile diseases, so measures must be taken to treat spasms without delay, or continuous spasms will lead to outward desertion of healthy qi that is fatal, or sequelae of paralysis, dementia, and blindness. Therefore, for the treatment of this pattern, aside from the prompt application of the above decoction, various spasm-relieving techniques should be carried out immediately, including acupuncture and moxibustion, physical cooling, and hospitalized treatment. As patients with spasms will often be unconscious, many Chinese patent medicines, such as *Zhì Bǎo Dān* (Supreme Jewel Elixir), *Zǐ Xuě Dān* (Purple Snow Elixir), and *Ān Gōng Niú Huáng Wán* (Peaceful Palace Bovine Bezoar Pill) are used together with this formula. The method of usage is as follows: each time, 1 pill should be infused with water and mixed with the decoction. It can also help awaken the mind and strengthen the effect of cooling the liver and extinguishing wind. If spasms persist, add *quán xiē*, *wú gong*, or *dì lóng* to enhance the spasm-relieving effect.

Although *Líng Jiǎo Gōu Téng Tāng* is established for exuberant heat stirring wind of externally contracted febrile diseases, it has efficacious properties on clearing heat, cooling the liver, and pacifying liver wind.

Cautions

Líng Jiǎo Gōu Téng Tāng is a classic formula for treating the excess–wind pattern. However, not all patterns of excess–wind can be treated exclusively by this formula; to prescribe *Líng Jiǎo Gōu Téng Tāng*, the disease must be stemmed from internal stirring of liver wind. The natures of various exuberant heat pathogens are different, including heat exuberance in the *yangming*, intestinal heat and bowel excess, and heat exuberance in the blood level, thus in order to achieve a favorable response on extinguishing wind and relieving spasms, methods of clearing and draining heat pathogens in the qi level, purging heat bind, and clearing heat to cool blood are often used in tandem.

Daily Exercises

1. What is the liver heat stirring wind pattern? What are its main symptoms and signs?
2. What are the ingredients of *Líng Jiǎo Gōu Téng Tāng*?
3. Mr. Zhang is a 16-year-old male. He has been having fever and headaches for 3 days. The fever has gradually worsened, with a burning sensation in the body and hands, restlessness, and extreme thirst triggering a compulsion for drinking cold water. His mouth odor is pungent and at certain times, he has also experienced unconsciousness. This afternoon, spasms suddenly occurred with symptoms of stiff extremities, lockjaw, and upturned pupils. They were relieved spontaneously several minutes later, but they relapsed again after 10 min. Other symptoms and signs are dry teeth, a red tongue with a dark greyish and dry coating with fissures, and a wiry, slippery, and rapid pulse. Please prescribe a Chinese medicinal formula for this case.

CHAPTER 9

The Qi Stagnation Pattern

DAY THREE

The qi stagnation pattern is a pattern of functional disorder caused by qi sluggishness in a part of the human body or in an organ. This pattern is a very common category in clinical practice, which can be observed either in externally contracted diseases or more often in diseases of internal damage.

Formation of Qi Stagnation

Qi is the manifestation of various functions of the human body. It is an essential substance, full of vigor, which flows all over the system, stimulates organs and tissues to perform their normal activities, and manages and induces blood circulation. The normal flow of qi is called qi movement. Only through the movement and nourishment of qi can the human body be sustained, grow, and defend against exogenous pathogens.

The movements of various qi are restricted to certain rules. For example, liver qi and spleen qi tend to ascend, stomach qi and intestinal qi tend to descend, while lung qi is for respiration — not only required to ascend and diffuse, but also to purify and descend. If normal qi movement is hindered, it will bring about diseases, manifesting as the qi stagnation pattern. It is thus evident that the qi stagnation pattern is caused when qi flow is inhibited. In addition, if qi that should ascend descends instead, or vice versa, it can also result in disorders. Factors that can affect qi movement are extensive, but the most important causes are the seven emotions, especially excessive anxiety, grief, and anger, all of which can inhibit qi movement and induce *zang–fu* hypofunctions. Moreover, pathological products of the body, such as water–dampness, phlegm–rheum, static blood, dry feces, and food stagnation, will inevitably block qi movement. Qi deficiency can also contribute to the weak force of qi flow, and thus it is accompanied by qi stagnation. For externally contracted febrile diseases, the constraint of heat may also cause qi stagnation. Therefore, a pattern that purely encompasses qi stagnation is rarely seen.

Features of the Qi Stagnation Pattern

Various parts of the *zang–fu* organs may be afflicted with qi stagnation, but their clinical manifestations have some common features — regions of qi stagnation will present distention, fullness, and pain, and is usually delocalized; the disease state is at times mild and at other times serious; and it is often closely related to emotional variations. The following factors can be concurrently taken into account during diagnosis: emotional fluctuations prior to the disease, symptoms of chest oppression, sighing, belching, frequent flatus, and a comfortable feeling after belching or farting.

Once the qi stagnation is initiated, it will become a pathological factor that affects the normal functions of the human body. For example, qi stagnation can influence the absorption, distribution, and discharge of body fluids, rendering water–dampness or phlegm–rheum. If qi stagnation influences blood flow, it leads to static blood. If it affects bowel movement, it will result in dry feces. Thus, qi stagnation and pathological products of water–dampness, phlegm–rheum, static blood, and dry feces are mutually the cause and result. They often occur simultaneously in the clinic, and in such cases, it is no longer a pure qi stagnation pattern.

Categories of the Qi Stagnation Pattern

The qi stagnation pattern is classified into many categories according to the location, nature, and degree of qi stagnation. Table 1 shows a summary of classification by location and nature. This section discusses the diagnosis and treatment of the liver and spleen qi stagnation pattern, qi

Table 1. Several categories of the qi stagnation pattern.

Location	Qi constraint in the liver channel
	Qi constraint in the liver and spleen
	Qi stagnation in the chest
	Qi stagnation in the lower body
	Spleen–stomach qi stagnation
	Lung qi stagnation
	Ascending counterflow of stomach qi
Nature	Dampness obstruction and qi stagnation
	Qi stagnation and blood stasis
	Binding obstruction of phlegm and qi
	Cold congealing and qi stagnation
	Yangming bowel
	Food and qi stagnation

stagnation in the chest pattern, and qi stagnation in the lower body pattern.

Treatment Methods of the Qi Stagnation Pattern

The key principle of treating the qi stagnation pattern is the rectification of the movement of qi. Rectifying qi means to free qi movement. Most medicinals that can rectify qi are acrid–warm and aromatic, which are potent in promoting digestion, stimulating smooth muscles, relieving spasms and pain, and have effects on regulating the digestive, cardiovascular, and nervous systems. In terms of locations, natures, and complicated pathogens of qi stagnation, methods of rectifying qi are various, including soothing the liver to rectify qi, soothing the liver and spleen, moving qi to resolve phlegm, soothing the liver to dispel cold, moving qi to resolve dampness, and lowering qi to reverse counterflow.

In application, the causes of qi stagnation must be considered. If it is caused by internal obstruction of qi movement, methods of removing stasis should be taken into account. If it results from cold congealing, methods of warming to unblock stagnation and dispel cold should be used together. If it is due to qi deficiency, boosting qi is a requisite. Solely applying qi-rectifying medicinals when there is qi stagnation is discouraged, as the targeted curative effect will not materialize. In addition, as qi-rectifying medicinals are acrid–warm and aromatic, they often cause dryness. Improper application tends to consume and impair body fluids, so it is not advisable to use them in large doses and for a long time. This is particularly pertinent to pregnant women, the elderly, or patients with yin deficiency.

Daily Exercises

1. How does the qi stagnation pattern develop?
2. What are the clinical features of the qi stagnation pattern?
3. What does it mean to rectify qi? What are the precautions to be noted when applying this method?

DAY FOUR

The Liver and Spleen Qi Stagnation Pattern

The liver and spleen qi stagnation pattern is a pattern of liver–spleen dysfunction caused by emotional constraints or latent pathogens that result in the inhibited flow of liver and spleen qi or by blood consumption in the liver that drives the counterflow of liver qi. This pattern can be seen in both externally contracted diseases and in diseases of internal damage. The liver governs the free flow of qi movement, so regardless of the seven emotions or external pathogens, if the liver's functions are affected, qi stagnation will be resulted. Furthermore, liver yin and blood deficiencies will trigger the loss of nourishment of liver qi and lead to the manifestation of exuberance, contributing to the counterflow of liver qi. Both liver qi constraint and counterflow can invade the spleen and stomach, rendering qi constraint and dysfunction of the spleen and stomach, a pathological change called "liver wood restricting earth," or briefly as "wood restricting earth." The liver and spleen qi stagnation pattern is primarily a pattern of wood restricting earth. This pattern is commonly seen in neurosis, anicteric hepatitis, chronic hepatitis, chronic cholecystitis, chronic gastritis, chronic enteritis, intercostal neuralgia, and so on.

Diagnosis

The main symptoms and signs of this pattern are chest and rib-side distention and fullness or delocalized pain, and gastric stuffiness. Other indications may include fever, cold limbs, belching, sighing, frequent flatus, feeling more comfortable after belching and farting, coughing, palpitations, inhibited urination, abdominal pain, diarrhea with the sensation of incomplete defecation, abdominal pain temporarily relieved after episodes of diarrhea, a thin and white tongue coating, and a wiry pulse.

The root cause of this pattern is the constraint or counterflow of liver qi, and as the liver channel runs along the chest and rib sides, there will be chest and rib-side distention and fullness or delocalized pain. Spleen and stomach qi stagnation causes gastric oppression or distention, or belching, sighing, frequent flatus, and feeling more at ease after belching and farting. As qi movement is stagnated and yang qi is blocked in the interior and fails to reach the extremities, the four limbs become cold. In externally contracted febrile diseases, this pattern may present hot sensations in the chest and abdomen, but not warmth in the four limbs, so it is also termed "counterflow cold of the four limbs." However, it is completely different from the counterflow cold of the four limbs due to yang qi declination, because the former belongs to heat syncope, while the latter pertains to cold syncope. Due to qi constraint in the liver and spleen, the spleen fails to transport and convert food substances, so abdominal pain and diarrhea occur. This type of diarrhea is usually accompanied by a sensation of incomplete defecation, or with abdominal urgency with rectal heaviness, and abdominal pain relieved after diarrhea, which is a sign of liver and spleen qi stagnation. A wiry pulse is a typical manifestation of qi stagnation.

In the past, the presence of counterflow cold of the four limbs in this pattern was emphasized, but not all patients may present this sign. Some may experience a feverish feeling in the palms and soles and a mild aversion to cold in the afternoon, which are also signs of internal constraint of yang qi and can serve as a reference for the diagnosis of this pattern.

Treatment method

Soothe the liver and rectify the spleen.

Formula and ingredients: Sì Nì Sǎn (*Frigid Extremities Powder*)

Dry-fried *gān cǎo* (Radix et Rhizoma Glycyrrhizae) 6 g; opened, soaked, and dry-fried *zhǐ shí* (Fructus Aurantii Immaturus) 6 g; *chái hú* (Radix Bupleuri) 6 g; *sháo yào* (Radix Paeoniae) 9 g.

Formula verse

Sì Nì Sǎn uses *chái hú*, *sháo yào zhǐ shí* and *gān cǎo;* specialized in treating counterflow cold of the four limbs due to yang constraint; it removes all constraint, stagnation, and counterflow by dredging.

Usage

Grind the ingredients into a fine powder. Take the powder orally with water, 1.5–3 g each time, 3 times a day. Alternatively, proportional doses of the above ingredients can be decocted in 1.2 L of water.

Analysis

Treatment of the liver and spleen qi stagnation pattern mainly involves soothing liver qi, hence in this formula, *chái hú* relieves constraint and stagnation by venting pathogens and raising yang, and soothes liver qi, being the chief medicinal. *Zhǐ shí* is added to cease qi constraint and is excellent in lowering qi. Its descent with *chái hú*'s ascent can restore normal qi movement. *Sháo yào* can nourish blood and supplement liver yin. Liver qi will be nourished when liver yin is sufficient, which is called "softening the liver," and can be supplemented with qi-freeing medicinals. *Zhì gān cǎo* is sweet and warm, which serves to boost the spleen and stomach. When the transportation and conversion functions of the spleen and stomach are restored, qi movement can be freed from stagnation. Although there are only four ingredients in the formula, it is efficacious in raising, lowering, supplementing, and purging, which can resolve qi constraint, soothe qi and blood, and spread yang qi.

According to modern pharmacological studies, *chái hú* and *sháo yào* can calm the mind and relieve pain, and are effective in treating various neuralgias and inhibiting bacteria and viruses. The combination of *chái hú* and *gān cǎo* is effective in protecting the liver. *Zhǐ shí* can stimulate the smooth muscles and promote gastrointestinal peristalsis. Studies in recent years have shown that the *zhǐ shí* preparation can increase blood pressure to prevent shock and clinically, it has been proven that it is curative in treating patients with heat syncope accompanied by cold limbs and a burning sensation in the chest and abdomen at the early stage of shock. This formula is also antibacterial and anti-inflammatory.

Treatment reference

Sì Nì Sǎn is a basic formula for rectifying liver–spleen qi movement and enhancing qi movement of the whole body. The counterflow cold of the four limbs can either be caused by nervous disorders of internal damage or by shock at the early stage of externally contracted febrile diseases, both of which can be treated by this formula. In addition, *Sì Nì Sǎn* can be applied to cure the liver–spleen qi stagnation pattern without the presence of counterflow cold of the four limbs. Clinically, this formula is applicable to chronic gastritis, intestinal spasms, hepatitis, cirrhosis, cholecystitis, gallbladder stones, hernia, intercostal neuralgia, bacillary dysentery, infectious dysentery, infectious shock, acute mammitis without pus, distending pain in the breasts, dysmenorrhea, amenorrhea, chronic adnexitis, hysteric syncope, and various neuroses.

In practice, proper modification according to the disease state is required and from which, many other qi-rectifying prescriptions are formulated. If it is accompanied by coughing, add *wǔ wèi zǐ* and *gān jiāng*. If there are palpitations, add *guì zhī*. If there is inhibited urination, add *fú líng* and *chē qián zǐ*. For cold abdominal pain, add cooked *fù zǐ*. For diarrhea with abdominal urgency and rectal heaviness, add *xiè bái* and *mù xiāng*. For liver qi constraint complicated with liver blood deficiency and failure of the spleen to transport and convert food, presenting rib-side pain, alternating chills and fever, headaches, dizziness, a dry mouth and throat, irregular menstruation, breast distention before menstruation, and a deficient and wiry pulse, remove *zhǐ shí* and add *dāng guī*, *bái zhú*, *fú líng*, *bò he*, and *shēng jiāng*, becoming *Xiāo Yáo Săn* (Free Wanderer Powder). For postpartum rib-side pain with alternating chills and fever or acute anicteric hepatitis, remove *zhǐ shí* and add *zhǐ qiào*, *chén pí*, *chuān xiōng*, and *xiāng fù*, becoming *Chái Hú Shū Gān Săn* (Bupleurum Liver-Soothing Powder), which can strengthen the effect of soothing the liver, rectifying qi, harmonizing blood, and unblocking collaterals.

Cautions

Tough *Sì Nì Săn* contains yin- and blood-supplementing ingredients; its focus is on dredging qi movement. Therefore, it is not advisable to apply this formula exclusively to treat qi stagnation due to qi deficiency in case of further consumption of healthy qi.

Daily Exercises

1. How does the liver and spleen qi stagnation pattern develop? What are its main symptoms and signs?
2. What are the ingredients of *Sì Nì Săn*? What is/are the action(s) of each ingredient?
3. Ms. Shan is a 48-year-old female. She has been suffering from chronic cholecystitis for many years. For the past 3 days, she has been experiencing rib-side pain together with paroxysmal abdominal pain, borborygmus, right rib-side pain extending to the back and left rib side, and distention in the stomach. She has a fairly red tongue with a thin and white coating, and a thin and wiry pulse. Please prescribe a Chinese medicinal formula for this case.

Additional Formulae

Xiāo Yáo Săn (*Free Wanderer Powder*)

Chái hú (Radix Bupleuri) 30 g; slightly dry-fried *dāng guī* (Radix Angelicae Sinensis) 30 g; *bái sháo* (Radix Paeoniae Alba) 30 g; *bái zhú* (Rhizoma Atractylodis Macrocephalae) 30 g; skinless *fú líng* (Poria) 30 g; *zhì gān căo* (Radix et Rhizoma Glycyrrhizae Praeparata cum Melle) 15 g.

   Grind into a fine powder and infuse 6–12 g each time with a bit of ginger and peppermint, 3 times a day. Alternatively, prepare the ingredients into pills for oral intake 6–9 g a time, 2 times a day, or decoct the ingredients with water using 20% of the original dosages.

Actions

Soothing the liver and resolving constraint; boosting the spleen and rectifying menstruation.

Indications

Liver constraint and blood deficiency presenting rib-side pain, alternating chills and fever, headaches, dizziness, a dry mouth and throat, mental fatigue, a poor appetite, irregular menstruation, breast distention before menstruation, a pale red tongue, and a deficient and wiry pulse.

Chái Hú Shū Gān Sǎn (Bupleurum Liver-Soothing Powder)

Vinegar-fried *chén pí* (Pericarpium Citri Reticulatae) 6 g; *chái hú* (Radix Bupleuri) 6 g; *chuān xiōng* (Rhizoma Chuanxiong) 4.5 g; *xiāng fù* (Rhizoma Cyperi) 4.5 g; *zhǐ qiào* (Fructus Aurantii) 4.5 g; *sháo yào* (Radix Paeoniae) 4.5 g; *zhì gān cǎo* (Radix et Rhizoma Glycyrrhizae Praeparata cum Melle) 1.5 g. Add water to decoct.

Actions

Soothing the liver and moving qi; harmonizing blood and relieving pain.

Indications

Rib-side pain, alternating chills and fever, gastric stuffiness and a poor appetite.

DAY FIVE

The Qi Stagnation in the Chest Pattern

This pattern occurs when yang qi in the chest lacks vigor and there is qi constraint in the same region. It is often seen in diseases of internal damage. Yang qi in the chest is related to heart and lung qi. If the function of the heart and lung becomes irregular, it is usually manifested as depressed chest yang qi, which can not only cause inhibited qi flow in the chest, but also lead to pathological changes such as the production of yin-cold qi, phlegm–turbidity obstruction in the middle, and congealing of static blood. Hence, this pattern is often complicated by such symptoms. This pattern is apparent in coronary disease, acute and chronic gastritis, ulcers, cholecystopathy, chest neuralgia, and some pulmonary diseases.

Diagnosis

The main symptoms and signs of this pattern are chest pain, fullness and oppression, with the possible spreading of the pain to the back. Other indications may include shortness of breath, panting, a sensation of gas running from the rib side to the heart, a white and greasy tongue coating, and a deep and wiry or deep and tight pulse.

This pattern falls into the scope of chest *bì* in Chinese medicine. As yang qi in the chest is not vigorous, qi movement in that area is inhibited and obstructed. The obstruction of qi movement causes chest pain, fullness, and oppression. Furthermore, as the organs and tissues in the chest are not warmed by yang qi, cold exuberance in the interior is resulted. Yang qi stagnation prevents fluids from being transported, transformed, and distributed, so phlegm is easily produced. Binding obstruction of the phlegm, cold, and qi blocks blood vessels and engenders static blood. If qi stagnation is complicated by phlegm and static blood, the blockage is much more severe and the chest pain will worsen and spread to the back or left shoulder. Due to chest yang qi blockage and together with phlegm–turbidity obstruction in the middle, the lung loses its normal functions of diffusing and descending, presenting shortness of breath, panting, or chest oppression. The ascending counterflow of gas in the rib side is a sign of abnormal qi movement. A white and greasy tongue coating and a deep and wiry or deep and tight pulse are signs of phlegm–turbidity obstruction in the middle and exuberance of cold in the interior.

Pain in the chest in this pattern can be located in the precordium, in the middle of chest, or in the rib sides. Regardless of the region, pain spreading to the back is the key indicator for pattern differentiation. The pain may either radiate to the left or right shoulder. Generally, precordium pain radiating to the left back and left shoulder is often a sign of angina in coronary disease, while right rib-side pain involving the right back and right shoulder is usually a sign of biliary colic due to cholecystitis or gallbladder stones.

Treatment method

Unblocking chest yang by warming, moving qi, and resolving phlegm.

Formula and ingredients: Guā Lóu Xiè Bái Bàn Xià Tāng (Trichosanthes, Chinese Chive, and Pinellia Decoction)

Guā lóu (Fructus Trichosanthis) 15 g; *xiè bái* (Bulbus Allii Macrostemi) 9 g; *bàn xià* (Rhizoma Pinelliae) 9 g; some white wine.

Formula verse

Guā Lóu Xiè Bái Bàn Xià Tāng is a formula with wine. It unblocks yang, regulates qi, and disperses masses; when there is chest *bì* or heart pain, apply it immediately.

Usage

Add 1.4 L of water to decoct until 600 mL are left. Remove the dregs and take the decoction warm, 200 mL each time, 3 times a day. White wine used in this formula is usually rice wine and its dose is 30–60 mL. If the patient refuses to drink wine, its dose can be reduced or it can be entirely removed.

Analysis

This pattern is mainly caused by depressed chest yang and qi movement obstruction in the chest, so *guā lóu* is applied to enhance qi, resolve phlegm, soothe the chest, and disperse masses. *Xiè bái* and *bàn xià*, both acrid–warm, are combined to unblock yang qi by warming, dissipating masses, and relieving pain. *Bàn xià* assists *guā lóu* in resolving phlegm. White wine is added to dredge qi and blood, invigorate chest yang by warming, and strengthen the effects of other ingredients. As a whole, this formula can unblock stagnation by warming, dispelling phlegm, and dissipating masses, hence it is more applicable to qi stagnation with exuberant phlegm–turbidity of chest *bì*.

Pharmacologically speaking *guā lóu* can relieve inflammation, dispel phlegm, and relax bowels, and is especially effective at dilating coronary arteries and capillaries and bringing down blood fat levels. It has definite curative effects on treating coronary sclerosis. *Xiè bái*, *bàn xià*, and white wine can enhance the effect of dilating blood vessels.

Treatment reference

Diseases treated by *Guā Lóu Xiè Bái Bàn Xià Tāng* usually involve the heart, lung, liver, gallbladder, and stomach. This formula is widely applied to cure bronchial asthma, coronary disease, costal neuralgia, acute and chronic cholecystitis, chronic hepatitis, acute and chronic gastritis, gastric and duodenal ulcers (especialy ulcers at the back wall of the stomach), and so on.

In practice, proper modification is required. For coronary disease or complication of static blood, add *dān shēn*, *chì sháo*, *dāng guī*, *hóng huā*, *chuān xiōng*, or *jiàng xiāng* to move qi and invigorate blood. For acute pain, add *rǔ xiāng, mò yào*, *tán xiāng*, or *yán hú suǒ*. If it is accompanied by coughing, add *xìng rén*, *mǎ dōu ling*, or *pí pá yè*. For chest and rib-side distention and fullness, add *yù jīn*, prepared *xiāng fù*, or *zhǐ qiào*. For severe phlegm–turbidity presenting a feeling of gas rushing upward from the rib side or severe chest oppression, shortness of breath, and a turbid and greasy tongue coating, add *guì zhī* and *zhǐ qiào*, or use *Zhǐ Shí Xiè Bái Guì Zhī Tāng* (Immature Bitter Orange, Chinese Chive, and Cinnamon Twig Decoction). For spitting of yellow sputum, a bitter taste in the mouth, a yellow and greasy tongue coating, and a slippery and rapid pulse, all of which are signs of constrained phlegm transforming into heat, add ginger-processed *tiān nán xīng*, *tiān zhú huáng*, *zhú rú*, or *huáng lián* to clear and dissolve hot phlegm. For severe chest oppression and pain, Chinese patent medicines can be combined. For example, *Sū Hé Xiāng Wán* (Storax Pill), 1 pill each time; *Sū Bīn Dī Wán* (Styrax and Borneol Drop Pill), 2–3 pills each time, 2 times a day; or *Shè Xiāng Bǎo Xīn Wán*

(Moschus Heart-Protecting Pill), 1–2 pills each time can be taken when the pain occurs.

Cautions

Chest *bì* consists of many patterns. If a pale complexion, palpitations, shortness of breath, apparent headaches, fatigue, a tongue bearing tooth marks, and an irregular pulse, which usually belong to a deficiency pattern, are observed, this formula is not appropriate. If angina remains after applying the previous therapies, myocardial infarction may occur and the patient is advised to visit a doctor.

Daily Exercises

1. What are the clinical features of the qi stagnation in the chest pattern?
2. What is the function of *Guā Lóu Xiè Bái Bàn Xià Tāng*? What are the precautions during its application?
3. Mr. Peng is a 46-year-old male. He has had angina of coronary disease for more than a decade. In recent years, its occurrences have become more frequent. In the most recent episode, it is accompanied by chest oppression, palpitations, shortness of breath, coughing, massive spitting of sputum, profuse sweating, dysphoria, inhibited bowel movement, and a wiry and slippery pulse. Please prescribe a Chinese medicinal formula for this case.

Additional Formulae

Zhǐ Shí Xiè Bái Guì Zhī Tāng (Immature Bitter Orange, Chinese Chive, and Cinnamon Twig Decoction)

Zhǐ shí (Fructus Aurantii Immaturus) 12 g; *hòu pò* (Cortex Magnoliae Officinalis) 12 g; *xiè bái* (Bulbus Allii Macrostemi) 9 g; *guì zhī* (Ramulus Cinnamomi) 3 g; *guā lóu* (Fructus Trichosanthis) 12 g. Add water to decoct.

Actions

Unblocking yang and dissipating masses; dispelling phlegm and lowering qi.

Indications

Chest *bì* with qi-binding in the chest presenting chest oppression, fullness and pain, gas rising from the rib side to the heart, a white and greasy tongue coating, and a deep, wiry, or tight pulse.

DAY SIX

The Qi Stagnation in the Lower Body Pattern

The qi stagnation in the lower body pattern refers to the stagnation of qi in the lower abdomen and genitals presenting swellings and pain. This pattern is related to the liver channel, because the liver channel runs along both sides of the lower abdomen and its collaterals are connected to the genitals. Besides having a direct association with the liver channel, the formation of this pattern is often related to cold and damp pathogens because binding of qi stagnation and cold–damp obstructs the lower part of the liver channel. Both this pattern and the liver–spleen qi stagnation pattern discussed in the previous section involve the disorder of the liver channel, although the disease location, complicating pathogen, and symptoms are different. This pattern often occurs in diseases of internal damage, and is much more common in acute and chronic inflammation of the testicle, spermatic cord, and adnexa (in women), hernia, and intestinal colic.

Diagnosis

The main symptom of this pattern are pain in the lower abdomen or its sides, radiating to the testicles, or swelling testicles. Other indications may include lower abdominal distention, aching pain, a cold appearance, a fear of cold, a pale tongue with a white coating, and a deep and slow or thin and wiry pulse.

This is a pattern of hernia. Hernia in Chinese medicine is defined as the projection of body contents out of body surface (such as the abdominal wall, groin, and scrotum) with pain, swellings, suppuration, or turbid exudates of the genitals, and acute pain in the lower abdomen with inhibited urination and defecation. These diseases are all in relation to cold congealing in the liver channel and qi stagnation. Blocked channel qi leads to pain in the lower abdomen that may spread to the testicles, or the testicles may prolapse with swelling and pain. Lower abdominal distention, a cold appearance, and a fear of cold are all caused by internal exuberance of cold and liver qi constraint and stagnation.

Treatment method

Moving qi and soothing the liver; dispelling cold and relieving pain.

Formula and ingredients: Tiān Tái Wū Yào Sǎn (Tiantai's Linderae Powder)

Wū yào (Radix Linderae) 6 g; *mù xiāng* (Radix Aucklandiae) 6 g; *xiǎo huí xiāng* (Fructus Foeniculi) 6 g; *qīng pí* (Pericarpium Citri Reticulatae Viride) 6 g; *gāo liáng jiāng* (Rhizoma Alpiniae Officinarum) 6 g; *bīng láng* (Semen Arecae) 9 g; *chuān liàn zǐ* (Fructus Toosendan) 12 g; *bā dòu* (Fructus Crotonis) 70 pieces.

Formula verse

Tiān Tái Wū Yào is formed by grinding *liàn huí xiāng*, *liáng jiāng bā dòu*, and *bīng láng*, and also *qīng pí* and *mù xiāng*, good for hernia due to cold stagnation and qi obstruction.

Usage

Crush *bā dòu* slightly and fry it with *chuān liàn zǐ* and wheat bran (scorched). Remove *bā dòu* and wheat bran, and add the other ingredients to be ground into powder. Take the powder 3 g each time orally with warm wine. Alternatively, fry *bā dòu* and *chuān liàn zǐ* (scorched), and remove *bā dòu*. Decoct *chuān liàn zǐ* with the other ingredients and water. Add a suitable amount of yellow wine in the decoction for oral intake.

Analysis

As this pattern is caused by cold congealing and qi stagnation in the liver channel, acrid–warm *wū yào* moves qi, disperses cold, and dredges the liver, being the chief ingredient. Warm, hot, and aromatic medicinals, such as *mù xiāng*, *qīng pí*, *gāo liáng jiāng*, and *xiǎo huí xiāng* are added to strengthen the effect of *wū yào*. The unique point of this formula lies in the combination of bitter–cold *chuān liàn zǐ* and extremely acrid and hot *bā dòu*. In usage, these two ingredients are fried together and then *bā dòu* is removed. In this way, the liver-dredging and qi-benefiting effects of *chuān liàn zǐ* are made used of, while its bitter and cold natures are suppressed. At the same time, it also absorbs the quick unblocking and mass dispersing effects of *bā dòu*, enhancing this formula's effect on dredging the liver and benefiting qi. *Bīng láng* can unblock the lower body and also functions to move qi and resolve stagnation.

According to current research, *wū yào*, *gāo liáng jiāng*, *xiǎo huí xiāng*, and *mù xiāng* contain various volatile oils and are potent in promoting intestinal peristalsis and relieving pain. *Chuān liàn zǐ* contains volatile fatty acids and has good pain-relieving effects as well. Therefore, this formula is well suited for diseases involving pain.

Treatment reference

Diseases treated by *Tiān Tái Wū Yào Sǎn* are often related to the reproductive system, such as testitis, spermatitis, hydrocele of testis, hernia of the small intestine, and adnexitis. In addition, it is suitable for some intestinal spasms and colic. All these diseases must pertain to cold congealing and qi stagnation.

As the qi stagnation in the lower body pattern is mainly due to cold congealing and qi stagnation, the treatment should be centered on rectifying liver qi and dispersing cold. In practice, flexible modification of the ingredients is necessary according to the state of cold congealing and qi stagnation. For severe qi stagnation with scattered pain without a fixed location at both sides of the lower abdomen, or radiating downward to the genitals, add *lì zhī hé* and *jú hé*. If cold congealing is severe and there is cold pain in the lower abdomen or genitals, add *wú zhū yú*, *ròu guì*, *bì bá*, and *fù zǐ*. If the disease is presented with static blood accumulation, leading to lower abdominal hardness, fullness, and pain, add *táo rén*, *hóng huā*, or *tǔ biē chóng* to invigorate blood and dissolve stasis as well as *kūn bù* and *hǎi zǎo* to soften hardness and dissolve masses. For this pattern, some Chinese patent medicines are also applicable. For instance, *Jú Hé Wán* (Tangerine Seed Pill) can be taken on an empty stomach with warm wine or light salty soup 6–9 g each time, 2 times a day. *Huí Xiāng Jú Hé Wán* (Fennel and Tangerine Seed Pill) can be taken 6–9 g each time, 2 times a day.

Cautions

There are many reasons that can account for the lower abdominal pain, among which are usually the inflammation of organs and tissues, tract obstruction, or spasms. If it pertains to damp–heat and heat toxins, do not prescribe *Tiān Tái Wū Yào Sǎn* and acrid–warm formulae. The presence of pathogenic heat typically presents abdominal pain aggravated by palpations, abdominal hardness, or genital pain, and swellings and a feverish sensation, by which it can be differentiated.

Daily Exercises

1. What are the clinical manifestations of the qi stagnation in the lower body pattern? What is its relation to hernia?
2. What are the ingredients of *Tiān Tái Wū Yào Sǎn*? What are its indications?
3. Mr. Shen is a 42-year-old male. Two days ago, he felt progressive pain in his left lower abdomen that gradually spread to the groin and testicle of the same side. There was tenderness in the left lower abdomen and it was accompanied by soreness and distention. There was a mild aversion to cold but his body temperature was normal. Other signs are a normal tongue with a white coating and a deep thin and wiry pulse. Please prescribe a Chinese medicinal formula for this case.

Additional Formulae

Jú Hé Wán (Tangerine Seed Pill)

Dry-fried *jú hé* (Semen Citri Reticulatae) 30 g, *hǎi zǎo* 30 g; *kun bù* 30 g; *hǎi dài cǎo* (Herba Zosterae Marinae); *chuān liàn zǐ* (Fructus Toosendan) 30 g; wheat bran-fried *táo rén* (Semen Persicae) 30 g; ginger-fried *hòu pò* (Cortex Magnoliae Officinalis) without rough skin 15 g; *chuān mù tōng*

(Caulis Clematidis Armandii) 15 g; wheat bran-fried *zhǐ shí* (Fructus Aurantii Immaturus) 15 g; dry-fried *yán hú suǒ* (Rhizoma Corydalis) 15 g; *ròu guì* (Cortex Cinnamomi) 15 g; *mù xiāng* (Radix Aucklandiae) 15 g.

Grind the ingredients into powder and make into small pills with wine. Take the pills 9 g each time on an empty stomach with wine or light salty soup, 2 times a day.

Actions

Moving qi to relieve pain, softening hardness, and dissipating masses.

Indications

Testicle swelling, a dragging sensation, stone-like hardness, or umbilicus and abdominal pain.

Huí Xiāng Jú Hé Wán (Fennel and Tangerine Seed Pill)

Salt-fried *xiǎo huí xiāng* (Fructus Foeniculi) 40 g; *bā jiǎo huí xiāng* (Fructus Anisi Stellati) 40 g; salt-fried *jú hé* (Semen Citri Reticulatae) 40 g; *lì zhī hé* (Semen Litchi) 80 g; salt-fried *bǔ gǔ zhī* (Fructus Psoraleae) 20 g; *ròu guì* (Cortex Cinnamomi) 16 g; *chuān liàn zǐ* (Fructus Toosendan) 80 g; vinegar-prepared *yán hú suǒ* (Rhizoma Corydalis) 40 g; vinegar-prepared *é zhú* (Rhizoma Curcumae) 20 g; *mù xiāng* (Radix Aucklandiae) 20 g; vinegar-prepared *xiāng fù* (Rhizoma Cyperi) 40 g; vinegar-prepared *qīng pí* (Pericarpium Citri Reticulatae Viride) 40 g; *kūn bù* (Thallus Laminariae) 40 g; *bīng láng* (Semen Arecae) 40 g; prepared *rǔ xiāng* (Olibanum) 20 g; *táo rén* (Semen Persicae) 16 g; prepared *chuān shān jiǎ* (Squama Manitis) 20 g.

Grind into a fine powder and mix with flour and water to make into pills; for oral intake 6–9 g each time, 2 times a day.

Actions

Dispersing cold and moving qi; relieving swelling and pain.

Indications

Testicular hardness, and swelling and pain due to cold.

THE 9TH WEEK

CHAPTER 10

The Static Blood Pattern

DAY ONE

This is a pattern formed by the chaotic and inhibited flow of blood or accumulation of blood stasis. It exists in externally contracted diseases or in diseases of internal damage, either manifesting in one area or all over the body.

Formation of Static Blood

Static blood results from pathological changes of the blood. Under normal circumstances, blood flows along the blood vessels with the aid of yang qi. Hence, if yang qi is in deficiency, blood flow will not be stimulated, leading to deceleration and further, stagnation. The constraint of qi can also affect blood flow and induce stasis. If pathogenic cold invades the blood vessels, blood will congeal, hence triggering stasis. For pathogenic heat invading the *ying*–blood levels, blood can bind with the heat pathogen to block blood flow, or alternatively, blood is heated, increasing its viscosity and decreasing its mobility, thus resulting in static blood. If blood deficiency is inherent, blood flow will become inhibited as well. If the blood vessels rupture and blood is leaked, its accumulation also results in static blood. Therefore, multiple factors, and multiple combinations of these factors, can be attributed to the formation of static blood. Static blood is regarded as a pathological product of the human body and once it emerges, it becomes a pathological factor that leads to a series of pathological changes, i.e., the static blood pattern.

Features of the Static Blood Pattern

Although the formation of static blood is triggered by numerous factors and its distribution spans across many regions in the body, the static blood pattern has several key symptoms which are the main indicators for diagnosis. The main characteristics of the static blood pattern are pain that is usually fixed, stabbing, and aggravated by palpations; lumps, purplish lips and fingertips, and a dry mouth with a desire for gargling but no desire to swallow; a dark purplish tongue, or a tongue bearing bluish spots and macules, and a thin and choppy pulse. Once static blood congeals in an organ or a tissue, it will influence the physiological functions of this organ or tissue, bringing forth various symptoms, which in turn provide evidence for the location of stasis.

This pattern exists in many disorders, such as various infectious diseases in the *ying*–blood level, coronary disease, shock, chronic pulmonary heart disease, stroke, peptic ulcers, cirrhosis, tumors, hemorrhagic diseases, trauma, sores, gynecological diseases, and so on. It is extremely common, and other patterns may also be complicated with static blood.

Categories of the Static Blood Pattern

As the site of stasis and the nature and cause of the pathogen are wide-ranging, the specific manifestations of static blood are very complicated. With respect to the disease location, some sub-patterns include: the static blood obstructing the heart pattern, the static blood obstructing the lung pattern, the stasis retention in the intestines and stomach pattern, the static blood obstructing the liver pattern, the blood stagnation in the uterus pattern, and the blood amassment in the lower *jiao* pattern. Based on the nature of the pathogen, sub-patterns include: the binding of heat and stasis pattern, the binding obstruction of the cold and stasis pattern, the binding obstruction of the phlegm and stasis pattern, and the binding of blood and water pattern. In terms of causes, there are the qi stagnation and blood stasis pattern, the qi deficiency and blood stasis pattern, the cold congealing and blood stasis pattern, and so on. This chapter mainly focuses on the diagnosis and treatment of the blood amassment in the lower *jiao* pattern, the qi stagnation and blood stasis pattern, the qi deficiency and blood stasis pattern, and the cold congealing and blood stasis pattern.

Treatment Methods of the Static Blood Pattern

The main principle of treatment for the static blood pattern is to dissolve stasis or invigorate blood and dissolve stasis. The method of dissolving stasis can be further classified in accordance to the different disease causes and pathogens. If static blood is resulted due to yang qi deficiency, it requires warming and unblocking yang qi to dissolve stasis. If it is caused by qi stagnation, stasis needs to be dissolved by moving qi. If the cause is cold congealing, the method to apply is to dissolve stasis by warming the channels and dispelling cold. For heat pathogens invading the blood, blood is dissolved by clearing heat. For yin consumption that leads to blood stasis, stasis is resolved by nourishing yin. For binding of static blood and phlegm–turbidity, phlegm needs to be removed and dissolved. For static blood and heat binding in the intestines and uterus, the stasis and heat should be purged via defecation.

By dissolving stasis, blood vessels are dilated, vessel elasticity is improved, blood viscosity is decreased, and blood flow is sped up. As blood-invigorating and stasis-dissolving formulae can regulate immunity, inhibit bacteria, calm the mind, relieve bleeding, and contract the uterus, such formulae cannot be applied in the same manner as the anticoagulatory and vascular-dilating medicines in modern practice.

In treatment, it is necessary to eliminate the disease cause right at the start, instead of only dissolving stasis. In addition, the blood-invigorating and stasis-dissolving formulae pertain to pathogen-removing therapies whose improper use may impair blood and healthy qi, so their doses must be moderate and should be stopped as soon as the disease has been alleviated. Sometimes, its application can be combined with qi-tonifying and blood-nourishing medicinals. Since the blood-invigorating and stasis-dissolving formulae can promote blood flow, women with profuse menstruation or with child should be cautioned when undergoing this therapy.

Daily Exercises

1. How does the static blood pattern develop?
2. What are the clinical features of the static blood pattern?
3. What are the curative effects of the stasis-dissolving method? Can the static blood pattern be cured by using only the stasis-dissolving method? Why or why not?

DAY TWO

The Blood Amassment in the Lower *Jiao* Pattern

The blood amassment in the lower *jiao* pattern is caused by static blood accumulation in the lower abdomen. There are two definitions for the lower *jiao*: (1) it is one of the six *fu* organs, i.e., the lower part of the *sanjiao* or (2) it refers to the liver and kidney. The lower *jiao* discussed here refers to the lower abdomen, including the bladder, uterus, and some parts of the intestines. This pattern is commonly seen at the late stage of externally contracted febrile diseases, gastrointestinal bleeding and schizophrenia from disorders of internal damage, irregular menstruation and amenorrhea of gynecology, and some external wounds. In externally contracted diseases, this pattern is manifested as the binding of static blood and pathogenic heat, while in other diseases, pathogenic heat is not necessarily present.

Diagnosis

The main symptoms and signs of this pattern are lower abdominal tension and cramps or hardness, fullness, and pain in response to pressure, and a purple tongue or a tongue bearing static spots and macules. Other indications are dysphoria, mania, amnesia, uninhibited urination, uninhibited bowel movements, dark-colored feces, fever, and a deep and choppy pulse.

This pattern concerns static blood accumulation in the lower abdomen, which will inevitably block the flow of qi movement, hence tension and cramps in the lower abdomen are triggered. If stagnation is severe, the lower abdomen will experience sensations of hardness, fullness, and pain in response to pressure, which reflect the presence of an excess pathogen in the interior. A purple tongue or a tongue bearing static spots and macules is one of the characteristics of the static blood pattern. If the binding of static blood and pathogenic heat obstructs the lower *jiao* and affects the heart, there will be some symptoms of mental disorder, such as amnesia or dysphoria in mild cases or weeping and hysterical laughter in severe cases. If static blood accumulates in the intestines or uterus, the bladder will be disconnected from direct regulation and influence, hence promoting smooth urination. If blood accumulates in the bladder, there will be hematuria, causing difficult and painful urination. Uninhibited bowel movements and dark-colored feces are obvious signs of static blood in the intestines. The obstruction by static blood leads to inhibited blood flow, thus causing the patient's pulse to be deep and choppy. In addition, some women may suddenly contract a cold or other febrile diseases during menstruation, which signifies that an external pathogen has invaded the interior, becoming a pattern of internal binding of static blood. Therefore, for women with fever, it is very important to note their state of menstruation.

Overall, apart from the basic manifestations of static blood, this pattern mainly affects the lower abdomen and produces evident mental symptoms.

Treatment method

Invigorating blood, dissolving stasis, and relaxing the bowels.

Formula and ingredients: *Táo Hé Chéng Qì Tāng* (Peach Kernel Qi-Guiding Decoction)

Táo rén (Semen Persicae) without skin and tip 12 g; *dà huáng* (Radix et Rhizoma Rhei) 12 g; *guì zhī* (Ramulus Cinnamomi) 6 g; *zhì gān cǎo* (Radix et Rhizoma Glycyrrhizae Praeparata cum Melle) 6 g; *máng xiāo* (Natrii Sulfas) 6 g.

Formula verse

Táo Hé Chéng Qì uses *xiāo huáng,* together with *guì zhī* and *gān cǎo.* For consumption during an emergency of blood amassment in the lower *jiao,* for expelling static blood and relieving fever and mania.

Usage

Add 1.4 L of water to decoct the first four ingredients until 500 mL are left. Remove the dregs and add *máng xiāo* to decoct with mild fire until the first signs of boiling are apparent. Take 100 mL of the decoction warm each time after meals, 3 times a day. After taking this decoction, there may be several episodes of loose stool.

Analysis

In the formula, *táo rén* is applied to invigorate blood, dissolve stasis, and moisten the intestines to promote defecation, while *dà huáng* is to relax the bowels and purge heat; it is a good herb for invigorating blood and dissolving stasis. A combination of these two ingredients can treat static heat and blood amassment in the lower *jiao*, being the chief medicinals. *Guì zhī* serves to diffuse and unblock yang qi and promote blood flow. *Máng xiāo* purges heat and softens hardness, which can strengthen the effect of relaxing the bowels to remove heat. *Gān cǎo* can attenuate the potent effect of the other ingredients in removing pathogens, thus protecting the healthy qi. This formula is in fact a blend of purgation and stasis expulsion. After taking this formula, static heat will be eliminated after experiencing a few days of loose stool.

Táo rén has significant effects on inhibiting blood coagulation, inflammation, and allergy. Among various blood-invigorating and stasis-resolving medicinals, it is the strongest in stimulating blood flow. *Guì zhī* can promote blood circulation and dilate blood vessels. *Máng xiāo* and *máng xiāo* can remove internal toxins by strengthening gastrointestinal peristalsis, improve intestinal blood circulation, decrease capillary permeability, and has favorable properties on inhibiting bacteria and boosting immunity. As a whole, this formula has multiple functions of improving blood circulation, relieving swellings and pain, and restoring the body to its normal state after impairment. However, there is little knowledge about the functional mechanism of this formula in treating mental disorders.

Treatment reference

Táo Hé Chéng Qì Tāng is a specialized formula for the blood amassment in the lower *jiao* pattern. Due to its elaborate composition, this formula is suitable for many diseases caused by static heat, such as local pain and inhibited bowel movement following falls and knocks; tearing and distending pain, red eyes, and swollen gums due to static heat and static blood accumulation in the head and eyes; dysmenorrhea, amenorrhea, lingering postpartum lochia, or vaginal hematoma due to internal blockage of static blood in women. This formula can also be used to treat mental disorders caused by internal binding of static heat, such as schizophrenia. In treating such diseases, it is advisable to add suitable amounts of *hŭ pò*, *hóng huā*, *yù jīn*, *qīng pí*, etc. Moreover, this formula is applicable to cerebral concussion, ileus, acute pelvic inflammation, and sores pertaining to internal binding of static heat. For acute bacillary dysentery (especially bloody dysentery with a greater amount of blood than pus), hemorrhagic enteritis, severe hepatitis, epidemic hemorrhagic fever at the oliguric level, etc., application of this formula can eliminate internal toxins rapidly by expelling stasis and relaxing the bowels, thus alleviating the general toxic symptoms. For menstrual irregularities, adnexitis, and dysmenorrhea, add some blood-invigorating medicinals like *dāng guī*, *hóng huā*, and *dān shēn*. For severe lower abdominal distention and fullness due to qi stagnation, add *xiāng fù*, *wū yào*, and *mù xiāng*. For high fever due to the binding of static blood and pathogenic heat, add *huáng lián*, *huáng qín*, and *mŭ dān pí*. For serious pain or amenorrhea due to internal binding of static blood, add *pú huáng*, *wŭ líng zhī*, *rŭ xiāng*, *mò yào*, *yán hú suŏ*, etc., or use *Xià Yū Xuě Tāng* (Static Blood-Purging Decoction).

To prescribe *Táo Hé Chéng Qì Tāng*, urination must uninhibited; if static obstruction occurs in the bladder, such as in prostatic hyperplasia, simple prostatitis, and strangury, and there is inhibited urination, this formula is still applicable. For the treatment of pain using this formula, keep the following key points of pattern differentiation in mind: fixed pain that is often stabbing and respond unfavorably to pressure or the discharge of dark purplish blood and clots, and a dark purplish tongue or a tongue bearing static spots are present.

Cautions

When this formula is applied to treat the blood amassment in the lower *jiao* pattern induced by externally contracted febrile diseases, it is inappropriate to solely prescribe this formula if the heat pathogen is exuberant as its heat-clearing effect is weak. If there are signs of the exterior pattern such as an aversion to cold with fever, exterior-releasing formulae must be applied first and after the exterior pattern has been relieved, *Táo Hé Chéng Qì Tāng* can then be used. Pregnant women must avoid taking this formula.

Daily Exercises

1. What are the clinical features of the blood amassment in the lower *jiao* pattern?
2. What are the ingredients of *Táo Hé Chéng Qì Tāng*? What are its actions?
3. Ms. Zhang is an 18-year-old female. She has been experiencing distending pain in the lower abdomen and has not had her menstruation for 5 months. However, it suddenly occurred on a rainy day when she was working on the farm. On that day, her menstruation came and she was drenched by the rain. The next day, she suffered from pain in the lower abdomen and her menstruation abruptly ceased. A physical examination showed hardness in the lower abdomen, a tight abdominal wall, difficult defecation, normal urination, a mild dark purplish tongue, and a thin and choppy pulse. Please prescribe a Chinese medicinal formula for this case.

Additional Formulae

Xià Yū Xuě Tāng (*Static Blood Purging Decoction*)

Dà huáng (Radix et Rhizoma Rhei) 9 g; *táo rén* (Semen Persicae) 9 g; dry-fried *zhé chóng* (Eupolyphaga seu Steleophaga) without feet 9 g.

Add water to decoct. Alternatively, grind the ingredients into a fine powder and make into 4 pills by mixing with honey. Then, decoct 1 pill with rice wine for oral intake.

Actions

Breaking up blood and purging static blood.

Indications

Static blood accumulation in the lower *jiao* presenting unbearable pain in the lower abdomen, masses detected by palpitations or fever, a dark purple tongue or a tongue bearing macules, a deep and choppy, or a deep and excessive pulse, or inhibited menstruation.

DAY THREE

The Qi Stagnation and Blood Stasis Pattern

The qi stagnation and blood stasis pattern is caused either by qi stagnation resulting in stasis or by static blood blockage influencing qi movement, becoming a state of co-existence between qi stagnation and blood stasis. Blood circulation depends on the normal movement of qi. If qi stagnation occurs, blood flow will be inhibited and static blood develops. After the formation of static blood, qi stagnation will become more severe; qi stagnation and blood stasis thus interact with each other, giving rise to the qi stagnation and static blood pattern. This pattern is commonly seen in various traumatic pain, intercostal pain, costal chondritis, angina, sequela of cerebral concussion, and various menstrual disorders.

Diagnosis

The main symptoms and signs of this pattern are prolonged, fixed, and needling pain in the chest, rib sides, head, or other places, and rib-side distention and fullness. Other indications may include belching, sighing, chronic hiccups, dry vomiting, vexing heat, palpitations, insomnia, impatience, irascibility, a dry mouth no desire for drinking, dark eyes, a dark red tongue bearing macules at the edges, and a thin and choppy pulse.

Although the location of the static blood pattern can be different, it is more common in the chest and rib sides, because qi stagnation is often caused by the constraint of liver qi as the liver channel runs along the chest and rib sides. Qi constraint in the chest and rib-sides is manifested as chest and rib-side pain, distention, and fullness. Since there is internal stagnation of static blood, the pain are fixed and difficult to treat. When static blood is not located in the chest and rib sides, the pain can be in other regions. The suppression of liver qi causes the patient to be impatient and irritable, with occasional belching or sighing. If liver qi invades the stomach and triggers the ascending counterflow of stomach qi, there will be hiccups and dry vomiting. Long-term constraint of static blood can transform into heat, showing some signs of internal heat, such as feverish sensations in palms and soles or in chest, and vexation. Internal obstruction by static blood together with internal production of constrained heat can influence the heart spirit and manifests as palpitations and insomnia. A dry mouth without any desire for drinking, dark eyes, a dark red tongue, and a choppy pulse are manifestations of internal obstruction by static blood.

Since this pattern is often caused by qi stagnation, the patient has to be questioned with regards to emotional changes, such as anger and anxiety. The pattern can also be caused by external injuries, falls, and knocks. The co-existence of qi stagnation and blood stasis can be determined according to its specific clinical manifestations and medical history of the patient.

Treatment method

Moving qi and invigorating blood; resolving stasis and relieving pain.

Formula and ingredients: Xuè Fǔ Zhú Yū Tāng (Blood Mansion Stasis-Expelling Decoction)

Táo rén (Semen Persicae) 12 g; *hóng huā* (Flos Carthami) 9 g; *dāng guī* (Radix Angelicae Sinensis) 9 g; *shēng dì* (Radix Rehmanniae) 9 g; *chuān xiōng* (Rhizoma Chuanxiong) 5 g; *chì sháo* (Radix Paeoniae Rubra) 6 g; *niú xī* (Radix Achyranthis Bidentatae) 9 g; *jié gěng* (Radix Platycodonis) 5 g; *chái hú* (Radix Bupleuri) 3 g; *zhǐ qiào* (Fructus Aurantii) 6 g; *gān cǎo* (Radix et Rhizoma Glycyrrhizae) 3 g.

Formula verse

Xuè Fǔ Zhú Yū uses *guī dì táo*, *hóng huā chì sháo zhǐ qiào cǎo,* and *chái hú xiōng jié niú xī*, relieving stubborn pain by resolving stasis and purgation.

Usage

Add 1.4 L of water to decoct until 250 mL are left. Take the decoction warm orally and add 800 mL of water to decoct the dregs again until 250 mL are left. Take the decoction warm, 2 times a day.

Analysis

This pattern is caused by qi stagnation and blood stasis, so the main treatment methods in this formula are to move qi and resolve stasis. Here, *táo rén*, *hóng huā*, *dāng guī*, *shēng dì*, *chuān xiōng*, and *chì sháo* are all blood-invigorating and stasis-dissolving herbs, especially the first two ingredients, which are the chief medicinals. As blood flow depends on qi, i.e., "when qi moves, the blood flows," qi-rectifying herbs such as *chái hú*, *zhǐ qiào*, *chì sháo*, and *gān cǎo* are added to this formula, which are the four ingredients of *Sì Nì Sǎn* (Frigid Extremities Powder), an important prescription for rectifying qi. *Jié gěng* serves to diffuse lung qi and thus is beneficial to the qi movement of the whole body. It can also direct the medicinal effect to the chest and head. *Niú xī* is added to unblock blood vessels and guide blood stasis downward. Its combination with *jié gěng* can dredge blood vessels through ascension and descension. Qi-rectifying ingredients can not only relieve symptoms caused by qi stagnation, but also help to eliminate static blood, while stasis-removing ingredients are beneficial to the uninhibited flow of qi after the static blood has been removed. Therefore, the methods of moving qi and removing stasis complement each other.

Táo rén, *hóng huā dāng guī*, *chì sháo*, *niú xī*, and *chuān xiōng* have anticoagulatory properties, dilating blood vessels and improving blood circulation. *Chái hú* calms the mind and relieves pain. Qi-moving and stasis-removing medicinals act in synergy and can enhance the above effects.

Treatment reference

Xuè Fǔ Zhú Yū Tāng is applicable to a variety of pain in the chest and rib sides. As it is integrated with liver-soothing and qi-rectifying *Sì Nì Sǎn*, it is very effective for treating intercostal neuralgia, costal chondritis, angina, and biliary colic. Furthermore, it is also used to treat stubborn hiccups of patients with a strong physique, liver and spleen enlargement, neurogenic headaches, headaches after cerebral concussion, insomnia, neurosis, and hypertension. For profuse menstruation, dysmenorrhea, and amenorrhea due to qi stagnation and blood stasis, this prescription is strongly encouraged if there are manifestations of breast distention, abdominal distention and pain, back soreness, and dark purple menstrual blood with clots.

If this formula is administered to treat the static blood pattern in other regions, modification is required. For headaches and dizziness due to static blood in the head, add *shè xiāng* and *cōng bái*, becoming *Tōng Qiào Huó Xuè Tāng* (Orifice-Unblocking and Blood-Moving Decoction). For liver and spleen enlargement due to static blood accumulation below the diaphragm, add *xiāng fù*, *yán hú suǒ*, and *wū yào* to move qi, becoming *Gé Xià Zhú Yū Tāng* (Expelling Stasis Below the Diaphragm Decoction). For irregular menstruation due to static blood obstruction in the lower *jiao*, add *xiǎo huí xiāng*, *ròu guì*, and *gān jiāng* to warm and rectify qi, becoming *Shào Fǔ Zhú Yū Tāng* (Lower Abdominal Stasis-Expelling Decoction). For amenorrhea and dysmenorrhea due to static blood, remove *jié gěng* from this formula and add *xiāng fù*, *wū yào*, and *yì mǔ cǎo*.

Cautions

Alhough *Xuè Fǔ Zhú Yū Tāng* is an excellent formula for removing stasis and relieving pain, it is not applicable to qi and blood deficiencies, or else qi and blood will be further consumed and damaged. It is also not indicated for pain where static blood is not the root cause.

Daily Exercises

1. What is the relationship between qi stagnation and blood stasis? What are the clinical features of the qi stagnation and blood stasis pattern?
2. What are the ingredients of *Xuè Fǔ Zhú Yū Tāng?* What are its main functions?
3. Mr. Sheng is a 45-year old male. He has been suffering from chest pain for more than 20 days, with accompanying chest and rib-side distention, fullness, and tenderness, dark red skin, dark eye orbits, purplish-red

tongue margins, and a thin and choppy pulse. Please prescribe a Chinese medicinal formula for this case.

Additional Formulae

Tōng Qiào Huó Xuè Tāng (Orifice-Unblocking and Blood-Moving Decoction)

Chì sháo (Radix Paeoniae Rubra) 3 g; *chuān xiōng* (Rhizoma Chuanxiong) 3 g; smashed *táo rén* (Semen Persicae) 9 g; *hóng huā* (Flos Carthami) 9 g; sliced *cōng bái* (Bulbus Allii Fistulosi) 3 sticks; *dà zǎo* (Fructus Jujubae) without core 7 pieces; fresh ginger 9 g; wrapped *shè xiāng* (Moschus) 0.1 g; yellow rice wine 250 g.

Usage

To be decocted with water and for *shè xiāng*, grind it into powder and take it infused.

Actions

Invigorating blood and unblocking the orifices.

Indications

Static blood obstruction in the head presenting headaches, dizziness, or deafness; hair loss, a purplish complexion, rosacea, and leukoderma; uterine tuberculosis; infantile malnutrition with accumulation presenting emaciation, abdominal enlargement with visible bluish veins, tidal fever, and so on.

Gé Xià Zhú Yū Tāng (Expelling Stasis Below the Diaphragm Decoction)

Dry-fried *wǔ líng zhī* (Faeces Trogopterori) 9 g; *dāng guī* (Radix Angelicae Sinensis) 9 g; *chuān xiōng* (Rhizoma Chuanxiong) 6 g; smashed *táo rén* (Semen Persicae) 9 g; *mǔ dān pí* (Cortex Moutan) 6 g; *chì sháo* (Radix Paeoniae Rubra) 6 g; *wū yào* (Radix Linderae) 6 g; *yán hú suŏ* (Rhizoma Corydalis) 3 g; *gān căo* (Radix et Rhizoma Glycyrrhizae) 9 g; *xiāng fù* (Rhizoma Cyperi) 5 g; *hóng huā* (Flos Carthami) 9 g; *zhĭ qiào* (Fructus Aurantii) 5 g.

Usage

To be decocted with water.

Actions

Invigorating blood and dissolving stasis, and moving qi to relieve pain.

Indications

Stasis below the diaphragm presenting liver and spleen enlargement, or localized abdominal pain.

Shào Fŭ Zhú Yū Tāng (*Lower Abdominal Stasis-Expelling Decoction*)

Dry-fried *xiăo huí xiāng* (Fructus Foeniculi) 1.5 g; *gān jiāng* (Rhizoma Zingiberis) 3 g; *yán hú suŏ* (Rhizoma Corydalis) 3 g; *mò yào* (Myrrha) 3 g; *dāng guī* (Radix Angelicae Sinensis) 9 g; *chuān xiōng* (Rhizoma Chuanxiong) 3 g; *ròu guì* (Cortex Cinnamomi) 3 g; *chì sháo* (Radix Paeoniae Rubra) 6 g; wrapped *pú huáng* (Pollen Typhae) 9 g; dry-fried *wŭ líng zhī* (Faeces Trogopterori) 6 g. Add water to decoct.

Actions

Invigorating blood and dissolving stasis, and warming the channels to relieve pain.

Indications

Static blood in the lower abdomen presenting lumps, pain, or distention and fullness; menstrual lumbar soreness and lower abdominal distention; several episodes of menstruation in a month with lingering dark or purple menstrual blood or with clots; flooding and spotting (*bēng lòu*, 崩漏) with lower abdominal pain; and so on.

DAY FOUR

The Qi Deficiency and Blood Stasis Pattern

The qi deficiency and blood stasis pattern is caused by healthy qi deficiency in which qi fails to propel normal blood flow, rendering the internal production of static blood which obstructs the collaterals. This pattern is commonly seen in stroke sequelae. Stroke, including various cerebrovascular accidents, is a result of the serious disorder of yin and yang of the *zang–fu* organs and abnormal flows of qi and blood, together with yin deficiency in the lower body and exuberant liver yang in the upper body. Blood follows the counterflow of qi, and when qi is complicated by phlegm and fire, static blood is resulted and rushes upward to the brain to cloud the spirit and drastically affect the channels, leading to sudden coma and hemiplegia. After an attack of stroke, aside from the obstruction of the collaterals by static blood and phlegm–turbidity, an extreme deficiency of original qi is resulted due to sudden coma, manifesting as the qi deficiency and blood stasis pattern. Therefore, in this pattern, cases of blood stasis caused by qi deficiency as well as cases of extreme deficiency of healthy qi due to static blood can be observed. This is evidently a deficiency–root and excess–branch pattern. The deficiency–root mainly lies in the deficiency of healthy qi and it may be accompanied by liver and kidney yin deficiency and spleen–stomach weakness. The excess–branch refers to static blood which may surface with phlegm–turbidity.

Diagnosis

The main symptoms and signs of this pattern are flaccid and weak limbs on one side which are unable to conduct movement and facial palsy. Other indications may include a sallow complexion, broken speech, slobbering, frequent urination or enuresis, numbness of limbs, a pale purple tongue, and a thin and choppy pulse or deficient and moderate pulse.

This pattern is caused by the obstruction of the collaterals of limbs by healthy qi deficiency and static blood, which prevents the tendons, pulse, and muscles from being nourished, hence resulting in hemiplegia and facial palsy. A tongue lacking nourishment presents broken speech and slobbering. A sallow complexion is a sign of qi deficiency. Frequent urination or enuresis is resulted from qi failing to control bladder due to deficiency. A pale purple tongue and a thin and choppy or deficient and moderate pulse are manifestations of qi deficiency and internal obstruction by static blood.

The main difference of this pattern and ascendant hyperactivity of liver yang caused by liver–kidney dysfunction after stroke is that for the latter, there are clinical indicators of dizziness, tinnitus, a red face and eyes, purplish-red lips, a bitter taste in the mouth, vexation, a deep red tongue, and a wiry, slippery, and rapid pulse. Blood pressure can also be taken into consideration. In ascendant hyperactivity of liver yang, blood pressure is usually high, while in this pattern, it is generally low.

Treatment method

Boosting qi and invigorating blood; dissolving stasis and unblocking collaterals.

Formula and ingredients: *Bǔ Yáng Huán Wǔ Tāng* (*Yang-Supplementing and Five-Returning Decoction*)

Huáng qí (Radix Astragali) 120 g; *dāng guī* (Radix Angelicae Sinensis) 6 g; *chì sháo* (Radix Paeoniae Rubra) 6 g; *dì lóng* (Pheretima) 3 g; *chuān xiōng* (Rhizoma Chuanxiong) 3 g; *hóng huā* (Flos Carthami) 3 g; *táo rén* (Semen Persicae) 3 g.

Formula verse

Bǔ Yáng Huán Wǔ uses *qí guī xiōng, táo rén chì sháo*, and *dì lóng*. Indicated for stroke with hemiplegia; it boosts qi, invigorates blood, and unblocks channels and collaterals.

Usage

Add 1.2 L of water to decoct until 300 mL are left. Take the decoction warm orally and add 800 mL of water to decoct the dregs again until 300 mL are left. Remove the dregs and take the decoction warm, altogether 2 times a day.

Analysis

The static blood present in this pattern is produced by the failure of qi to drive blood flow due to weakness, and if the qi-deficient state cannot be rectifed after static blood is formed, the static blood can be difficult to remove. Therefore, this formula is based chiefly on the medicinal *huáng qí* for promoting blood flow by significantly boosting spleen–stomach qi. Its dosage is 20–40 times more than other blood-invigorating and stasis-removing ingredients. *Dāng guī, chì sháo, chuān xiōng, hóng huā*, and *táo rén* are all herbs that can invigorate blood, dissolve stasis, and dredge collaterals. *Dì lóng* is added to dissolve phlegm, extinguish wind, dredge channels and collaterals, and assist stasis-removing ingredients to completely eliminate substantial excess pathogens.

Bŭ Yáng Huán Wŭ Tāng can relieve myocardial ischemia, correct arrhythmia, improve blood flow in the brain and limbs, resist blood vessel contraction caused by noradrenaline, and reduce blood cholesterol levels. Therefore, this formula demonstrates curative effects on cardiovascular and related diseases.

Treatment reference

Clinically, *Bŭ Yáng Huán Wŭ Tāng* is used to treat paralysis following various cerebrovascular accidents or acute contagious diseases, such as epidemic encephalitis B, epidemic cerebrospinal meningitis, and leptospirosis. It can also be used to treat facial paralysis, acute myelitis, progressive muscular dystrophy, acute myocardial infarctions, infantile convulsions, thromboangiitis obliterans, sciatica, ankylosing spondylitis, amenorrhea, and other diseases with qi deficiency and static blood.

In practice, proper modification is required according to different patient conditions. For impaired speech, add *shí chāng pú* and *yuăn zhì*. For hemiplegia and facial palsy, add prepared *tiān nán xīng, bái fù zĭ, bái jiāng cán*, and so on. For numbness of limbs, add *wū shāo shé, sāng zhī, rŭ xiāng, guì zhī*, and *jī xuè téng*. For paralysis of the upper limb on one side, add *guì zhī* and *sāng zhī*. For paralysis of the lower limb on one side, add *xù duàn, sāng jì shēng, niú xī*, and *gŏu jĭ*. For urinary incontinence, add *jīn yīng zĭ, sāng piāo xiāo, yì zhì rén*, and *shān zhū yú*. For paralysis with cold limbs, add cooked *fù zĭ, guì zhī*, and so on. For fatigue, a lack of strength, shortness of breath, and a reluctance to speak, add *dǎng shēn* and *bái zhú*. If the disease is complicated with phlegm–turbidity presenting chest and gastric stuffiness and oppression, and a greasy tongue coating, add prepared *bàn xià*, *bái fù zǐ*, and *tiān zhú huáng*. If the disease persists, add *tǔ biē chóng*, *shuǐ zhì*, *méng chóng*, and *dān shēn*.

Cautions

Bǔ Yáng Huán Wǔ Tāng uses qi-boosting *huáng qí* as the chief medicinal, but improper application will intensify pathogenic fire, hence serious consideration is required if it is used to treat ascendant hyperactivity of liver yang. Be cautious when applying this formula for patients with high blood pressure.

Daily Exercises

1. What are the clinical features of the qi deficiency and blood stasis pattern?
2. What are the ingredients of *Bǔ Yáng Huán Wǔ Tāng*? What are the unique points of its medicinal dosage? What are the main modifications in clinical practice?
3. Mr. Sun is a 55-year-old male. Three days ago before getting up in the morning, he found that he could not freely move his limbs on the left side and progressively, he was unable to lift them. This was accompanied by lateral numbness, facial palsy, unclear speech, general fatigue, a pale complexion, a pale tongue with a yellow and turbid coating, and a thin and choppy pulse. His blood pressure was recorded as 126/84 mmHg. Please prescribe a Chinese medicinal formula for this case.

DAY FIVE

The Cold Congealing and Blood Stasis Pattern

The cold congealing and blood stasis pattern is caused by a pathogenic cold attack on the blood vessels, resulting in congealed blood becoming static blood. This pattern may occur in different locations. In this section, the main focus is on the attack of cold on the uterus which leads to static blood. It is commonly observed in menstrual irregularities, amenorrhea, postpartum abdominal pain, and infertility.

Diagnosis

The main symptoms and signs of this pattern are cold pain in the lower abdomen and dark purplish menstrual blood with clots. Other indications may include scant menstruation, delayed menstruation, early menstruation, amenorrhea, dribbling menstrual blood, lower abdominal cramps and fullness, infertility, dry lips and tongue, vexing heat in the five centers, fever at dusk, and a deep and thin pulse.

The lower abdomen is attacked by pathogenic cold, which congeals and hinders qi and blood flows. As a result, there is cold pain in the lower abdomen with cramps, distention, and fullness. Pathogenic cold together with qi stagnation and static blood in the uterus causes menstrual irregularities or amenorrhea. Dark purplish menstrual blood with clots is the key manifestation of pathogenic cold and static blood. The binding obstruction of the uterus by these two factors will lead to infertility. If static obstruction persists, the transformation and production of blood will be affected, causing blood deficiency that is presented with yin deficiency and symptoms of feverish sensations and vexing heat in the palms and soles, or fever in the evening. Deficiency–heat symptoms are not necessarily indicative of this pattern, but if feverish signs are detected, it generally is not a simple cold congealing and blood stasis pattern, but more likely a complex pattern of cold, heat, stasis, and deficiency.

Treatment method

Warming the channels and dissipating cold; dissolving stasis and nourishing blood.

Formula and ingredients: Wēn Jīng Tāng (Channel-Warming Decoction)

Wú zhū yú (Fructus Evodiae) 9 g; *dāng guī* (Radix Angelicae Sinensis) 9 g; *sháo yào* (Radix Paeoniae) 6 g; *chuān xiōng* (Rhizoma Chuanxiong)

6 g; *rén shēn* (Radix et Rhizoma Ginseng) 6 g; *guì zhī* (Ramulus Cinnamomi) 6 g; *ē jiāo* (Colla Corii Asini) 9 g; *mǔ dān pí* (Cortex Moutan) 6 g; *shēng jiāng* (Rhizoma Zingiberis Recens) 6 g; *gān cǎo* (Radix et Rhizoma Glycyrrhizae) 6 g; *bàn xià* (Rhizoma Pinelliae) 6 g; *mài dōng* (Radix Ophiopogonis) without core 9 g.

Formula verse

Wēn Jīng Tāng contains *yú guì xiōng* and *guī sháo dān pí jiāng xià dōng*; also *shēn cǎo* to boost the spleen and nourish blood. It rectifies channels by focusing on warming the uterus.

Usage

Add 2 L of water to decoct until 600 mL are left. Remove the dregs and take the decoction warm, 200 mL each time, 3 times a day.

Analysis

The static blood of this pattern is due to pathogenic cold congealing in the lower body, so *wú zhū yú* and *dāng guī*, being the chief ingredients, are used to warm the uterus, dissipate cold, remove stasis, and nourish blood. *Guì zhī* is added to strengthen the formula's channel-warming and blood-invigorating functions. *Chuān xiōng*, *sháo yào*, and *mǔ dān pí* serve to enhance the invorigation of blood and dissolution of stasis. Since this pattern may be accompanied by blood deficiency, *rén shēn* and *gān cǎo* are added to supplement spleen qi, thus fortifying the source of blood production. After spleen qi reaches sufficient levels, the spleen's blood-managing function can be strengthened. In the formula, *ē jiāo* and *mài dōng* are combined with *dāng guī* and *sháo yào* to nourish yin and blood. Apart from revitalizing blood, *mǔ dān pí* can clear heat produced from deficiency. Static blood obstruction can induce internal retention of water dampness and form phlegm–damp, so *bàn xià* is used to warm and dry phlegm–damp. Moreover, it can lower stomach qi and disperse constraints due to its pungent nature. Overall, this formula functions by regulating menstrual diseases through dissipating cold, removing stasis, and nourishing blood.

Wú zhū yú can not only fortify the stomach, relieve pain, check vomiting, reduce gastric acid production, and inhibit bacteria, but also constrict the uterus. *Dāng guī*, *chuān xiōng*, and *sháo yào* are effective in relieving spasms and pain and dilating blood vessels. *Dāng guī*, *rén shēn*, and *ē jiāo* can stimulate erythrocyte production and increase the volume of hemoglobin in the blood. Therefore, this formula is excellent in regulating channels and menstruation.

Treatment reference

Clinically, emphasis is placed on either cold congealing or static blood, because in some cases of this pattern, the main pathological change is in the attack of the cold pathogen on the uterus in tandem with static blood, while in other cases, the main disorder lies in internal obstruction due to static blood accompanied by cold congealing. For a condition mainly with cold congealing in the uterus, the clinical manifestations include significant cold sensations in the lower abdomen, cold sensations that are aggravated during periods, cold sensations throughout the day, and even cold limbs; a sallow complexion, fatigue, a lack of strength, or loose leukorrhea; and dark menstrual blood. Here, it is advisable to remove *mǔ dān pí* and *mài dōng* from the formula and add *ài yè*, prepared *xiāng fù*, *páo jiāng*, and *xiǎo huí xiāng*, or simply use *Ài Fù Nuǎn Gōng Wán* (Mugwort and Cyperus Palace Warming Pill) instead. For a condition primarily concerned with internal obstruction due to static blood, clinical manifestations include menstrual blood with dark purplish clots, lower abdominal cramps, hardness, and fullness, and a dark red tongue or a tongue bearing macules. In this case, add *táo rén*, *hóng huā*, *rǔ xiāng*, *mò yào*, *dān shēn*, and so on. If it is accompanied by phlegm–damp obstruction, presenting chest and gastric stuffiness and oppression and a greasy and dirty tongue, add *cāng zhú*, *chén pí*, and *chuān pò*. For cold lower abdominal pain and an absence of lochia due to postpartum binding of cold and stasis in the uterus, *Shēng Huà Tāng* (Engendering and Transforming Decoction) can be alternatively prescribed to warm channels, invigorate blood, and relieve pain.

Cautions

The types of menstrual diseases are extensive, and hence are their causes. *Wēn Jīng Tāng* is not indicated for patterns without the presence of cold congealing and blood stasis. This formula is also not appropriate for cases of vexing heat caused by qi constraint transformed into fire, internal accumulation of damp–heat, or internal exuberance of fire–heat.

Daily Exercises

1. What are the main symptoms and signs of the cold congealing and blood stasis in the uterus pattern?
2. What are the ingredients of *Wēn Jīng Tāng*? What are the functions of each ingredient in the formula?
3. Ms. Cao is a 28-year-old female. She has been suffering from dysmenorrhea for 10 years. Her menstruation is regular, but is profuse and dark purple in color. During her period, she experiences cold pain in the waist and abdomen, and there are manifestations of cold sweat, lower abdominal distention not adverse to pressure, a warm, thin, and white tongue coating, and a deep and thin pulse. Please prescribe a Chinese medicinal formula for this case.

Additional Formulae

Ài Fù Nuǎn Gōng Wán (*Mugwort and Cyperus Palace Warming Pill*)

Ài yè (Folium Artemisiae Argyi) 90 g; *xiāng fù* (Rhizoma Cyperi) 180 g; *wú zhū yú* (Fructus Evodiae) 90 g; *chuān xiōng* (Rhizoma Chuanxiong) 90 g; wine-fried white *sháo yào* (Radix Paeoniae) 90 g; *huáng qí* (Radix Astragali) 90 g; *xù duàn* (Radix Dipsaci) 45 g; wine-fried *shēng dì* (Radix Rehmanniae) 30 g; *ròu guì* (Cortex Cinnamomi) 15 g; wine-washed *dāng guī* (Radix Angelicae Sinensis) 90 g.

Grind the above ingredients into a fine powder and add vinegar and flour to make into paste-like pills. Take the pills 6 g orally each time with light vinegar soup. Avoid consuming cold and raw foods and maintain a good mood.

Actions

Warming the uterus and channels, and nourishing and invigorating blood.

Indications

Uterine deficiency–cold presenting white and turbid leukorrhea, a sallow complexion, limbs with pain, fatigue, a lack of strength, a poor appetite, inhibited channels, occasional abdominal pain, and chronic infertility.

Shēng Huà Tāng (Engendering and Transforming Decoction)

Dāng guī (Radix Angelicae Sinensis) 24 g; *chuān xiōng* (Rhizoma Chuanxiong) 9 g; *táo rén* (Semen Persicae) without skin and core 6 g; dark blast-fried *gān jiāng* (Rhizoma Zingiberis) 1.5 g; *zhì gān cǎo* (Radix et Rhizoma Glycyrrhizae Praeparata cum Melle) 1.5 g. Decoct with water or yellow wine.

Actions

Invigorating blood and dissolving stasis, and warming the channels to relieve pain.

Indications

Inhibited postpartum lochia.

CHAPTER 11

The Food Accumulation Pattern

DAY SIX

In the food accumulation pattern, the intestines and stomach fail to function normally in transporting and converting food substances due to local food accumulation. This pattern clearly pertains to diseases of internal damage, and food accumulation can be regarded as a substantial pathogen that is produced internally. For externally contracted diseases, food accumulation can be a supplementary disorder.

Formation of the Food Accumulation Pattern

The human body relies on the spleen and stomach to digest food and circulate substances and waste products after digestion. It also depends on the dredging function of the liver and gallbladder, the transporting and distributing functions of the heart and lung, and transportation of the large intestine and small intestine. If food intake surpasses the capacity of the body to transport and convert food or if this capacity is reduced (examples of causes include spleen–stomach weakness, failure of the liver and gallbladder to dredge, and failure of the intestines to transport food residues), food will stagnate in the stomach or intestines, giving rise to the food accumulation pattern. The buildup of food will further affect spleen–stomach transportation and conversion of food and hinder qi movement in the stomach and intestines, both of which tend to be accompanied by the qi stagnation pattern (Chapter 9). Long-term food accumulation will generate pathogenic heat or form phlegm–damp, bringing forth the binding of food accumulation and damp–heat.

287

Features of the Food Accumulation Pattern

Regardless of the cause of the food accumulation pattern, its occurrence in the intestines and stomach will present some common symptoms, such as gastric and abdominal distention and fullness, swallowing of acid, pungent belching, nausea and vomiting, and loose stool with sour and foul odors. These are the primary indicators of diagnosing this pattern. In addition, the nutritional history of the patient, e.g., engorgement or excessive food intake, can be taken into account. A greasy tongue coating and a slippery pulse are signs of internal food accumulation. If it is complicated by pathogenic heat, there will be bad breath, hot and pungent belching, a preference for cold, an aversion to heat, a tongue with a yellow and greasy coating, and a slippery and rapid pulse. If food accumulation is accompanied by the congealing of cold, the manifestations will include vomiting of clear fluids, a preference for heat, an aversion to cold, a white and greasy tongue coating, and a thin and moderate pulse.

Categories of the Food Accumulation Pattern

Although the concept of the food accumulation pattern is relatively simple to grasp, it can be further categorized according to different disease causes and complications by other pathogens. Based on the former, sub-patterns include the food accumulation in the stomach and intestines pattern and the food accumulation due to spleen deficiency pattern. In terms of supplementary pathogens, there are the food accumulation and damp–heat pattern, the qi stagnation and food accumulation pattern, and the cold congealing and food accumulation pattern. In this chapter, we will mainly discuss the diagnosis and treatment of the food accumulation in the stomach and intestines pattern, the food stagnation and damp–heat pattern, and the food accumulation due to spleen deficiency pattern.

Treatment Methods of the Food Accumulation Pattern

To treat the food accumulation pattern, the key method is to promote digestion and direct food stagnation outward. These two techniques belong to the dispersion method, which is one of the eight methods employed in

Chinese medicine. This is mainly to assist the digestion and absorption of food, thus eliminating food accumulation. The medicinals administered by this method often have properties of promoting the secretion of gastric juices and gastrointestinal peristalsis, and relieving gastroenteritis. As the occurrence of food accumulation is usually related to the hypofunction of the spleen and stomach in food transportation and conversion, spleen qi-boosting medicinals are added to treat food accumulation. Further, the food accumulation pattern is usually complicated by qi stagnation and damp–heat, so qi-rectifying and damp–heat-clearing medicinals are often supplemented. In summary, treatment methods include promoting digestion to resolve food stagnation, clearing damp–heat to resolve food stagnation, and boosting the spleen to resolve food stagnation.

In application, it is important to eliminate the root causes of the food accumulation pattern. For instance, boosting the spleen to assist transportation should be used simultaneously with medicinals that disperse and supplement for food accumulation due to spleen–stomach weakness, or spleen–stomach qi will be impaired. Food accumulation in the stomach and intestines will affect the uninhibited flow of qi and encourage the breeding of damp–heat, hence the technqiues of promoting digestion and directing food stagnation outward are often combined with methods of rectifying qi and clearing damp–heat. If food accumulation is complicated by internal obstruction by pathogenic cold, medicinals with warming and unblocking properties should be added.

Daily Exercises

1. How does the food accumulation pattern develop?
2. What are the main clinical manifestations of the food accumulation pattern?
3. What does "promoting digestion and directing food stagnation outward" mean? What are its specific treatment methods?

THE 10TH WEEK

DAY ONE

The Food Stagnation in the Stomach and Intestines Pattern

The food stagnation in the stomach and intestines pattern is a syndrome of gastrointestinal disorder due to excessive food intake and internal food accumulation. Food stagnation in the stomach and intestines not only includes dyspepsia, but also poor appetite, vomiting, diarrhea, and abdominal pain caused by various intestinal diseases. This pattern is seen in indigestion, acute gastroenteritis, chronic gastritis, and chronic colitis.

Diagnosis

The main symptoms and signs of this pattern are gastric and abdominal distention and fullness, vomiting, diarrhea, and a sour and putrid odor of the discharged contents. Other indications may include belching, swallowing of acids, a lack of appetite, abdominal pain, a thick and greasy tongue coating, and a slippery pulse.

This pattern is caused by engorgement or by excessive daily food intake which encumbers the spleen and stomach, resulting in failure to transport and transform. As a result, food stagnates in the stomach and intestines and hinders the flow of qi, with gastric and abdominal distention and fullness and even pain. Abnormal digestion, absorption, and discharge of food, together with dysfunctional ascending and descending functions of the stomach and spleen, lead to symptoms of vomiting and diarrhea with undigested food. In the process of food fermentation in the stomach and intestines, a sour and foul odor is produced. Internal food accumulation also affects the transportation and conversion of the stomach and spleen, leading to a poor appetite. Diagnosis of this pattern is not much of a difficulty if patient history of dietary irregularities is taken into account.

Treatment method

Promoting digestion and resolving food stagnation.

Formula and ingredients: Bǎo Hé Wán (Harmony-Preserving Pill)

Shān zhā (Fructus Crataegi) 180 g; *shén qū* (Massa Medicata Fermentata) 60 g; *bàn xià* (Fú Líng Wán) 90 g; *fú líng* (Poria) 90 g; *chén pí* (Pericarpium Citri Reticulatae) 30 g; *lián qiào* (Fructus Forsythiae) 30 g; *lái fú zǐ* (Semen Raphani) 30 g.

Formula verse

Bǎo Hé uses *shén qū, shān zhā, chén qiào líng xià*, and *fú zǐ*. It promotes digestion and resolves food stagnation, and for decoction, *mài yá* can be added.

Usage

The ingredients are made into powder and cooked into pills the size of firmiana seeds. Seventy to 80 pills (6–9 g) should be taken orally each time with warm water, 2–3 times a day. Alternatively, use 10% of the original dosage for decoction in water.

Analysis

Bǎo Hé Wán combines *shān zhā, shén qū*, and *lái fú zǐ*, the chief ingredients, to promote digestion and resolve food stagnation. *Shān zhā* can assist the spleen and strengthen the stomach in promoting digestion. It is especially potent at eliminating stagnation of fatty and greasy foods and infantile milk accumulation. *Shén qū* can also promote digestion and resolve food stagnation, and is particularly effective at dispelling stagnation of grain and wine. Aside from promoting digestion, *lái fú zǐ* can move qi, resolve phlegm, and unblock the stomach and intestines. *Chén pí* and *bàn xià* are added to move qi, resolve food stagnation, harmonize the stomach, and check vomiting. *Fú líng* serves to fortify the spleen and harmonize the middle. If food accumulation is complicated by internal binding of phlegm–damp, *fú líng, chén pí*, and *bàn xià* are used to remove dampness, dispel phlegm, and rectify qi. As food accumulation tends to induce heat production, *lián qiào* is used to clear heat. *Mài yá* can be added during the decoction of this formula, because its stomach-boosting and digestion-promoting effects can be utilized to remove food stagnation.

Shén qū has been discovered to contain many digestive enzymes, and *shān zhā*, *lái fú zǐ*, and *mài yá* can promote digestion. *Shān zhā* also dilates blood vessels to improve blood circulation of the alimentary tract. Moreover, *shān zhā* and *lián qiào* can sanitize the digestive tract and eliminate infection. Therefore, *Bǎo Hé Wán* is effective in treating dyspepsia and digestive inflammation.

Treatment reference

Bǎo Hé Wán is a typical formula for food accumulation. Clinically, besides dyspepsia, it is also applied to treat many gastrointestinal diseases, such as infantile malnutrition and acute and chronic enteritis.

In practice, proper modification is required. For food accumulation due to excessive intake of rice, flour, and fruit, it is encouraged to add *mài yá* or use its decoction when taking the formula pills. For severe food accumulation, add appropriate amounts of *zhǐ shí*, *bīng láng*, and *gǔ yá*. For severe constrained heat presenting a bitter taste in the mouth, a tongue with a yellow coating, and a rapid pulse, add *huáng lián* and *huáng qín*. For severe abdominal distention and pain as well as tenesmus, add *mù xiāng*, *bīng láng*, and so on. For abdominal pain with constipation, add *zhǐ shí* and *dà huáng*. For food stagnation due to spleen–stomach weakness, add *bái zhú*, becoming *Dà Ān Wán* (Great Tranquility Pill), a dispersion formula incorporated with the aim supplementation.

Cautions

Bǎo Hé Wán is mainly used for dispersion. If dyspepsia or food accumulation is caused by spleen–stomach weakness, it is not applicable.

Daily Exercises

1. What are the diagnostic criteria of the food accumulation in the stomach and intestines pattern?
2. What are the ingredients of *Bǎo Hé Wán*? What is/are the function(s) of each ingredient?

3. Mr. Song is a 34-year-old male. Recently, he attended many banquets and food intake is often excessive. For the past 2 days, he has been feeling gastric and abdominal distention and fullness and pain around the navel. He has had diarrhea with a putrid odor, occasional acid regurgitation, a thick and greasy tongue coating, and a wiry and slippery pulse. Please prescribe a Chinese medicinal formula for this case.

Additional Formulae

Dà Ān Wán (Great Tranquility Pill)

Ingredients of *Bǎo Hé Wán* together with *bái zhú* (Rhizoma Atractylodis Macrocephalae) 60 g. The usage is similar to that of *Bǎo Hé Wán*.

Actions

Promoting digestion and boosting the spleen.

Indications

Food accumulation complicated by spleen deficiency and infantile food accumulation.

DAY TWO

The Food Stagnation with Damp–Heat Pattern

This pattern occurs when food accumulation in the stomach and intestines breeds damp–heat or binds with the initial damp–heat to obstruct qi movement. This pattern can be formed under two circumstances: (1) food accumulates in the stomach and intestines to produce damp–heat and food accumulation binds with the damp–heat and (2) the damp–heat exists inherently in the intestines and stomach and as the spleen and stomach are weak in food transportation and conversion, food stagnates in the stomach and intestines, inducing the binding of food accumulation and damp–heat. The former circumstance exists in diseases of internal damage, while the latter can be seen in both diseases of internal damage or in externally contracted febrile diseases, particularly those which are damp–heat-natured, such as acute gastroenteritis, dysentery, intestinal typhoid, and leptospirosis.

Diagnosis

The main symptoms and signs of this pattern are gastric and abdominal distending pain, and constipation or loose stool, incomplete defecation, tenesmus, and yellowish stool with a foul odor. Other indications may include fever, a pungent breath, burning abdominal pain, yellow and scant urine, a red tongue with a yellow and greasy coating, and a deep, slippery, and powerful pulse.

This pattern is caused by the binding of food buildup and damp–heat and qi stagnation, hence the coexistence of food accumulation, damp–heat, and qi stagnation manifests as gastric and abdominal pain. If food accumulation obstructs the intestinal tract, constipation occurs. If damp–heat travels downward, diarrhea is induced. Since food accumulation in the intestines and qi stagnation inevitably lead to inhibited intestinal assimilation, incomplete defecation and tenesmus are fairly common. Food accumulation together with damp–heat produce stool, with a color not unlike soy sauce and a pungent odor, which is significantly different from common diarrhea. Damp–heat accumulation in the intestines and stomach is reflected through fever, and is especially severe in the chest and abdomen. This symptom is more noticeable in externally contracted febrile diseases. Yellow and scant urine is a sign of interior heat. A yellow and greasy tongue coating and a deep, slippery, and powerful pulse are symptoms of the binding obstruction of damp–heat and food accumulation.

Treatment method

Promoting digestion and relieving accumulation; clearing heat and removing dampness.

Formula and ingredients: Zhǐ Shí Dǎo Zhì Wán (*Immature Bitter Orange Stagnation-Moving Pill*)

Dà huáng (Radix et Rhizoma Rhei) 30 g; bran-fried *zhǐ shí* (Fructus Aurantii Immaturus) 15 g; dry-fried *shén qū* (Massa Medicata Fermentata)

15 g; *fú líng* (Poria) 9 g; *huáng qín* (Radix Scutellariae) 9 g; *huáng lián* (Rhizoma Coptidis) 9 g; *bái zhú* (Rhizoma Atractylodis Macrocephalae) 9 g; *zé xiè* (Rhizoma Alismatis) 6 g.

Formula verse

Zhǐ Shí Dǎo Zhì uses *qū lián qín, dà huáng zhú zé,* and *fú líng.* For constraint of heat produced by the binding of food and dampness; it treats abdominal distention and constipation.

Usage

Grind the above ingredients into a fine powder and make into pills the size of firmiana seeds by soaking and steaming. Take 50–70 pills (6–9 g) orally each time with warm water on an empty stomach. The dosage of each ingredient can be modified according to the state of the disease. The method of preparation can also be modified into a decoction. In such a case, add *dà huáng* at the end.

Analysis

As intestinal assimilation is affected by food accumulation and damp–heat in the intestines, *dà huáng, zhǐ shí,* and *shén qū* are added as the chief ingredients. *Dà huáng* relaxes the bowels to expel heat, guiding damp–heat and food accumulation in the stomach and intestines downward and triggering defecation. *Zhǐ shí* moves qi and relieves gastric and abdominal distention and fullness. *Shén qū* promotes digestion to eliminate internal accumulation. The combination of the above three ingredients can dispel food accumulation, damp–heat, and qi stagnation. For the internal obstruction by damp–heat, *huáng lián* and *huáng qín* are used to clear heat and dry dampness, and are especially applicable to patients with diarrhea. *Fú líng, zé xiè,* and *bái zhú* are added to fortify the spleen and drain dampness. This achieves the effect of eliminating food accumulation and damp–heat without impairing healthy qi.

Dà huáng can relax the bowels, inhibit bacteria, and fortify the stomach, exerting favorable effects on treating gastrointestinal inflammation. *Zhǐ shí* can enhance gastrointestinal peristalsis. *Huáng qín* and *huáng lián* are relatively potent at inhibiting bacteria. *Shén qū* is a good herb for promoting digestion. This formula demonstrates efficacy in treating infectious inflammation of the stomach and intestines with dyspepsia.

Treatment reference

The pattern of the binding of damp–heat and food accumulation can be seen either in externally contracted febrile diseases or in diseases of internal damage. In the former, the formation of this pattern is not necessarily related to dietary irregularity, but may be resulted from the steaming of damp–heat in the interior which weakens stomach–intestine functions — a condition where damp–heat binds with residues in the intestines, causing the food accumulation with damp–heat pattern. In such a case, *Zhǐ Shí Dǎo Zhì Tāng* (Immature Bitter Orange Stagnation-Moving Decoction) is much more suitable. Here, *lián qiào*, *zǐ cǎo*, and *huáng lián* are applied to clear heat and resolve toxins; *dà huáng*, *hòu pò*, *bīng láng*, and *chuān mù tōng* are used to scatter accumulation; and *shén qū* and *shān zhā* are to remove food stagnation. Purgation is the key method in treating the food accumulation with damp–heat pattern. As the damp pathogen is characterized by stickiness and difficulty in being removed, several stagnation-moving ingredients are prescribed to completely drain the pathogens in the stomach and intestines. Therefore, the formula should be applied repeatedly, so-called the "frequent use of mild methods." If qi stagnation is significant, presenting obvious distending abdominal pain, tenesmus, and feces with red and white mucus as dysentery, a Chinese patent medicine, *Mù Xiāng Bīng Láng Wán* (Costus Root and Areca Pill), can be used. After proper modification, this formula can be prescribed to treat enteroplegia due to heat bind in the interior. For damp–heat bind in the interior with potent heat toxins, add *bái tóu wēng*, *jīn yín huā*, *dì jǐn cǎo*, *là liào*, and so on.

Cautions

The causes of abdominal pain and diarrhea are extensive, but this formula is only indicated for those with the internal binding of damp–heat and food accumulation. For the cold and deficiency patterns, this formula should never be applied. In clinical practice, do not unsystematically administer heavy formulae with the aim of rapid treatment, or healthy qi will be impaired while increasing the difficulty of removing the damp–heat pathogen.

Daily Exercises

1. How does the food accumulation with damp–heat pattern develop? What are its main symptoms and signs?
2. What are the functions of *Zhǐ Shí Dǎo Zhì Wán*? What are the ingredients?
3. Mr. Wang is a 24-year-old male. He complains of abdominal distention and fullness, borborygmus, mild tenderness, defecation following abdominal pain, stool with foams and a sour odor, a burning sensation around the anus, and a feeling of incomplete defecation. His tongue coating is yellow and greasy, and his pulse is thin and slippery. Please prescribe a Chinese medicinal formula for this case.

Additional Formulae

Zhǐ Shí Dǎo Zhì Tāng (*Immature Bitter Orange Stagnation-Moving Decoction*)

Zhǐ shí (Fructus Aurantii Immaturus) 6 g; wine-washed raw *dà huáng* (Radix et Rhizoma Rhei) 4.5 g; *shān zhā* (Fructus Crataegi) 9 g; *bīng láng* (Semen Arecae) 4.5 g; *chuān pò* (Cortex Magnoliae Officinalis) 4.5 g; *huáng lián* (Rhizoma Coptidis) 1.8 g; *shén qū* (Massa Medicata Fermentata) 9 g; *lián qiào* (Fructus Forsythiae) 4.5 g; *zǐ cǎo* (Radix Arnebiae) 9 g; *chuān mù tōng* (Caulis Clematidis Armandii) 2.4 g; *gān cǎo* (Radix et Rhizoma Glycyrrhizae) 1.5 g. Add water to decoct.

Actions

Promoting digestion and relaxing bowels, and clearing and resolving damp–heat.

Indications

Food accumulation with damp–heat in the intestines presenting burning pain in the chest and abdomen, nausea, loose stool, incomplete defecation, yellow- and red-colored stool, a yellow and greasy tongue coating, and a soggy and rapid pulse.

Mù Xiāng Bīng Láng Wán (Costus Root and Areca Pill)

Mù xiāng (Radix Aucklandiae) 30 g; *bīng láng* (Semen Arecae) 30 g; *qīng pí* (Pericarpium Citri Reticulatae Viride) 30 g; *chén pí* (Pericarpium Citri Reticulatae) 30 g; *é zhú* (Rhizoma Curcumae) 30 g; *zhǐ qiào* (Fructus Aurantii) 30 g; *huáng lián* (Rhizoma Coptidis) 30 g; *huáng bǎi* (Cortex Phellodendri Chinensis) 30 g; *dà huáng* (Radix et Rhizoma Rhei) 15 g; dry-fried *xiāng fù* (Rhizoma Cyperi) 60 g; *qiān niú zǐ* (Semen Pharbitidis) 60 g.

The ingredients are made into powder and fried with water to make pills the size of firmiana seeds. Take the pills 3–6 g orally each time with warm water, 2–3 times a day.

Actions

Moving qi and removing food stagnation; expelling accumulations and purging heat.

Indications

Internal accumulation of food and damp–heat presenting gastric and abdominal fullness and distention; gastric and abdominal distending pain, red- and white-colored stool like dysentery, tenesmus, a yellow and greasy tongue coating, a deep and excessive pulse; or constipation.

DAY THREE

The Food Accumulation and Spleen Deficiency Pattern

The food accumulation and spleen deficiency pattern is defined as the internal stagnation of food due to spleen–stomach weakness that results in the weakening of food transportation and conversion. This pattern usually follows severe or chronic diseases, or occurs in patients with spleen–stomach qi deficiency. Together with improper food intake or consumption of food that are difficult to digest, a deficiency–excess complex pattern emerges. This pattern can also result from prolonged dietary irregularities that frequently cause damage and waning spleen–stomach qi. This pattern is commonly seen in various chronic dyspepsia, infantile malnutrition, chronic enteritis, gastrointestinal neurosis, convalescence of acute febrile diseases, and many more.

Diagnosis

The main symptoms and signs of this pattern are gastric distention, fullness, and softness, which are aggravated following excessive food intake, and a poor appetite. Other indications may include general fatigue, a lack of strength, loose stool, chest and abdominal fullness, a white and greasy tongue coating, and a weak pulse.

Due to spleen–stomach weakness, food is poorly transported and converted, leading to fullness and distention in the stomach, and aggravation following excessive food intake. Spleen deficiency with food accumulation in the interior results in a poor appetite, and spleen deficiency alone triggers the indigestion of food and internal production of water–dampness, thus stool produced is loose. If food stagnation is severe, the stool will emit a foul odor. If spleen deficiency is severe, the stool can be loose or mucous. General fatigue, a lack of strength, and a weak spleen are signs of spleen–stomach qi deficiency. A white and greasy tongue coating is a reflection of dampness encumbering the spleen.

Treatment method

Fortifying the spleen and promoting digestion.

Formula and ingredients: Jiàn Pí Wán (Spleen-Fortifying Pill)

Dry-fried *bái zhú* (Rhizoma Atractylodis Macrocephalae) 75 g; *mù xiāng* (Radix Aucklandiae) 20 g; wine-fried *huáng lián* (Rhizoma Coptidis) 20 g; *gān cǎo* (Radix et Rhizoma Glycyrrhizae) 20 g; skinless *fú líng* (Poria) 60 g; *rén shēn* (Radix et Rhizoma Ginseng) 45 g; dry-fried *shén qū* (Massa Medicata Fermentata) 30 g; *chén pí* (Pericarpium Citri

Reticulatae) 30 g; *shā rén* (Fructus Amomi) 30 g; dry-fried *mài yá* (Fructus Hordei Germinatus) 30 g; *shān zhā* (Fructus Crataegi) flesh 30 g; *shān yào* (Rhizoma Dioscoreae) 30 g; oil-free *ròu dòu kòu* (Semen Myristicae) 30 g.

Formula verse

Jiàn Pí uses *shēn zhú líng cǎo chén*, *ròu kòu xiāng lián*, and *shā rén*, and also *zhā* flesh *shān yào* and dry-fried *qū mài*; able to disperse and supplement without impairing healthy qi.

Usage

All the ingredients are ground into a fine powder, which is steamed and made into pills the size of mung beans. Take 50 pills (6–9 g) orally each time with stocked rice soup or warm water on an empty stomach, 2 times a day. *Rén shēn* in the formula can be replaced by *dǎng shēn* (Radix Codonopsis).

Analysis

This pattern is resulted from spleen–stomach weakness, so the treatment focuses on boosting spleen and stomach qi. In the formula, *rén shēn*, *bái zhú*, *fú ling*, and *gān cǎo* are the four ingredients of *Sì Jūn Zǐ Tāng* (Four Gentlemen Decoction) for treating qi deficiency, which is fundamental in *Jiàn Pí Wán*. *Bái zhú* and *fú líng* are heavily used to enhance the effect of fortifying the spleen and percolating dampness and both of them also assist *shān yào* and *ròu dòu kòu* to arrest diarrhea by fortifying the spleen. *Shān zhā*, *shén qū*, and *mài yá* serve to promote digestion and dispel stagnation. As spleen deficiency and food accumulation usually cause inhibited qi movement, *mù xiāng*, *shā rén*, and *chén pí* are added to liberate qi flow and assist in strengthening spleen–stomach qi. Food stagnation will generate dampness and produce heat, so *huáng lián* is added to clear heat and dry dampness. Therefore, this formula is of both dispersion and supplementation; on one hand, it boosts qi and fortifies the spleen and on the other hand, it promotes digestion, moves qi, and clears damp–heat.

Rén shēn (or *dǎng shēn*) and *bái zhú* can strengthen functions of digestive organs, improve digestion, absorption, and metabolism, stimulate the nervous system, and strengthen body resistance, and when combined with other spleen-fortifying and qi-boosting medicinals, it is effective in treating chronic diseases of the digestive system. *Mù xiāng*, *shā rén*, and *chén pí* can improve intestinal peristalsis, and relieve pain and diarrhea as well.

Treatment reference

Clinically, the food accumulation with spleen deficiency pattern is relatively common, and there are many formulae which can be prescribed. The application of *Jiàn Pí Wán* is based on the principle of identifying the severity of spleen deficiency and food accumulation. For a primary spleen deficiency and secondary food accumulation, boosting spleen–stomach qi and using qi-rectifying and digestion-promoting ingredients for assistance should be emphasized. In such a case, remove *huáng lián* and *ròu dòu kòu* from this formula, reduce the dosages of digestion-promoting ingredients, such as *shān zhā*, *shén qū*, and *mài yá,* or apply the Chinese patent medicine *Zhǐ Zhú Wán* (Immature Bitter Orange and Atractylodes Macrocephala Pill) instead. For a condition primarily caused by food stagnation, promoting digestion and applying spleen qi-boosting ingredients for supplementation should be highlighted. If this pattern is without damp–heat or with cold signs, such as cold limbs, loose stool, a bland taste in the mouth, and an absence of thirst or excessive secretion of saliva, remove *huáng lián* and add appropriate amounts of *gān jiāng* and *fù zǐ* to warm the center and dispel cold.

Cautions

The effect of *Jiàn Pí Wán* is moderate; it is not regarded as a strong supplementary and purgative formula. As it contains digestion-promoting and damp–heat-clearing ingredients, it is strongly discouraged to apply this formula to treat pure spleen–stomach weakness presenting stomach stuffiness and fullness with emptiness and softness under palpitations.

Daily Exercises

1. How does the food accumulation with spleen deficiency pattern develop? What are its main symptoms and signs?
2. What are the ingredients of *Jiàn Pí Wán*?
3. Ms. Cai is a 45-year-old female. Half a month ago, she recovered from a fever caused by intestinal typhoid. However, she still feels a general lack of strength, stuffiness and fullness of the chest and stomach, and a poor appetite. Two days ago, she managed to consume a lot of food, but later, she suffered from gastric distention, fullness and discomfort, belching, loose stool, and frequent farting. Her tongue coating is thin, white, and greasy, and her pulse is thin and weak. Please prescribe a Chinese medicinal formula for this case.

Additional Formulae

Zhǐ Zhú Wán (Immature Bitter Orange and Atractylodes Macrocephala Pill)

Bran-fried *zhǐ shí* (Fructus Aurantii Immaturus) 30 g; *bái zhú* (Rhizoma Atractylodis Macrocephalae) 60 g.

The ingredients are made into a fine powder, wrapped with a lotus leaf, cooked with rice, and then made into pills the size of firmiana seeds. Take the pills 5–10 g orally each time with warm water, 2–3 times a day.

Actions

Fortifying the spleen and promoting digestion.

Indications

Spleen–stomach weakness and food accumulation presenting chest and stomach stuffiness and fullness, a lack of appetite, indigestion, or abdominal fullness and diarrhea.

CHAPTER 12

The Wind–Damp Pattern

DAY FOUR

The wind–damp pattern is characterized by joint pain, cramps, and swellings due to an exogenous wind–damp pathogen attacking the muscles, channels and collaterals, and bones and tendons. It is therefore an external contraction that rarely involves any disorder of the internal organs. However, if the wind–damp pattern lasts for a long time, it can be transmitted to the internal organs, especially the heart and kidney. Such a scenario is beyond a pure wind–damp pattern, but falls within the scope of diseases of internal organs.

Features of the Wind–Damp Pattern

The wind–damp pathogen originates from an external source, possessing pathogenic natures of both wind and dampness. Its manifestations are extensive, but there are some common symptoms, including joint and muscle pain that are aggravated during cloudy, rainy, or cold days, potentially enlarged joints, inhibited stretching and bending of limbs, cramps, and occasional numbness and weakness of limbs. In addition, there is often a history of wind, cold, and dampness contraction before the occurrence of this pattern. Since pathogenic dampness is sticky and difficult to be drained, the disease usually lingers and becomes challenging to treat.

The Wind–Damp Pattern and *Bì* Syndrome (痹证)

In Chinese medicine, the pattern of aching pain, heaviness, numbness, inhibited movement, and the swelling of muscles, joints, and tendons caused by the contraction of external wind, cold, dampness, and heat is termed *bì* syndrome. Evidently, the wind–damp pattern is closely related to *bì* syndrome and thus, it is also known as the wind–damp *bì* pattern. However, aside from wind–damp pathogens, many other factors, such as cold and heat pathogens, can cause *bì* syndrome. Moreover, the pathological change of *bì* syndrome at the late stage is not only limited to wind–damp, but also in relation to phlegm, static blood, etc. This chapter covers a few patterns of *bì* syndrome.

The wind–damp pathogen is also the cause of the exterior wind–damp pattern, which is associated with *bì* syndrome caused by damp–heat, but the former is characterized by temporary fever, an aversion to cold, headaches, and body pain, while the latter manifests as lasting muscular and joint pain that are difficult to treat. Therefore, these patterns are different, and the wind–damp exterior pattern will not be discussed in this chapter.

Categories of the Wind–Damp Pattern

The wind–damp pattern is caused by the exogenous contraction of wind–damp, but in some cases, the wind pathogen is the primary factor, while in others, the damp pathogen is the main cause. The wind–damp pattern is often complicated by pathogenic cold or heat and becomes a wind–cold–damp pathogen or a wind–heat–damp pathogen, each having its own features. During pattern development, the wind–damp pathogen impairs qi and blood or fluids of the liver and kidney, or produces phlegm–damp and static blood. Accordingly, the wind–damp pattern can be further categorized into the wind–cold–damp pattern, the wind–heat–damp pattern, the wind phlegm–stasis–damp pattern, and the healthy qi deficiency and wind–damp pattern.

Treatment Methods of the Wind–Damp Pattern

The removal of wind–damp is the key principle in treatment of this pattern. Most wind–damp-removing medicinals are warm and pungent, able to unblock and disperse. Some can also relax the tendons, relieve pain, and strengthen the tendons and bones. The wind–damp-removing method has multiple effects, such as relieving pain, suppressing inflammation and allergy, promoting local blood circulation, reducing joint exudates, allaying fever, and improving body constitution.

As there are many categories of the wind–damp pattern, different treatment methods need to be specifically applied; the major techniques include dispelling wind and dispersing cold, removing dampness and unblocking collaterals, dispelling wind and removing dampness, clearing heat and unblocking collaterals, eliminating wind and resolving phlegm, draining stasis and unblocking collaterals, and reinforcing healthy qi and removing dampness. The phlegm- and stasis-removing methods are often used to treat lingering wind–damp pattern with the internal production of phlegm and stasis. The healthy qi-reinforcing method is administered to treat prolonged wind–damp pattern with healthy qi deficiency, usually by nourishing blood, boosting qi, and fortifying the liver and kidney.

The medicinals for dispelling wind–damp are usually warm- and dry-natured, and improper use of them tend to induce serious damage to yin and blood, thus an overdose or long-term usage should be avoided. When using them for patients with a blood-deficient physique, extra care should be taken, otherwise add appropriate amounts of qi- and blood-supplementing ingredients to suppress the negative effects.

Daily Exercises

1. Are all diseases caused by the wind–damp pathogen within the scope of *bì* syndrome? What are the main symptoms and signs of the wind–damp pattern?
2. What pathogens may be involved in the pathological changes of the wind–damp pattern?
3. What does the treatment principle "removing wind–damp" mean? What are its specific methods?

DAY FIVE

The Wind–Cold–Damp Pattern

The wind–cold–damp pattern presents pain, numbness, and inhibited movement due to the external contraction of wind, cold, and dampness, in which pathogens reside in the muscles, channels and collaterals, and joints. The occurrence of this pattern is often related to humid environmental conditions, wading, being drenched by rain, and suffering from a cold for a long time. It is commonly observed in various arthritis and rheumatic diseases.

Diagnosis

The main symptoms of this pattern are joint or muscle pain, or numbness and heaviness, and inhibited joint movement. Other clinical manifestations include cold limbs, a fear of cold, pain aggravated on rainy and cold days, a white and slippery tongue coating, and a tight or floating and wiry pulse.

As the channels and collaterals are obstructed by wind, cold, and damp pathogens, qi and blood flows are inhibited. Consequently, the joints and muscles affected by the pathogens experience localized pain and numbness. However, the severity of contracted wind, cold, and damp pathogens are not level, so the clinical manifestations are different. For a condition primarily triggered by a wind pathogen, the pain is usually delocalized and sometimes accompanied by signs of the exterior pattern, such as fever and an aversion to wind and cold, and is termed migratory *bì* (wind *bì*). For a cold pathogen, the pain is acute and often localized, and usually appears with joint stiffness, a fear of cold in the affected region that can be relieved by warming but aggravated by coldness, and cold limbs, called painful *bì* (cold *bì*). For a damp pathogen, it is often manifested as limb numbness, aching pain, sweating, chest and stomach stuffiness and oppression, a white and greasy tongue coating, and a soggy and moderate pulse, termed fixed *bì* (dampness *bì*).

Treatment method

Dispelling wind and dispersing cold; removing dampness and unblocking collaterals.

Depending on the severity of wind, cold, and dampness, methods of dispelling wind, dispersing cold, and removing dampness should be applied accordingly.

Formula and ingredients: *Fáng Fēng Tāng (Ledebouriella Decoction)*

Fáng fēng (Radix Saposhnikoviae) 6 g; *gān cǎo* (Radix et Rhizoma Glycyrrhizae) 6 g; *dāng guī* (Radix Angelicae Sinensis) 6 g; *chì fú líng* (Poria Rubra) 6 g; *xìng rén* (Semen Armeniacae Amarum) 6 g; *ròu guì* (Cortex Cinnamomi) 6 g; *huáng qín* (Radix Scutellariae) 2 g; *qín jiāo* (Radix Gentianae Macrophyllae) 2 g; *gé gēn* (Radix Puerariae Lobatae) 2 g; *má huáng* (Herba Ephedrae) 3 g.

Formula verse

Fáng Fēng Tāng contains *guī cǎo líng, xìng rén ròu guì,* and *huáng qín,* and also *qín jiāo, gé gēn,* and *má huáng.* By decocting with jujubes and ginger, it is effective in treating migratory *bì.*

Usage

Grind the above ingredients into a crude powder and administer 15 g each time for decocting with 5 pieces of ginger, 3 pieces of jujubes, water, and wine.

Analysis

The wind–cold–damp pattern is resulted from the collective contraction of pathogenic cold, wind, and dampness, so in *Fáng Fēng Tāng, fáng fēng, qín jiāo, gé gēn,* and *má huáng* are applied to dispel wind and disperse cold. *Ròu guì* is added to strengthen the effect of dispersing cold. *Fú líng* fortifies the spleen and percolates dampness. *Qín jiāo* and *fáng fēng* dispel wind and remove dampness as well. As the wind, cold, and damp pathogens block the channels and collaterals and lead to inhibited qi and blood flows, *dāng guī* is used to harmonize blood and unblock collaterals. For ginger, jujubes, and *gān cǎo,* they serve to harmonize the spleen, stomach, and blood. Wine added in the decocting process to enhance the effects of warming, dispersing, and unblocking. Long-term qi and blood stagnation can produce internal heat, so *huáng qín* is used to clear this heat. If there are no signs of heat, it can be removed. This formula is mainly indicated for migratory *bì* (wind *bì*) presenting delocalized joint and muscle pain. It can also disperse cold and remove dampness.

Fáng fēng has been shown to inhibit experimental arthritis of animals and has some effects on relieving pain. *Qín jiāo* is able to relieve pain, calm the mind, and inhibit inflammation; it can also suppress allergic reactions and reduce capillary permeability. *Ròu guì*, *gé gēn*, *dāng guī*, and *má huáng* can dilate blood vessels, improve blood circulation, relieve pain and inflammation, and inhibit bacteria. Hence, this formula can be applied to treat various pain and swellings due to arthritis.

Treatment reference

The clinical manifestations of the wind–cold–damp pattern are complicated and extensive. This formula is more applicable to migratory *bì* that is marked by a relatively exuberant wind pathogen. In practice, modification of the formula or application of other suitable formulae is needed according to different disease locations, the severity of the cold, wind, and damp pathogens, and other accompanying pathogens. For instance, in the early stage of the contraction of the wind, cold, and damp pathogens, they mainly reside on the body surface presenting joint pain and stiffness, or exterior signs of an aversion to cold with fever and headaches, thus pungent and dispersing medicinals, such as *qiāng huó* and *dú huó*, should be added to disperse the wind–damp in the exterior. Alternatively, *Qiāng Huó Shèng Shī Tāng* (Notopterygium Dampness-Drying Decoction) can be used instead. For pain predominantly located in the upper limbs, add *qiāng huó*, *bái zhǐ*, *piàn jiāng huáng*, or *wēi líng xiān* to strengthen the effect of dispelling wind and unblocking collaterals. For those in the lower limbs, add *dú huó*, *niú xī*, *fáng jǐ*, *bì xiè*, or *cāng zhú* to enhance the potency of removing dampness and unblocking collaterals. For fixed pain with a preference for warmth and a fear of cold, add channel-warming and cold-dispersing medicinals, such as *zhì chuān wū*, cooked *fù zǐ*, and *gān jiāng*, or apply *Wū Tóu Tāng* (Aconiti Decoction). For skin numbness and heaviness with a greasy tongue coating, which is due to the exuberance of pathogenic dampness, add *yì yǐ rén*, *hǎi tóng pí*, *xī xiān cǎo*, *lù lù tōng*, and *cāng zhú* to remove dampness and unblock collaterals. For chronic diseases accompanied by lumbar and back pain, which are often due to kidney qi deficiency, add *yín yáng huò*, *dù zhòng*, *chuān xù duàn*, or *sāng jì shēng*. For qi and blood insufficiencies presenting mental fatigue, a lack of strength, general aching, a pale tongue, and a weak pulse, add *huáng qí*, *dǎng shēn*, and *jī xuè téng* to boost qi and blood, and assist healthy qi to expel pathogens.

Cautions

The ingredients of this formula are relatively warm and dry, so it is disencouraged for use on treating blood insufficiency or fairly severe internal heat, lest fluids are excessively consumed, resulting in strengthening the heat pathogen.

Daily Exercises

1. What are the main symptoms and signs of *bì* syndrome caused by pathogenic wind, cold, and dampness? What are the main characteristics of the migratory *bì* (wind *bì*), painful *bì* (cold *bì*), and fixed *bì* (dampness *bì*)?
2. What are the ingredients of *Fáng Fēng Tāng*? What are its indications? What are the different modifications that can be done according to the disease conditions?
3. Ms. Su is a 43-year-old female. She has been suffering from delocalized joint pain for 3 years, with the legs being the predominant site of pain. The pain is aggravated on cold or rainy days, and there is no visible color change of the skin on the affected region and no obvious swelling. Other manifestations are an absence of thirst, limbs lacking warmth, a white and slightly greasy tongue coating, and a deep and thin pulse. Please prescribe a Chinese medicinal formula for this case.

Additional Formulae

Qiāng Huó Shèng Shī Tāng
(Notopterygium Dampness-Drying Decoction)

Qiāng huó (Rhizoma et Radix Notopterygii) 9 g; *dú huó* (Radix Angelicae Pubescentis) 9 g; *gǎo běn* (Rhizoma Ligustici) 4.5 g; *fáng fēng* (Radix Saposhnikoviae) 4.5 g; *zhì gān cǎo* (Radix et Rhizoma Glycyrrhizae

Praeparata cum Melle) 4.5 g; *chuān xiōng* (Rhizoma Chuanxiong) 4.5 g; *màn jīng zǐ* (Fructus Viticis) 3 g. Decoct the ingredients with water and take the decoction warm.

Actions

Dispelling wind and overcoming dampness.

Indications

Wind–damp in the exterior presenting headaches, head heaviness, pain and heaviness in the waist and back, or general pain and difficulty in turning the body, a white tongue coating, and a floating pulse.

Wū Tóu Tāng (Aconiti Decoction)

Prepared *chuān wū* (Radix Aconiti) 10 g; *huáng qí* (Radix Astragali) 10 g; *má huáng* (Herba Ephedrae) 6 g; *bái sháo* (Radix Paeoniae Alba) 6 g; *zhì gān cǎo* (Radix et Rhizoma Glycyrrhizae Praeparata cum Melle) 6 g; honey 60 g. Add water to decoct.

Actions

Dispersing cold and relieving pain, and boosting qi and blood.

Indications

Painful *bì* (cold *bì*) occurring in temperate conditions, acute pains all over the body, inhibited movement, and a white and greasy tongue coating. *chuān wū* is toxic, and should be decocted first for 30 min to 1 h.

DAY SIX

The Wind–Heat–Damp Pattern

The wind–heat–damp pattern presents swelling and pain due to the external contraction of wind, heat, and dampness, which reside in the muscles, channels and collaterals, and joints, blocking qi and blood flows. This pattern is often caused by the infection of pathogenic wind, dampness, and heat, or by the internal exuberance of damp–heat with the contraction of external wind–damp that transforms into wind-, damp-, and heat-natured pathogens with relative ease, or by the constraint of wind, cold, and damp that converts heat to wind-, damp-, and heat-natured pathogens. This pattern is commonly observed in acute rheumatic fever, rheumatic arthritis, gout, and other immunological diseases, such as lupus erythematosus.

Diagnosis

The main symptoms and signs of this pattern are burning joint pain and reddish swelling. Other indications may include fever, thirst, vexation, restlessness, perspiration, a red tongue with a yellow coating, and a slippery and rapid pulse.

As this pattern is essentially heat-natured, it is also termed heat *bì*, and there are signs of heat. Its clinical manifestations, such as burning joint pain and reddish swelling, are resulted from damp–heat accumulation in joins, which blocks the flows of qi and blood. Its symptoms are similar to sores in external medicine, but pus is not produced. Fever, perspiration, thirst, and vexation are a reflection of exuberant heat.

The key point in pattern differentiation to distinguish it from the wind–cold–damp pattern is to note the manifestation of a burning sensation and localized reddish swelling. The wind–cold–damp pattern may also present symptoms of internal heat constraint, but no signs of burning pain and localized reddish swelling will be detected. Specifically, although pain in the joints is experienced, the color of the skin remains the same and there is no burning sensation, and even if swelling occurs, it is not severe. In addition, this pattern is extreme and develops quickly, with significant general symptoms. It may also affect the heart and other organs, so special attention must be given when a patient is diagnosed with this pattern.

Treatment method

Dispelling wind, removing dampness, clearing heat, and unblocking collaterals.

Formula and ingredients: Xuān Bì Tāng
(Painful Obstruction-Resolving Decoction)

Fáng jǐ (Radix Stephaniae Tetrandrae) 15 g; *xìng rén* (Semen Armeniacae Amarum) 15 g; *huá shí* (Talcum) 15 g; *lián qiào* (Fructus Forsythiae) 9 g; *zhī zǐ* (Fructus Gardeniae) 9 g; *yì yǐ rén* (Semen Coicis) 15 g; vinegar-fried *bàn xià* (Rhizoma Pinelliae) 9 g; *cán shā* (Faeces Bombycis) 9 g; skin of *chì xiǎo dòu* (Semen Leveloli) 9 g.

Formula verse

Xuān Bì Tāng contains the skins of *chì dòu*, *yǐ rén xìng rén*, and *fáng jǐ*, and also *zhī zǐ xià huá* and *cán shā*, which are good for joint pain of *bì* syndrome.

Usage

Add 1.4 L of water to decoct until 400 mL are left. Remove the dregs and take it warm 3 times, 2–3 times a day.

Analysis

This pattern mainly targets the wind, damp, and heat pathogens, so besides heat-clearing medicinals, warm- and dry-natured ingredients for expelling wind and removing dampness should be avoided. In the formula, *fáng jǐ*, *cán shā*, *yì yǐ rén*, and *chì xiǎo dòu* are all wind-dispelling, dampness-removing, and channel-unblocking medicinals with a cool nature instead of being pungent and warm. They can clear heat and drain dampness when *lián qiào*, *zhī zǐ*, and *huá shí* are added. The usage of *xìng rén* is to restore qi flow of the whole body by ventilating lung qi, a technique that removes dampness as well as frees channels and collaterals. *Bàn xià* is acrid and resolves dampness. Though its nature is relatively warm and dry, its combination with heat-clearing medicinals can suppress its warm dryness.

Studies have shown that *fáng jǐ* and *cán shā* can inhibit inflammation and relieve pain. *Fáng jǐ* contains ingredients that can activate the adrenal cortex and relieve allergy. *Cán shā*, *lián qiào*, and *zhī zǐ* can inhibit bacteria.

It has also been revealed that this formula has certain effects on rheumatic fever, rheumatic arthritis, and lupus erythematosus.

Treatment reference

The varying disease locations and severities of pathogenic wind, damp, and heat of this pattern result in extensive clinical profiles and corresponding treatment methods. For diseases located mainly in the upper limbs, add *piàn jiāng huáng*, or use *Bái Hǔ Jiā Guì Zhī Tāng* (White Tiger plus Cinnamon Twig Decoction) instead. For diseases located mainly in the lower limbs, add *cāng zhú, huáng bǎi, chuān niú xī, chē qián zǐ*, and *bì xiè*. For severe qi and blood stagnation presenting acute pain, add *hǎi tóng pí, wēi líng xiān*, and *chì sháo*. For severe local red swellings and burning pain, or a general feverish sensation, vexation, thirst, a yellow tongue coating, and a slippery and rapid pulse (i.e., a case of exuberant heat), add *shí gāo, zhī mǔ, jīn yín huā*, and *qīng fēng téng*. For red swellings on joints, acute pain especially at night, fever, vexing thirst, a deep red tongue with a scant and dry coating (i.e., toxic fire driving the blood level), add *shuǐ niú jiǎo, huáng lián, shēng má, mǔ dān pí*, and *shēng dì*. For skin erythema or red lumps, which are induced by toxic heat and static blood accumulation in the skin, add *zǐ cǎo, mǔ dān pí, dì fū zǐ, chì sháo, shēng dì*, and *táo rén* to cool and invigorate blood. For patients with exuberant heat that impairs yin, add some yin-nourishing medicinals.

Cautions

This formula is relatively cold and cool, hence it should not be used to treat *bì* syndrome with lingering cold pathogens. Cold signs seen in the tendons, bones, muscles, and joints with interior heat signs often pertain to the wind–cold–damp pattern with constrained heat. In this condition, pattern differentiation should be accurate and application of this formula should be meticulous. Moreover, since *bì* syndrome caused by wind, heat, and damp tends to affect the heart as well, close attention should be paid to the cardiac functions of the patient. An electrocardiogram (ECG) should be recorded when necessary.

Daily Exercises

1. What are the main symptoms and signs of *bì* syndrome caused by pathogenic wind, heat, and dampness? What are the main differences from the wind–cold–damp pattern?
2. What are the ingredients of *Xuān Bì Tāng*? What is/are the function(s) of each ingredient?
3. Ms. Jin is an 18-year-old female. She has been complaining of fever with an aversion to cold for 5 days, accompanied by headaches, a sore throat, and aching pains all over her body. After taking some antipyretics and analgesics, her fever and aversion to cold were relieved, but there was spontaneous sweating, an occasional aversion to wind, worsening pain in the knees and elbows with reddish skin, swollen knees with a burning sensation when pressure was applied, and pain aggravated when walking. Six red and hard nodes in the shank were detected, and are painful under pressure. Other clinical manifestations include a bitter taste and dryness in the mouth, vexation, yellow urine, a red tongue with a pale yellow and greasy coating, and a thin, slippery and rapid pulse. Please prescribe a Chinese medicinal formula for this case.

THE 11TH WEEK

DAY ONE

The Wind–Damp and Phlegm Stasis Pattern

This pattern is caused by the external contraction of wind–damp which causes persistent blockage of qi and blood circulation, forming turbid phlegm and static blood that combine with pathogenic wind and damp to obstruct channels and collaterals. This pattern is usually due to the wind–damp pattern left untreated for a long time, and hence these external pathogens block the channels and collaterals, tendons, bones, and muscles. Therefore, the flows of qi, blood, and fluids are inhibited; accumulation of fluids becomes turbid phlegm, and blockage of blood vessels produces static blood. Once phlegm and static blood develop, they bind to the external pathogens to further obstruct channels and collaterals, tendons, bones, and muscles. Thus, it is more difficult to expel the resulting pathogens, which finally advance into a chronic and persistent disorder. This pattern is commonly seen in various kinds of lasting arthritis or related relapses, especially prolonged rheumatoid arthritis presenting joint swellings, deformation, and dysfunction.

Diagnosis

The main symptoms of this pattern are joint pain that remain mild or acute for years, long-term joint swellings or deformation, stiffness, and inhibited movement. Other clinical manifestations are a dark red or dark purple tongue or a tongue bearing macules, a white and greasy tongue coating, and a thin and choppy pulse.

This pattern is triggered by the substantial amassment of phlegm and static blood in channels and collaterals, thus joint swellings cannot be easily relieved, and if it lingers for a long time, complete recovery will be difficult and normal movement of the joints may never be restored. If the hand is affected, there will be finger cramps, deformation, and muscle atrophy (even into a chicken claw-like structure). If it occurs in the vertebral chest joints, the vertebrae will fail to bend and a humped back is observed. Signs of a dark red or purple tongue and a thin and choppy pulse are evidences of the presence of static blood and phlegm–turbidity.

The key feature of this pattern is the dysfunction of joint movement due to joint deformation and stiffness, and is difficult to treat. This is different from joint movement inhibition caused by joint pain or temporary swellings in the wind–cold–damp pattern and the wind–heat–damp pattern.

Treatment method

Dispelling wind and dissolving phlegm; removing stasis and unblocking collaterals.

Formula and ingredients: Shēn Tòng Zhú Yū Tāng (Generalized Pain Stasis-Expelling Decoction)

Qín jiāo (Radix Gentianae Macrophyllae) 3 g; *chuān xiōng* (Rhizoma Chuanxiong) 6 g; *táo rén* (Semen Persicae) 9 g; *hóng huā* (Flos Carthami) 9 g; *gān cǎo* (Radix et Rhizoma Glycyrrhizae) 6 g; *qiāng huó* (Rhizoma et Radix Notopterygii) 3 g; *mò yào* (Myrrha) 6 g; *dāng guī* (Radix Angelicae Sinensis) 9 g; dry-fried *wǔ líng zhī* (Faeces Trogopterori) 6 g; *xiāng fù* (Rhizoma Cyperi) 3 g; *niú xī* (Radix Achyranthis Bidentatae) 9 g; cleaned *dì lóng* (Pheretima) 6 g.

Formula verse

Shēn Tòng Zhú Yū contains *qín jiāo xiōng, táo hóng mò guī xī dì lóng*, and *qiāng huó xiāng fù gān wǔ líng*, effective for body pain due to wind, damp, stasis, and phlegm.

Usage

Add 1.4 L of water to decoct until 250 mL are left. Take the decoction warm orally and add 800 mL of water to decoct the dregs again until 250 mL are left. Take the decoction warm, altogether 2 times a day.

Analysis

In this formula, *dāng guī* and *chuān xiōng* can nourish and invigorate blood. *Táo rén, hóng huā, wǔ líng zhī, mò yào*, and *niú xī* are added to revitalize blood and dispel stasis. Through such a combination, the body is supplemented with the simultaneous expulsion of pathogens and removal of static blood without impairing blood. Also, the static blood in this pattern is formed in the lengthy course of external wind and dampness in channels and collaterals; *qiāng huó*, *dì long*, and *qín jiāo* are applied to resolve wind–damp and unblock channels and collaterals. The binding of static blood and wind–damp inevitably influences qi flow, so *xiāng fù* is added to liberate and move qi. Freed qi flow is beneficial to the elimination of static blood and wind–damp. Though no phlegm-dissolving ingredients are used, turbid phlegm is spontaneously removed following the liberation of qi and blood by dredging channels and collaterals.

Research has shown that *táo rén*, *hóng huā*, *dāng guī*, *niú xī*, *qín jiā*, *mò yào*, and *chuān xiōng* are able to dilate blood vessels and improve local blood circulation. Furthermore, some of them can relieve pain, calm the mind, suppress inflammation, reduce proliferation of connective tissues, and allay allergy. Therefore, aside from being anti-inflammatory and analgesic, this formula has extensive pharmacological applications and can improve local locomotion.

Treatment reference

The wind–damp and phlegm–stasis pattern is persistent. As joint deformation occurs, the route to recovery is arduous and the duration of the treatment course is long. Flexible modification is required for this formula according to the state of pathogenic wind, damp, phlegm, and stasis as well as the health constitution of the patient. If the pain are acute due to severe wind–damp, add *qiāng huó*, *fáng fēng*, *wū shāo shé*, *bái huā shé*, and *guì zhī*. If there is excessive accumulation of static blood while joint deformation is obvious, add *jī xuè téng*, *tǔ biē chóng*, and *chuān shān jiǎ* to strengthen the effect of invigorating blood and unblocking collaterals. If phlegm turbidity is severe and common wind–damp-dispelling and blood-invigorating medicinals are not potent, add *bái jiè zǐ* and *dǎn nán xīng*. If it is accompanied by signs of cold triggering a fear of cold and preference for warmth in the affected regions, and limbs lacking warmth, add *fù zǐ*, *ròu guì*, *zhì chuān wū*, *lù jiǎo*, and *yín yáng huò*.

Cautions

Long-term joint pain induce the overproduction of phlegm and stasis, and can also cause healthy qi deficiency. This formula is indicated for the excess pattern due to the binding of the phlegm stasis and wind–damp. If there is obvious healthy qi deficiency, supplementary ingredients should be added.

Daily Exercises

1. What are the main clinical features of the wind–damp and phlegm–stasis pattern?
2. What are the ingredients of *Shēn Tòng Zhú Yū Tāng?* What is/are the function(s) of each ingredient in the formula?
3. Mr. Chen is a 41-year-old male. His chief complaint is recurring general joint pain for more than 4 years. The pain is mainly located in the fingers and toes, with the small joints swollen with inhibited movement. His condition worsens during cold or rainy days, but the color of the skin of the affected regions remains the same. His tongue is pale purple and his pulse is deep and thin. Please prescribe a Chinese medicinal formula for this case.

DAY TWO

The Wind–Damp and Healthy Qi Deficiency Pattern

This pattern occurs due to the long-term contraction of external wind–damp, while presenting deficiency of qi, blood, kidney and liver in the interior. This is evidently a pattern of healthy qi deficiency and pathogenic excess, and a complex of deficiency and excess. Usually, healthy qi deficiency exists in other cases of *bì* syndrome in varying degrees (mild cases will not be discussed in this section). The formation of this pattern begins from the accumulation of external wind, cold, damp, and heat pathogens in the tendons, vessels, muscles, and joints, which may inhibit the flows of qi and blood with time. Such a consequence not only produces phlegm and static blood, but also affects the transformation and generation of qi and blood, leading to the insufficiency of both essential life components.

As the tendons and bones are closely associated with the liver and kidney, i.e., the liver governing tendons and the kidney controlling bones, long-term illness of the tendons and bones will cause the liver and kidney to lack nourishment, presenting kidney and liver deficiency. Since the wind–damp pathogen remains after the development of healthy qi deficiency, it hence becomes a healthy qi deficiency and pathogenic excess pattern. This pattern is commonly seen in various kinds of arthritis, systemic lupus erythematosus (SLE), gout and several other chronic diseases.

Diagnosis

The main symptoms of this pattern are relapsing joint pain that persists for years, fatigue, weakness of the back and waist, a pale tongue, and a weak pulse. Other clinical manifestations include a sallow and lusterless complexion, inhibited movement of limbs or numbness, palpitations, shortness of breath, a fear of cold, a preference for warmth, and a white tongue coating.

This pattern often develops after repeated occurrences or a chronic episode of *bì* syndrome, turning it from the pathogenic excess pattern into the healthy qi deficiency and pathogenic excess pattern. As qi and blood fail to nourish the body due to deficiency, fatigue, a lack of strength, a sallow and lusterless complexion, limb numbness, palpitations, and shortness of breath are observed. Because the liver governs the tendon and the kidney controls the bone, impairment of the liver and kidney causes the tendons and bones to lack nourishment, manifesting as back and waist weakness and inhibited flexing and stretching movements.

Treatment method

Dispelling wind and dampness, supplementing qi and blood, and boosting the liver and kidney.

Formula and ingredients: Dú Huó Jì Shēng Tāng (Pubescent Angelica and Mistletoe Decoction)

Dú huó (Radix Angelicae Pubescentis) 9 g; *sāng jì shēng* (Herba Taxilli) 6 g; *dù zhòng* (Cortex Eucommiae) 6 g; *niú xī* (Radix Achyranthis

Bidentatae) 6 g; *xì xīn* (Radix et Rhizoma Asari) 6 g; *qín jiāo* (Radix Gentianae Macrophyllae) 6 g; *fú líng* (Poria) 6 g; *ròu guì* (Cortex Cinnamomi) 6 g; *fáng fēng* (Radix Saposhnikoviae) 6 g; *chuān xiōng* (Rhizoma Chuanxiong) 6 g; *rén shēn* (Radix et Rhizoma Ginseng) 6 g; *gān cǎo* (Radix et Rhizoma Glycyrrhizae) 6 g; *dāng guī* (Radix Angelicae Sinensis) 6 g; *sháo yào* (Radix Paeoniae) 6 g; *gān dì huáng* (Radix Rehmanniae Recens) 6 g.

Formula verse

Dú Huó Jì Shēng contains equal doses of *jiāo fáng xīn*, *guī xiōng dì sháo guì líng*, and also *dù zhòng niú xī rén shēn* and *cǎo*, treating stubborn cold and wind *bi*.

Usage

Grind the above ingredients into a crude powder and add 2 L of water to decoct until 600 mL are left. Remove the dregs and take the decoction warm, 200 mL each time, 3 times a day. Keep warm and do not catch a cold during the treatment process.

Analysis

This pattern originates from lingering wind–damp and deficient qi, blood, kidney, and liver, so *dú huó* is applied as the chief ingredient to dispel wind, disperse cold, and remove dampness due to its warm and dry natures. Meanwhile, *qín jiāo*, *fáng fēng*, and *xì xīn* are added to strengthen the effect of dispelling wind, dispersing cold, and removing dampness. As healthy qi has been in deficiency, *rén shēn* and *fú líng* are used to boost qi and the spleen. *Dāng guī*, *chuān xiōng*, *dì huáng*, and *bái sháo* serve to nourish and invigorate blood. *Ròu guì* warms and unblocks blood vessels to disperse cold. *Gān cǎo* harmonizes the actions of all medicinals in the formula. In summary, this formula boosts healthy qi as well as dispels pathogens, both of which are supplementary to each other.

According to modern pharmacological studies, *dú huó*, *qín jiāo*, *chuān xiōng*, *xì xīn*, *fáng fēng*, *and dù zhòng* can suppress inflammation and alleviate pain. *Rén shēn*, *fú líng*, *dāng guī*, *dì huáng*, and *bái sháo* can regulate the immunity, inhibit allergic reactions, fortify the body, and increase the number of erythrocytes. If *ròu guì* is used with *chuān xiōng* and *dāng guī*, blood vessels are dilated and blood circulation improved. Such a combination is curative on the pain and swellings caused by various chronic inflammations.

Treatment reference

Dú Huó Jì Shēng Tāng has moderate effects on simultaneously boosting healthy qi and dispelling pathogens. In practice, ingredient and dosage modifications are needed according to the state of healthy qi deficiency and pathogenic excess. For severe qi and blood deficiency presenting general weakness, a fear of cold, and spontaneous sweating, add *zhì huáng qí*, *gǒu qǐ zǐ*, and *bái zhú*, or apply *Sān Bì Tāng* (Three Impediments Decoction) instead. For severe deficiency of the liver and kidney presenting waist and knee weakness, add *chuān xù duàn*, *gǒu jǐ*, and *yín yáng huò*. For extreme signs of cold presenting cold joint pain and limbs lacking warmth, add *fù zǐ*, *gān jiāng*, and *bā jǐ tiān*. For severe pathogenic dampness presenting joint heaviness and skin numbness, add *cāng zhú*, *fáng jǐ*, and *hǎi tóng pí*. For extreme pain, add *zhì chuān wū*, *bái huā shé*, and *dì lóng*. When the pattern is complicated with excess pathogens such as phlegm and stasis, add *rǔ xiāng*, *táo rén*, *hóng huā*, and *bái jiè zǐ*.

Cautions

This formula contains medicinals that can boost qi, blood, the liver, and the kidney. If there are no obvious signs of healthy qi deficiency, it should not be prescribed. Hence, this is not a formula suitable for all cases of *bì* syndrome.

Daily Exercises

1. How does the wind–damp and healthy qi deficiency pattern develop? What are its main clinical features?
2. What are the ingredients of *Dú Huó Jì Shēng Tāng*? What is/are the function(s) of each ingredient?

3. Ms. Huang is a 36-year-old female. She has had joint pain for more than 10 years, especially in the knees. Her other clinical manifestations are a sallow complexion, cold limbs, fatigue, a lack of strength, waist and knee weakness, dizziness, tinnitus, a poor appetite, a bland taste in the mouth, a pale red tongue with a white coating, and a thin and weak pulse. Please prescribe a Chinese medicinal formula for this case.

Additional Formulae

Sān Bì Tāng (Three Impediments Decoction)

Ingredients of *Dú Huó Jì Shēng Tāng* without *sāng jì shēng* and with larger doses of *huáng qí* and *xù duàn*, and additional ginger.

Actions

Boosting qi and nourishing blood; dispelling wind and overcoming dampness.

Indications

Congealing qi and blood presenting limb cramps, wind *bì*, and so on.

CHAPTER 13

The Deficiency Pattern

DAY THREE

The deficiency pattern arises due to weak healthy qi, namely weakness of yin and yang, qi, blood, fluids, *zang–fu* organs, and tissues. In Chinese medicine, all disease patterns can be classified under either the deficiency pattern or the excess pattern, with those presenting the main manifestations of healthy qi deficiency belonging to the former, while others with symptoms of pathogenic excess to the latter. Accordingly, there can also be patterns with both healthy qi deficiency and pathogenic excess.

Formation of the Deficiency Pattern

Many factors can contribute to insufficient healthy qi. Generally, they originate from two sources: (1) constitutional healthy qi deficiency, which includes innate weakness (such as hereditary diseases and disorders in pregnancy and delivery stages) and improper postnatal regularities (such as a large appetite or malnutrition), and (2) food irregularities, emotional disorders, and the contraction of various pathogens by a patient already having consumed or impaired healthy qi, especially after serious or prolonged illness. Therefore, for cases of the deficiency pattern, some are mainly due to constitutional healthy qi weakness, usually manifesting as pure deficiency, while some others are resulted from other diseases, often presenting deficiency–excess complex as the root disease still remains.

Features of the Deficiency Pattern

Since the categories of healthy qi deficiency are extensive and the locations are different, its clinical manifestations are extremely complicated. In general, the main features of the deficiency pattern are a pale or sallow complexion, dispiritedness, fatigue, a lack of strength, feeling flustered, shortness of breath that is aggravated after exertion, fear of cold, limbs lacking warmth, or vexing heat in the five centers (i.e., chest, palms, and soles), tendency to perspire, loose stool, urinary incontinence, a scant tongue coating, and a feeble pulse. With respect to yin, yang, qi, and blood, some symptoms are shared by each type of deficiency. For yin and blood deficiency, as the yin and yang are imbalanced, symptoms of yang hyperactivity are often present, called deficiency heat. For yang and qi deficiency, especially yang deficiency, various signs of cold will manifest due to the loss of the warming function of yang qi, called deficiency–cold (the cold pattern is discussed in Chapter 5).

The deficiency pattern exists in a variety of diseases. For example, it occurs in infectious diseases at the recovery or chronic stage, organ functional failure stage of internal diseases, many kinds of malnutrition, hypoglycemia, hypotension, anemia, degenerative endocrine functions, chronic leukemia, neurosis, and so on. For the deficiency–excess complex pattern, it may occur in nearly all diseases, although the severity of healthy qi deficiency and pathogenic excess varies individually, which should be distinguished by their clinical manifestations.

Categories of the Deficiency Pattern

The deficiency pattern can be further categorized in accordance with the state of yin, yang, qi, blood, as well as the *zang–fu* organs, namely yin deficiency, yang deficiency, qi deficiency, and blood deficiency of the corresponding *zang–fu* organs. Common and individual manifestations of all these categories are listed in Table 1.

Aside from the above patterns, there are cases of simultaneous deficiencies of yin, yang, qi, blood, or several *zang–fu* organs, such as deficiencies of both qi and blood, deficiency of both yin and yang, yang and qi

Table 1. Manifestations of the deficiency pattern.

Pattern	Manifestations
Yin deficiency	Tidal fever
	Vexing heat in the five centers
	Night sweat
	Dry mouth and throat
	Reddish tongue with scant coating
	Thin and rapid pulse
Lung yin deficiency	Dry cough with minimal sticky sputum
	Hoarse voice
Heart yin deficiency	Palpitations
	Insomnia
	Vexation
	Restlessness
	Sores in the mouth and tongue
Stomach yin deficiency	Lack of appetite
	Epigastric upset
	Dry stool
	Dry vomiting
	Hiccups
Liver yin deficiency	Dizziness
	Blurred vision
	Tinnitus
	Dry eyes
	Lusterless nails
Kidney yin deficiency	Waist and knee weakness
	Vertigo
	Tinnitus
	Emaciation
	Seminal emission
	Scant menses
Intestinal fluid deficiency	Dry stool
	Constipation

(Continued)

Table 1.   (*Continued*)

Pattern	Manifestations
Yang deficiency	Fatigue
	Weak breathing
	Cold appearance
	Preference for resting
	Limbs lacking warmth
	Clear and profuse urine
	Pale complexion
	Pale and bulgy tongue
	Weak pulse
Heart yang deficiency	Palpitations
	Spontaneous sweating
	Oppression or pain in the chest and
	heart regions Cyanotic lips and tongue
	Slow pulse
Spleen yang deficiency	Loss of appetite
	Loose stool
	Borborygmus
	Abdominal pain
	Vomiting
	Diarrhea
	Excess secretion of drool in the mouth
	White tongue coating
	Thin and weak pulse
Kidney yang deficiency	Waist and knee weakness and coldness
	Seminal emission
	Impotence
	Profuse urine or urination incontinence
	Indigested food in the stool
	Edema,
	White tongue coating
	Deep and thin pulse
Qi deficiency	Fatigue
	Lack of strength
	Reluctance to speak
	Low voice
	Pale tongue
	Weak pulse

(*Continued*)

Table 1. (*Continued*)

Pattern	Manifestations
Lung qi deficiency	Shortness of breath
	Spontaneous sweating that is aggra-vated after exertion
	Coughing and panting; lack of strength
	Fear of cold
	Deathly pale complexion
Spleen qi deficiency	Lack of appetite
	Loose stool
	Postcibal abdominal distention
	Sallow complexion
Heart qi deficiency	Palpitations
	Shortness of breath that worsens after exertion
	Insomnia
Exterior deficiency	Perspiration
	Fear of wind
	Susceptible to colds
Blood deficiency	Dizziness
	Flowery vision
	Lusterless complexion
	Pale lips and tongue
	Thin and week pulse
Heart blood deficiency	Palpitations
	Amnesia
	Insomnia
	Dreaminess
Liver blood deficiency	Rib-side pain
	Numbness of limbs
	Nails lacking nourishment
	Tendon cramps
	Dry eyes
	Blurred vision

deficiencies, yin and blood deficiency, yang deficiency of both the heart and kidney, qi deficiency of both the lung and kidney, yin deficiency of both the lung and stomach, yin deficiency of both the liver and kidney, qi deficiency of both the spleen and stomach, yang deficiency of both the spleen and kidney, qi deficiency of both the spleen and lung, qi deficiency of both the heart and lung, and deficiency of both the heart and spleen. In this chapter, the diagnosis and treatment of the exterior deficiency pattern, the yin deficiency of the lung and stomach pattern, the yin deficiency of the liver and kidney pattern, the qi deficiency pattern, the center qi sinking pattern, the deficiency of both qi and yin pattern, the blood deficiency pattern, and the deficiency of both qi and blood pattern will be discussed.

Treatment Methods of the Deficiency Pattern

The main principle to treat the deficiency pattern is supplementation, which pertains to the supplementing method in the eight methods. Supplementation means to apply medicinals for the replenishment of healthy qi. Specifically, it boosts qi, blood, yin, and yang to eliminate various symptoms of weakness or to prevent aging. In addition, for cases of extreme healthy qi deficiency with other lingering pathogens, supplementation can build up the body's defenses and expel the pathogens by boosting healthy qi, i.e., "boosting healthy qi to eliminate pathogens." The functions of the supplementary medicinals are not only to complement various vitamins, nutrients, amino acids, and trace elements, but more importantly, regulate body immunity, improve its healthy state, neutralize toxins, and even inhibit bacteria and viruses. Therefore, supplementary medicinals are *not* equivalent to nutriment products.

Since the categories of deficiency pattern are broad, the clinical application of supplementation is not the same under different conditions. For example, this method can be categorized into supplementing qi, supplementing blood, supplementing yin, and supplementing yang. The main mechanism lies in enhancing specific *zang–fu* organs. In this chapter, we will review the supplementary methods of boosting qi to consolidate the exterior, nourishing the lung and stomach, boosting the liver and kidney, fortifying the center and boosting qi, boosting qi and nourishing yin, nourishing heart blood, boosting qi and nourishing blood, and so on. For treatment methods of boosting yang qi, see Chapter 5.

In the application of supplementing methods, it is necessary to differentiate the true and false natures of the deficiency and excess patterns. Under some circumstances, pathogenic factors are extremely exuberant and the excess pattern can present manifestations similar to those of a deficiency pattern. For such a case, supplementation methods should not be applied. Instead, the patient's spleen and stomach functions should be focused on. For patients with severe spleen–stomach weakness, the supplementary medicinals cannot be absorbed but burden the spleen and stomach, called "deficiency failing to be supplemented." For this, regulate and treat the spleen and stomach first. Furthermore, many supplementary medicinals are greasy and heavily flavored, which can affect food conversion and transportation in the spleen and stomach, thus medicinals that can fortify the spleen and harmonize the stomach, rectify qi, and assist digestion are applied.

Daily Exercises

1. How does a deficiency pattern develop? What are the diagnostic criteria of this pattern?
2. What are the main clinical manifestations of the qi deficiency, blood deficiency, yin deficiency, and yang deficiency patterns?
3. Explain the treatment principle of "supplementation." What are its main functions?
4. What aspects should be noted when applying the supplementing method?

DAY FOUR

The Exterior Deficiency Pattern

The exterior deficiency pattern refers to a disease pattern due to weakness of defensive qi and loose skin that render frequent perspiration or contraction of external pathogens. The lung is closely associated with the skin, whose functions on opening and closing sweat pores and defending external pathogens are governed by the lung, i.e., "the lung is connected to the skin and body hair." Therefore, the exterior deficiency pattern is often related to the deficiency of lung qi. Lung qi deficiency, lung illness, and serious diseases weakening lung qi can all contribute to its hypofunction in regulating the skin, thus causing the opening of sweat pores and continuous discharge of sweat, which is known as spontaneous sweating. As the *wei*–exterior qi fails to resist external pathogens due to weakness, the patient is extremely susceptible to external pathogens. This pattern is commonly seen in autonomic nervous disorders and metabolic disorders of patients with constitutional weakness or after illness or delivery.

Diagnosis

The main symptoms and signs of this pattern are frequent sweating especially after exertion and susceptibility to the common cold. Other indications include an aversion to wind, a lusterless complexion, fatigue, a lack of strength, shortness of breath, a reluctance to speak, and a thin and weak pulse.

The loosening of skin results in loss of control in the opening and closing of sweat pores, which leads to spontaneous sweating. Exertion consumes qi, triggering further loosening of skin and more severe sweating. Sweating consumes yang qi in the exterior, so the body surface lacks warmth and nourishment, causing an aversion to wind and development of cold sensations. Patients with *wei*–exterior qi deficiency are predisposed to catching a cold. As lung qi fails to nourish the body, a lusterless complexion, fatigue, a lack of strength, shortness of breath, and a reluctance to speak are observed.

The main feature of the exterior deficiency pattern is spontaneous sweating, but not all cases of spontaneous sweating pertain to this pattern. For instance, spontaneous sweating is also a main symptom of the exterior deficiency–cold pattern, but that is due to the contraction of wind–cold with many accompanying symptoms of the exterior pattern. The *yangming* qi heat pattern presents spontaneous sweating as well due to exuberant heat driving fluids outward, but in contrast, there are also interior heat symptoms. Hence, though the above two patterns and the exterior deficiency pattern have the common manifestation of spontaneous sweating, they can be differentiated by other symptoms.

Treatment method

Boosting qi to consolidate the exterior.

Formula and ingredients: Yù Píng Fēng Sǎn
(Jade Wind Barrier Powder)

Huáng qí (Radix Astragali) 180 g; *bái zhú* (Rhizoma Atractylodis Macrocephalae) 60 g; *fáng fēng* (Radix Saposhnikoviae) 60 g.

Formula verse

Yù Píng Fēng Sǎn contains *zhú qí fáng*, favorable to exterior deficiency, qi weakness, and profuse sweating.

Usage

Grind the above ingredients into a crude powder and take 6–9 g each time infused with water, 2 times a day. Alternatively, decoct the ingredients 10% of the original dosages with water.

Analysis

Spontaneous sweating of the exterior deficiency pattern is caused by lung qi deficiency, hence *huáng qí* is applied as the chief ingredient to boost lung qi and consolidate the body surface. *Bái zhú* is added to strengthen the spleen, as this organ is the source of qi and blood production and lung qi can be replenished if spleen qi is strong. Moreover, *bái zhú* itself can check sweating and its combination with *huáng qí* is able to optimize both effects. As this is a deficiency pattern and *wei*–exterior qi is weak, external pathogens tend to attack and are difficult to be removed. Therefore, *fáng fēng* is used to remove pathogens in the exterior. Its combination with *huáng qí* contains both supplementation and dispersion properties, replenishing the exterior without retaining the pathogens, and eliminating pathogens without impairing healthy qi.

Huáng qí is a proven effective agent in promoting or regulating body fluids and cellular immunity to strengthen the cells' vitality and resistance. *Yù Píng Fēng Sǎn* has a bi-directional regulatory function on the immune system — boosting weakness and suppressing overactivity.

336 Introduction to Formulae of Traditional Chinese Medicine

Treatment reference

Aside from being effective in resolving spontaneous sweating due to exterior deficiency, *Yù Píng Fēng Sǎn* is a typical formula for fortifying the immunity and treating upper respiratory diseases, especially for those with lung qi deficiency. In addition, this formula is applicable to repeated occurrences of glomerulonephritis and rheumatic diseases due to the common cold.

In practice, proper modification according to the specific disease state is required. For profuse sweating or even continuous sweating throughout the day, add *fú xiǎo mài*, *nuò dào gēn xū*, *wǔ wèi zǐ*, and *mǔ lì* to restrain leakage, consolidate the exterior, and check sweating. For serious qi deficiency, add *dǎng shēn*, *fú líng*, and *huáng jīng* to assist *huáng qí's* qi-boosting function. To counter the contraction of exogenous pathogens due to exterior deficiency and lingering exterior pathogens, add *guì zhī* and *bái sháo* to release wind–cold in the body surface and regulate qi at the *ying* and *wei* levels. If this formula is applied to treat repeated occurrences of chronic rhinitis or allergic rhinitis belonging to exterior deficiency, add *xīn yí* and *cāng ěr zǐ* to scatter wind and unblock the orifices. If there are spontaneous sweating and night sweat due to qi deficiency, *Mǔ Lì Sǎn* (Oyster Shell Powder) can also be used.

Cautions

This formula is chiefly prescribed to supplement and is only indicated for spontaneous sweating due to exterior qi deficiency. If exogenous pathogens are exuberant, do not use this formula, or the pathogens will be boosted and difficult to eliminate. Sweating in the night due to yin deficiency with internal heat is not an indication of this formula either.

Daily Exercises

1. What is the exterior deficiency pattern? What are the main symptoms and signs of this pattern? What are its main differences from the exterior deficiency–cold pattern?
2. What are the ingredients of *Yù Píng Fēng Sǎn*? What are its functions?

3. Ms. Chen is a 23-year-old female. She has been suffering from spontaneous sweating for 2 years after giving birth. It occurs even on cold winter days and an aversion to wind after sweating is observed. Since her clothes are easily drenched due to sweating, she catches a cold quite frequently. She often feels fatigued and sweating becomes much more profuse after slight exertion. Other clinical manifestations are a lusterless complexion, a poor appetite, loose stool, a pale red tongue with a white and thin coating, and a thin and weak pulse. Please prescribe a Chinese medicinal formula for this case.

Additional Formulae

Mǔ Lì Sǎn (Oyster Shell Powder)

Huáng qí (Radix Astragali) 30 g; má huáng gēn (Radix et Rhizoma Ephedrae) 30 g; calcined mǔ lì (Concha Ostreae) 30 g.

Grind the ingredients into a crude powder. Take 9 g of the powder each time and decoct 30 g of xiǎo mài (Fructus Tritici) or fú xiǎo mài (Fructus Tritici Levis) with water. Remove the dregs and take the decoction warm. Alternatively, use half of the original dosages for decoction and consumption.

Actions

Securing the exterior to check sweating.

Indications

Spontaneous sweating (aggravated in the night), palpitations, fright, shortness of breath, vexation, fatigue, a pale red tongue, and a thin and weak pulse.

DAY FIVE

The Lung–Stomach Yin Deficiency Pattern

Due to yin and fluid insufficiencies in the lung and stomach, this pattern occurs with some symptoms of dryness. Body fluids, blood, and essence are a few of the fluidal substances in our system, whose functions are to nourish and moisten organs and tissues. The main source of fluids lies in the nutrients of food, that is, stomach yin is the foundation of general fluids. Sufficient stomach yin can nourish lung yin, while stomach yin insufficiency or consumption of stomach yin after illness subsequently leads to lung yin deficiency. In turn, lung yin deficiency can also involve stomach yin. Therefore, the simultaneous impairment of lung and stomach yin is clinically frequent and a pattern emerges, which often exists in various infectious diseases of the lung (tuberculosis, pneumonia, etc.), contagious diseases of the respiratory tract (diphtheria, scarlet fever, etc.) at the late stage, and chronic gastritis.

Diagnosis

The main symptoms and signs of this pattern are a dry mouth and throat, dry cough with scant sputum, and a slippery and red tongue with a scant coating. Other clinical manifestations may include mild fever, a lack of appetite, heartburn, dull gastric pain, epigastric upset, dry stool, dry vomiting, and a thin and rapid pulse.

Since the lung and stomach fluids are unable to moisten the upper body due to insufficiency, there are feelings of a dry mouth and throat. Fluid insufficiency causes the loss of normal digestive function of the stomach, hence accounting for the lack of appetite and epigastric upset. The stomach also fails to moisten itself and the intestines, rendering dry vomiting, dry stool, and dull pain in that region. If it is accompanied by heartburn, it is almost certain caused by stomach yin insufficiency, which leads to deficiency heat. Due to lung yin insufficiency and the ascending counterflow of lung qi, dry cough and scant sputum are present. A slippery and red tongue with a scant coating and a thin and rapid pulse are signs of lung yin deficiency.

Clinically, the manifestations of this pattern may be specific to lung yin impairment or stomach yin impairment. Generally, for the former, dry coughing and chest pain can be serious, while for the latter, epigastric upset, dull pain, and a slippery and red tongue are observed. This pattern can be seen either in diseases of internal damage or in externally contracted diseases, whose manifestations are those concerning the lung in particular, and lingering pathogens are often in attendance, presenting mild fever.

Treatment method

Nourishing the lung and stomach.

Formula and ingredients: Shā Shēn Mài Dōng Tāng
(Adenophorae and Ophiopogon Decoction)

Shā shēn (Radix Adenophorae seu Glehniae) 9 g; *yù zhú* (Rhizoma Polygonati Odorati) 6 g; *gān cǎo* (Radix et Rhizoma Glycyrrhizae) 3 g; winter-collected *sāng yè* (Folium Mori) 4.5 g; *mài dōng* (Radix Ophiopogonis) 9 g; raw *biǎn dòu* (Semen Lablab Album) 4.5 g; *tiān huā fěn* (Radix Trichosanthis) 4.5 g.

Formula verse

Shā Shēn Mài Dōng contains *biǎn dòu shā*, *yù zhú huā fěn*, and *gān cǎo*, most favorable to lung–stomach yin impairment with epigastric upset and dry cough.

Usage

Add 1.4 L of water to decoct until 400 mL are left. Remove the dregs and take it warm, 2 times in a day.

Analysis

As this pattern is typically resulted from lung–stomach fluid impairment, *shā shēn*, *mài dōng*, *yù zhú*, *tiān huā fěn*, and other such sweet, cold, and fluid-generating medicinals are applied to nourish lung–stomach fluids. *Biǎn dòu* and *gān cǎo* are added to boost stomach qi because restoration of the stomach triggers spontaneous production of fluids. *Sāng yè*, light and diffusing, serves to remove lingering pathogens in the lung. The whole formula is specially indicated for impaired lung–stomach yin chiefly presenting dry cough. It can replenish lung yin and remove lingering pathogens to stop dry cough.

According to modern pharmacological studies, *shā shēn*, *mài dōng*, and *yù zhú* have functions of relieving fever, removing sputum, checking cough, inhibiting bacteria, and regulating immunity to a certain extent.

Treatment reference

Shā Shēn Mài Dōng Tāng is indicated for both lung yin deficiency and stomach yin deficiency, but in application, modification is required according to the particularity in each kind of deficiency. For a dominant deficiency of stomach, add *shí hú* and use a large dose of *yù zhú* and *mài dōng*, while for that of lung yin, use a large dose of *běi shā shēn* and pear skin. For dull pain in the stomach, add *bái sháo*, which in combination with *gān cǎo* in the formula can produce and nourish yin through its acid and sweet natures, as well as relax spasms and alleviate pain. For stomach yin deficiency with stomach qi stagnation presenting gastric distention and aggravation after meals, add *hòu pò huā*, *méi gui huā*, *fó shǒu*, and so on. For dry, constipated stool, add *huǒ má rén*, *guā lóu rén*, *bǎi zǐ rén*, and so on. For lingering lung heat with chronic cough, add *dì gǔ pí* and *pí pá yè*. For lung yin insufficiency with a distressing cough and scant phlegm, add *guā lóu pí*, *hǎi gé qiào*, and *chuān bèi mǔ*. For chronic impairment of lung yin, stew *bǎi hé* with tremella separately for consumption. In addition, stomach yin deficiency tends to induce weak food conversion and transportation in the spleen and stomach, and qi movement is also prone to stagnation. Therefore, in the duration of applying lung–stomach yin-nourishing medicinals, it is advisable to add some qi-freeing and digestion-promoting herbs, such as *chén pí* and *shā rén*, and also to avoid sweet and cold nourishing ingredients that hinder spleen–stomach functions.

Cautions

The functions of the spleen and stomach should be closely monitored when this formula is applied to treat the disease. For severe lung heat presenting a dry cough and throat, do not administer this formula in case pathogens are retained by the nourishing and greasy ingredients.

Daily Exercises

1. What are the main symptoms and signs of the lung–stomach yin deficiency pattern?
2. What are the ingredients of *Shā Shēn Mài Dōng Tāng*? What are its indications?

3. Mr. Jin is a 27-year-old male. He has been suffering from lobar pneumonia for 2 weeks. His body temperature has been back to normal after treatment, but he complains of hot sensations in the face in the afternoon, feverish feelings in palms and soles, dry coughing, chest oppression and pain, a poor appetite, dry stool, yellow urine, a red tongue with a scant coating, and a thin and rapid pulse. An X-ray examination shows shadows of lesions of pneumonia. Please prescribe a Chinese medicinal formula for this case.

DAY SIX

The Liver–Kidney Yin Deficiency Pattern

The liver–kidney yin deficiency pattern occurs due to yin and fluid insufficiencies in the liver and kidney, with some symptoms of malnourished essence, internal stirring deficiency fire, and so on. Kidney yin, also called kidney essence or genuine yin, is the prenatal foundation for body structure and functions. Liver yin is originated from kidney yin, thus kidney yin insufficiency usually leads to liver yin insufficiency and accordingly, consumption of liver yin results in kidney yin insufficiency. Therefore, the simultaneous impairment of liver and kidney yin is clinically common and forms a pattern. Under normal circumstances, kidney yin and kidney yang mutually regulates each other to maintain a balance. If kidney yin is insufficient, hyperactivity of yang fire may occur, which is termed ministerial fire. Likewise, liver yin insufficiency can also cause hyperactivity of liver yang, bringing about various symptoms of deficiency–heat. In addition, along with kidney yin, stomach yin, the postnatal foundation, is rooted in kidney yin and constantly nourishes and replenishes kidney yin. Severe or prolonged deficiency of stomach yin hence induces depletion of kidney yin. This pattern is commonly seen in acute infectious diseases at the late stage, various chronic diseases such as hypertension, diabetes, *xiāo kě* ("wasting-thirst," 消渴), neurosis, chronic nephritis, chronic pyelonephritis, tuberculosis, and various gynecological diseases.

Diagnosis

The main symptoms and signs of this pattern are waist and knee weakness, vertigo, tinnitus, feverish sensations in the chest, palms, and soles, and a red tongue. Other indications may include amnesia, insomnia, flowery vision, a dry mouth and throat, red cheeks, night sweat, thirst with a compulsion for drinking, seminal emission, scant menses or amenorrhea, or flooding and spotting (*bēng lòu*, 崩漏) in females, and a thin and rapid pulse.

The liver and kidney respectively control the tendons and bones. Liver–kidney yin and fluid insufficiencies cause depletion of nourishment in the waist and knees, resulting in weakness in those regions. Liver and kidney yin deficiency leads to deficiency–fire disturbing the upper body, hence presenting vertigo, tinnitus, amnesia, and flowery vision. Vexing heat in the chest, palms, and soles, reddish cheeks, night sweat, and a red tongue are all signs of deficiency–heat. A dry mouth and throat, and a thirst with desire for drinking reflect fluid deficiency. Insufficient essence and blood lead to scant menses or amenorrhea in females, but if there is internal exuberance of deficiency–heat, the blood will flow frenetically due to heat, causing flooding and spotting (*bēng lòu*, 崩漏). Deficiency–fire disturbing the heart spirit causes insomnia, and if it disrupts the essence chamber, seminal emission occurs.

Since the kidney governs the bone and produces marrow, and the brain is the center of marrow (thus also known as "the sea of marrow") and is dependent on kidney yin for nourishment, there is a close relationship between the brain and clinical manifestations of the liver–kidney yin deficiency pattern. Moreover, the kidney also regulates urinary and reproductive functions, hence diseases in these systems often present the liver–kidney yin deficiency pattern. In this respect, it differs from the lung–stomach yin deficiency pattern, which often occurs in respiratory and digestive diseases. For liver–kidney yin deficiency at the late stage of externally contracted febrile diseases, it usually arises following critical conditions and aside from the above related symptoms, there are other manifestations of malnourished tendons and vessels and internal stirring of deficiency–wind, such as lingering mild fever, and cramps and stiffness in the hands and feet.

Treatment method

Nourishing the liver and kidney.

Formula and ingredients: Liù Wèi Dì Huáng Wán (Six-Ingredient Rehmannia Pill)

Shú dì huáng (Radix Rehmanniae Praeparata) 24 g; *shān zhū yú* (Fructus Corni) 12 g; *shān yào* (Rhizoma Dioscoreae) 12 g; *zé xiè* (Rhizoma Alismatis) 12 g; skinless *fú líng* (Poria) 9 g; *mǔ dān pí* (Cortex Moutan) 9 g.

Formula verse

Liù Wèi Dì Huáng Wán boosts the kidney and liver, with a combination of *shān yào dān zé yú* and *líng*.

Usage

The ingredients are made into a powder and cooked with honey into pills the size of firmiana seeds. Take 6–9 g each time with warm water or light salt water on an empty stomach, 3 times a day. Alternatively, similar doses of the above ingredients can be decocted in 1.5 L of water.

Analysis

The treatment focused on the liver–kidney yin deficiency pattern lies in boosting kidney yin. When kidney yin has been replenished, liver yin production will resume. Therefore, *shú dì huáng* is applied as the chief ingredient to nourish kidney yin. *Shān zhū yú* assists *shú dì huáng* in enhancing kidney yin and supplements liver yin as well. Moreover, as it is sour and astringent, it can restrain leakages, so it is especially applicable to frequent urination, seminal emissions, profuse menstruation, continuous sweating, and other incontinent symptoms. *Shān yào* fortifies spleen and stomach qi. By strengthening the conversion and transportation functions of the spleen and stomach, sufficient food essence will be produced to replenish liver and kidney yin, i.e., "boosting the postnatal foundation to restore the prenatal root." Traditionally, *shān yào* can supplement spleen yin as well. Since liver and kidney yin fluid insufficiency causes hypofunction or disorder of the liver and kidney, deficiency–heat-clearing *mǔ dān pí* and dampness-removing *zé xiè* and *fú líng* are added to eliminate pathological products and rectify the *zang–fu* organs, which are beneficial to the restoration of liver and kidney fluids. In the past, this formula was considered as a method of supplementation with drainage, which can boost without retaining pathogens due to the lack of greasy properties. Indeed, with its main function to nourish and boost, the dosages of boosting medicinals in this formula are relatively large.

Liù Wèi Dì Huáng Wán has been shown to significantly strengthen cellular immunity by stimulating and enhancing the formation of antibodies. In addition, it possesses properties of supplementation. This formula can also promote urea discharge, so it is indicated for chronic nephritis. Furthermore, it is effective in reducing renal hypertension, improving renal functions, ameliorating the nervous system and sexual glands, delaying senility, and inhibiting tumor growth. *Shú dì huáng* in the formula is able to bring down blood sugar, strengthen the heart, promote urination, and inhibit allergy. A large dose of *shān zhū yú* exerts bidirectional regulation through enhancing and reducing blood pressure levels to prevent shock and treat pathological hypertension, respectively. *Shān yào* is rich in nutrients and amylases, which can boost and nourish the body and help in digestion. *Mǔ dān pí* can dilate blood vessels and improve capillary permeability. *Zé xiè* reduces blood fat levels, alleviates atherosclerosis, and ameliorates renal functions. *Fú líng* is able to promote urination and strengthen cellular immunity. The above-mentioned properties of this formula prove that it is effective for rectifying body immunity and treating disorder of multiple organs.

Treatment reference

Liù Wèi Dì Huáng Wán is a classical formula for nourishing kidney and liver yin. It covers a wide spectrum of indications in the clinic. It is applicable to yin deficiency with a yang hyperactivity pattern of hypertension, esophageal epithelial hyperplasia, diabetes, insipidus, chronic prostatitis, functional uterine bleeding, central retinitis, sudden deafness, infantile malnutrition, bradygenesis, sores in the mouth and tongue, aplastic anemia, and many more.

In practice, proper modification is required. For significant yin deficiency and vigorous fire presenting vexing heat in the five centers, night sweat, and sores and ulcers in the mouth and tongue, replace *shú dì huáng* with *shēng dì* to strengthen the effect of cooling blood and clearing heat, or add *zhī mǔ* and *huáng bǎi* to clear deficiency heat, becoming *Zhī Bǎi Dì Huáng Wán* (Anemarrhena, Phellodendron, and Rehmannia Pill). For failure of the kidney to receive qi which causes the ascending counterflow of kidney qi presenting panting and hiccups due to kidney yin deficiency, add *wǔ wèi zǐ* to astringe kidney qi and check panting and hiccups, becoming *Dū Qì Wán* (Qi-Restraining Pill). For failure of the liver and kidney to nourish the head and eyes due to yin deficiency presenting significant dizziness, tinnitus, flowery vision, or dry eyes, add *gǒu qǐ zǐ* and *jú huā*, becoming *Qǐ Jú Dì Huáng Wán* (Lycium Berry, Chrysanthemum, and Rehmannia Pill). For severe deficiency-type panting due to kidney yin insufficiency with lung yin deficiency, add *mài dōng* and *wǔ wèi zǐ*, becoming *Bā Xiān Cháng Shòu Wán* (Eight-Immortal Longevity Pill). Aside from liver yin insufficiency, if there is liver yang deficiency, which is manifested as cold sensations in the lower part of the body, clear and profuse urine, lower limb edema, and a pale bulgy tongue, add *guì zhī* (or *ròu guì*) and *fù zǐ*, becoming *Shèn Qì Wán* (Kidney Qi Pill).

At the late stage of externally contracted febrile diseases, the presence of the liver–kidney yin deficiency pattern due to consumption of liver and kidney fluids is usually accompanied by lingering pathogenic heat. For such a case, the medicinals for supplementing the liver and kidney should not be too greasy and astringent, so *shú dì huáng* and *shān zhū yú* are inappropriate. Instead, *Jiā Jiǎn Fù Mài Tāng* (Pulse-Restoring Variant Decoction) is often prescribed. In this formula, *gān dì huáng*, *mài dōng*, and *bái sháo* serve to nourish and supplement kidney yin, and *má rén* and *zhì gān cǎo* boost healthy qi and moisten dryness. If the patient also presents profuse sweating and is extremely flustered, add raw *lóng gǔ* and *mǔ lì*. If cramps, stiffness, and wriggling of the extremities are also observed, which is a case of internal stirring of deficiency–wind, add raw *mǔ lì*, *biē jiǎ*, and *guī bǎn* to nourish yin and extinguish wind.

Cautions

Though *Liù Wèi Dì Huáng Wán* is a supplementary formula with drainage properties, it is chiefly used for boosting. If the liver–kidney yin deficiency pattern is accompanied by obvious dampness, deficiency–fire, turbid phlegm, and static blood, pathogen-removing medicinals should be accordingly added.

Daily Exercises

1. What are the main symptoms and signs of the liver–kidney yin deficiency pattern? What is the relationship between kidney yin and liver yin?
2. What are the ingredients of *Liù Wèi Dì Huáng Wán*? What is/are the main function(s) of each ingredient?
3. List at least three formulae modified according to *Liù Wèi Dì Huáng Wán*.
4. Ms. Chen is a 36-year-old female. She has been suffering from renal tuberculosis for more than a year. After treatment, a routine urine test showed no abnormal findings, but she still feels aching pain in the lumbar region and is unable to sit or stand for long. Her other clinical manifestations are feverish feelings in palms and soles, emaciation, mildly red cheeks, vexation, insomnia, thirst at night, a dry feeling in the eyes, a red and thin tongue with a scant coating and dry surface, and a thin and rapid pulse. Please prescribe a Chinese medicinal formula for this case.

Additional Formulae

Zhī Bǎi Dì Huáng Wán (*Anemarrhena, Phellodendron, and Rehmannia Pill*)

Ingredients of *Liù Wèi Dì Huáng Wán* (Six-Ingredient Rehmannia Pill) together with *zhī mǔ* (Rhizoma Anemarrhenae) and *huáng bǎi* (Cortex Phellodendri Chinensis). The ingredients are made into pills. Take the pills 3–6 g orally each time, 2–3 times a day.

Actions

Nourishing yin and purging fire.

Indications

Yin deficiency resulting in vigorous fire presenting steaming bone fever, tidal fever, night sweat, nocturnal emission, and dark urine.

Dū Qì Wán (Qi-Restraining Pill)

Ingredients of *Liù Wèi Dì Huáng Wán* (Six-Ingredient Rehmannia Pill) together with *wǔ wèi zǐ* (Fructus Schisandrae Chinensis). The ingredients are made into pills. Take the pills 3–6 g orally each time, 2–3 times a day.

Actions

Astringing the lung and supplementing the kidney.

Indications

Deficiency of both the lung and kidney presenting panting and coughing.

Qǐ Jú Dì Huáng Wán (Lycium Berry, Chrysanthemum, and Rehmannia Pill)

Ingredients of *Liù Wèi Dì Huáng Wán* (Six-Ingredient Rehmannia Pill) together with *gǒu qǐ zǐ* (Fructus Lycii) and *jú huā* (Flos Chrysanthemi). The ingredients are made into pills. Take the pills 3–6 g orally each time, 2–3 times a day.

Actions

Nourishing yin and supplementing the kidney; nourishing the liver and brightening the vision.

Indications

Liver and kidney deficiencies presenting headaches, dizzy vision, weakened eyesight, or diplopia, and dry and painful eyes.

Shèn Qì Wán (Kidney Qi Pill)

Gān dì huáng (Radix Rehmanniae Recens) 24 g; *shān yào* (Rhizoma Dioscoreae) 12 g; *shān zhū yú* (Fructus Corni) 12 g; *zé xiè* (Rhizoma

Alismatis) 9 g; *fú líng* (Poria) 9 g; *mǔ dān pí* (Cortex Moutan) 9 g; *guì zhī* (Ramulus Cinnamomi) 3 g; *fù zǐ* (Radix Aconiti Lateralis Praeparata) 3 g.

Usage

The ingredients are made into powder and cooked with honey into pills. Take the pills 6–9 g orally each time with warm water or salt water, 1–2 times a day. Alternatively, decoct the above ingredients in similar dosages with water.

Actions

Warming and supplementing kidney yang.

Indications

Kidney yang insufficiency presenting lumbar pain, leg weakness, cold feelings in the lower part of the body, cramps in the lower abdomen, restlessness due to vexing heat, inhibited or frequent urination, a pale bulgy tongue, and a deficient and weak pulse with a deep and fine feeling in the *chǐ* section.

Jiā Jiǎn Fù Mài Tāng (Pulse-Restoring Variant Decoction)

Zhì gān cǎo (Radix et Rhizoma Glycyrrhizae Praeparata cum Melle) 18 g; *gān dì huáng* (Radix Rehmanniae Recens) 18 g; raw *bái sháo* (Radix Paeoniae Alba) 18 g; *mài dōng* (Radix Ophiopogonis) with the core 15 g; *ē jiāo* (Colla Corii Asini) 9 g; *má rén* (Fructus Cannabis) 9g.

Usage

Add 1.2 L of water to decoct until 900 mL are left. Remove the dregs and take the decoction warm, 3 times a day.

Actions

Nourishing yin and blood, and supplementing the liver and kidney.

Indications

Pathogenic heat consuming liver and kidney yin and fluids presenting persistent mild fever, feverish feelings in the palms and soles, a dry mouth and lips, vexation, palpitations, and a large deficient or hasty pulse.

THE 12TH WEEK

DAY ONE

The Qi Deficiency Pattern

The qi deficiency pattern is primarily caused by spleen–lung qi deficiency. Broadly speaking, qi deficiency indicates insufficient qi of the whole body, so all *zang–fu* organs may potentially suffer from the qi deficiency pattern. However, since the spleen is the source of qi and blood production and the lung governs qi movement of the body, both of which are also closely related, qi deficiency is chiefly manifested as spleen and lung qi deficiency, and hence generally, the qi deficiency pattern refers to the qi deficiency in these two organs if there is no specific explanation. This pattern is commonly seen in various chronic diseases, such as chronic gastritis, chronic enteritis, chronic nephritis, chronic hepatitis, anemia, malnutrition, and neurosis. It may also occur in the convalescence from acute febrile diseases.

Diagnosis

The main symptoms and signs of this pattern are a pale or sallow complexion, fatigue, a lack of strength, a poor appetite, and loose stool. Other manifestations may include weak breathing, a reluctance to speak, a low voice, a pale tongue with a thin coating, and a thin and moderate or soft pulse.

Qi of the human body is vital for the nourishment of the system and maintenance of life. Deficiency leads to a pale or sallow complexion, a lack of strength, fatigue, dispiritedness, and a pale tongue. As spleen qi fails to transport and convert food due to insufficiency, a poor appetite and loose stool result. Lung qi insufficiency renders weak breathing and a low voice. The deficiency of qi also causes weakness in blood circulation, which is presented as a thin and moderate or soft pulse.

Both the qi deficiency pattern and yang deficiency pattern have manifestations of weakened body functions. In general, the yang deficiency pattern is accompanied by symptoms of qi deficiency, and for the qi deficiency pattern, if it develops further, it will turn into the yang deficiency pattern. The main differences of these two patterns lie in the fact that for the yang deficiency pattern, since there is insufficient yang qi, symptoms of cold such as a fear of cold, cold limbs, and feeling comfortable in a warm surrounding are presented, while the qi deficiency pattern has no obvious cold signs.

Treatment method

Supplementing qi and fortifying the spleen.

Formula and ingredients: Sì Jūn Zǐ Tāng (Four Gentlemen Decoction)

Rén shēn (Radix et Rhizoma Ginseng) 10g; *bái zhú* (Rhizoma Atractylodis Macrocephalae) 9g; skinless *fú líng* (Poria) 9g; *zhì gān cǎo* (Radix et Rhizoma Glycyrrhizae Praeparata cum Melle) 6g.

Formula verse

Sì Jūn Zǐ Tāng fortifies the spleen, containing *shēn*, *zhú*, *fú ling*, and *gān cǎo*.

Usage

Grind the ingredients into powder. Take 6g each time to be decocted with 800mL of water until 200mL are left. Remove the dregs and take the decoction warm at any time. Alternatively, decoct the same dosages of the above ingredients with water. *Rén shēn* in the formula can be replaced by *dǎng shēn* (Radix Codonopsis), but the latter's function is relatively inferior.

Analysis

In *Sì Jūn Zǐ Tāng*, *rén shēn* serves as a power supplement to boost basal qi and also fortifies the spleen and lung, being the chief ingredient of this formula. *Bái zhú* and *fú líng* are added to strengthen the spleen and dry dampness. *Zhì gān cǎo* can fortify the spleen and stomach to harmonize the actions of all medicinals. As a whole, this formula enhances the source of qi and blood production by boosting spleen qi and restoring transportation and conversion functions. Consequently, weak qi can be replenished.

According to modern pharmacological studies, this formula can increase the synthesis of hepatic glycogen, enhance thymosin activity, and improve cellular and humoral immunity. Moreover, this formula can also rectify gastrointestinal functions and promote marrow blood production, especially the production of red blood cells. Therefore, this formula is often used in blood-supplementing therapies to strengthen the effect of enhancing blood. In addition, this formula can increase blood pressure levels to rescue patients from shock by regulating the nervous system, heart functions, and endocrine secretion. In this formula, *rén shēn* is able to increase the number of red blood cells, hemoglobin, and white blood cells, promote metabolism, strengthen the nervous system, adrenal cortex, and heart functions, decrease blood sugar levels, and prevent allergy. *Bái zhú* can protect the liver, prevent the decrease of hepatic glycogen, and promote urination. Aside from inducing urination, *fú líng* and *bái zhú* can also improve the immunity of the body, which is similar to that of *rén shēn*. *Gān cǎo* is effective in increasing the production of adrenocortical hormones, removing toxins, relieving spasms, as well as protecting the stomach mucous membrane.

Treatment reference

Sì Jūn Zǐ Tāng is the fundamental formula for supplementing qi, applicable to patients with a qi-deficient physique, improper nursing after illness, or qi deficiency due to chronic illness. It is suitable for long-term oral intake. Clinically, this formula is applied to treat various chronic digestive diseases, anemia, chyluria, insipidus, infantile malnutrition, vomiting during pregnancy, neurosis, and many more.

Many qi-supplementing formulae devised in the past are based on *Sì Jūn Zǐ Tāng*. For example, if *chén pí* is added to this formula, it becomes *Yì Gōng Sǎn* (Special Achievement Powder), which is more suitable in treating spleen–stomach weakness with qi stagnation presenting gastric and abdominal distention and fullness. If *chén pí* and *bàn xià* are added, it becomes *Liù Jūn Zǐ Tāng* (Six Gentlemen Decoction), which is more appropriate for spleen–stomach weakness with internal obstruction by phlegm–damp presenting nausea, vomiting, a productive cough with loose and white phlegm, and a greasy tongue coating. If *xiāng fù* (or *mù xiāng*) and *shā rén* are added to *Liù Jūn Zǐ Tāng*, it becomes *Xiāng Shā Liù Jūn*

Zǐ Tāng (Costusroot and Amomum Six Gentlemen Decoction), whose functions of supplementing qi, boosting the spleen, rectifying qi, dissolving phlegm, and removing dampness are all-rounded. If *biǎn dòu*, *yì yǐ rén*, *shān yào*, *lián zǐ*, *shā rén*, and *jié gěng* are added to *Sì Jūn Zǐ Tāng*, it is called *Shēn Líng Bái Zhú Sǎn* (Ginseng, Poria, and Atractylodes Macrocephalae Powder), which is indicated for spleen–stomach weakness presenting vomiting, diarrhea, weakness in limbs, or the poor development of a child. This formula is safe for long-term intake.

Cautions

Sì Jūn Zǐ Tāng is a mild formula and rarely has side effects, thus it is called "Four Gentlemen Decoction." It is prescribed mainly for supplementation and has little effect in eliminating pathogens, so for patients with qi deficiency and persistent pathogens, this formula is not appropriate as a single prescription.

Daily Exercises

1. What are the main clinical symptoms of the qi deficiency pattern?
2. What are the ingredients of *Sì Jūn Zǐ Tāng*? What are the functions of this formula?
3. Mr. Wang is a 31-year-old male. Since young, he has been extremely susceptible to illnesses. In the past 6 months, he has had a poor appetite, loose stool for 2 to 3 times a day, a lack of strength, dizziness, feeling flustered, liability to sweat after exertion, difficulty in concentrating in tasks, an absence of taste, an absence of thirst, a pale tongue with a white coating, and a thin, soft, and weak pulse. Please prescribe a Chinese medicinal formula for this case.

Additional Formulae

Yì Gōng Sǎn (Special Achievement Powder)

Ingredients of *Sì Jūn Zǐ Tāng* with *chén pí* (Pericarpium Citri Reticulatae) 6 g.

Usage

Grind the ingredients into a fine powder. Take 6 g each time to be decocted with 5 pieces of ginger and 2 pieces of date as well as water. Remove the dregs and take the decoction warm. Alternatively, directly decoct the ingredients of the original dosages with water.

Actions

Boosting qi and fortifying the spleen; rectifying qi and promoting transportation.

Indications

Spleen–stomach qi deficiency with qi stagnation presenting a poor appetite, chest and epigastric stuffiness, oppression and distress, vomiting, and diarrhea.

Liù Jūn Zǐ Tāng (Six Gentlemen Decoction)

Ingredients of *Sì Jūn Zǐ Tāng* with *chén pí* (Pericarpium Citri Reticulatae) 6 g and *bàn xià* (Rhizoma Pinelliae) 6 g. Add water to decoct.

Actions

Boosting qi and fortifying the spleen; drying dampness and dissolving phlegm.

Indications

Spleen–stomach qi deficiency with phlegm–damp presenting a poor appetite, loose stool, chest and epigastric oppression and distress, productive cough with whitish phlegm, nausea, and vomiting.

Xiāng Shā Liù Jūn Zǐ Tāng (Costusroot and Amomum Six Gentlemen Decoction)

Ingredients of *Liù Jūn Zǐ Tāng* together with *xiāng fù* (Rhizoma Cyperi) 6 g and *shā rén* (Fructus Amomi) 6 g. Currently, *xiāng fù* is often replaced by *mù xiāng* (Radix Aucklandiae). Add water to decoct.

Actions

Boosting qi and supplementing the middle, fortifying the spleen and harmonizing the stomach, and rectifying qi and relieving pain.

Indications

Spleen–stomach qi deficiency with obstruction by dampness and qi stagnation presenting a poor appetite, belching, abdominal distention, fullness, or pain, vomiting, and diarrhea.

Shēn Líng Bái Zhú Sǎn (Ginseng, Poria, and Atractylodes Macrocephalae Powder)

Skinless *lián zǐ* (Semen Nelumbinis) 10 g; *yì yǐ rén* (Semen Coicis) 10 g; *shā rén* (Fructus Amomi) 5 g; dry-fried until deep yellow *jié gěng* (Radix Platycodonis) 10 g; ginger juice-soaked and slightly fried *bái biǎn dòu* (Semen Lablab Album) without skin 15 g; *fú líng* (Poria) 20 g; *rén shēn* (Radix et Rhizoma Ginseng) 10 g; dry-fried *gān cǎo* (Radix et Rhizoma Glycyrrhizae) 5 g; *bái zhú* (Rhizoma Atractylodis Macrocephalae) 10 g; *shān yào* (Rhizoma Dioscoreae) 20 g.

Grind the ingredients into a fine powder and take 6–9 g each time for oral intake with jujube soup. Alternatively, decoct the ingredients in water.

Actions

Boosting qi and fortifying the spleen; harmonizing the stomach and percolating dampness.

Indications

Spleen–stomach qi deficiency with dampness presenting limb weakness, emaciation, indigestion, or vomiting, or diarrhea, chest and epigastric distress and distention, a sallow complexion, a pale tongue with a white and greasy coating, and a deficient and moderate pulse.

DAY TWO

The Center Deficiency with Qi Sinking Pattern

This is a disease pattern where the spleen and stomach lose their function of raising due to qi deficiency. The raising function of these two organs is mainly reflected by their functions of transportation, conversion, and distribution of food substances. Food substances can only be distributed throughout the body by the lung under normal circumstances of raising. Many organs and tissues that are localized are also dependent on the raising function of the spleen and stomach. Therefore, when this property becomes dysfunctional, pathological changes of sinking can be triggered, and is termed center deficiency and qi sinking. Its specific manifestations are associated with the disorder of food conversion, transportation, and distribution in that food essence is discharged from the urine and stool instead of being distributed upward, generating diarrhea and chyluria. In addition, some organs and tissues, especially the stomach, liver, kidney, rectum, anus, and uterus, will sink and may even become prolapsed. This pattern is commonly seen in various kinds of chronic enteritis, dysentery, functional disorders of the intestines, rectal prolapse, uterine prolapse, gastroptosis, hepatoptosis, nephroptosis, profuse menstruation, abortion, chyluria, and so on. From the above, this pattern is actually representative of only one type of the qi deficiency pattern, namely qi deficiency presenting symptoms of the lack of strength to raise and sinking center qi.

Diagnosis

The main symptoms and signs of this pattern are a sagging and distending stomach or abdomen, sagging or prolapse of anus, uterus, and other organs, and persistent diarrhea. Other indications include fatigue, a lack of strength, shortness of breath, a reluctance to speak, dizziness, flowery vision, a pale tongue with a white coating, and a thin and weak pulse.

Due to center qi sinking and a lack of strength to raise, there will be gastric or abdominal sagging, distention, and fullness, and also symptoms of sagging or prolapse of the anus and other organs. Due to general qi deficiency, there may be fatigue, a lack of strength, shortness of breath, and a reluctance to speak. Since clear yang qi is unable to ascend, dizziness and flowery vision occur. As this pattern is chiefly manifested as head heaviness, it is different from the swirling sensation of dizziness caused by liver–kidney yin deficiency.

Treatment method

Supplementing the spleen and stomach, raising center qi.

Formula and ingredients: Bǔ Zhōng Yì Qì Tāng (Center-Supplementing and Qi-Boosting Decoction)

Huáng qí (Radix Astragali) 3 g; *zhì gān cǎo* (Radix et Rhizoma Glycyrrhizae Praeparata cum Melle) 1.5 g; *rén shēn* (Radix et Rhizoma Ginseng) 1 g; wine-baked or sun-dried *dāng guī* (Radix Angelicae Sinensis) 0.6 g; *chén pí* (Pericarpium Citri Reticulatae) 1 g; *shēng má* (Rhizoma Cimicifugae) 1 g; *chái hú* (Radix Bupleuri) 1 g; *bái zhú* (Rhizoma Atractylodis Macrocephalae) 1 g.

Formula verse

Bǔ Zhōng Yì Qì contains *qí zhú chén, shēn chái shēng cǎo*, and *dāng guī*. Good at treating fatigue and internal damage, also excellent for qi deficiency with sinking.

Usage

Grind the above ingredients into a crude powder and add 600 mL of water to decoct until 200 mL are left. Remove the dregs and take the decoction warm on an empty stomach, 2 times a day. Alternatively, decoct 5 times of the above dosages with water or make into pills for oral intake with warm water or ginger soup, 6–12 g a time, 2–3 times a day.

Analysis

This formula prescribes *huáng qí* as the chief ingredient to supplement spleen–stomach qi, and when it is combined with raising and dispersing medicinals such as *shēng má* and *chái hú*, it is able to lift center qi, which is a feature of the this formula combination. *Rén shēn, bái zhú*, and *zhì gān cǎo* are used to fortify qi and the spleen, strengthening the qi-boosting effect of this formula. *Chén pí* is an assistant ingredient to prevent supplementing products from stagnating qi movement. As qi and blood can be mutually generated, *dāng guī* is included to nourish blood. Sufficient blood is beneficial to the transformation and production of qi. In conclusion, this formula can supplement the spleen and stomach, and lift sinking qi at the same time. It is indicated for center deficiency with sinking qi presenting prolonged diarrhea, bleeding, sagging organs, or prolapse.

Researches have shown that *Bǔ Zhōng Yì Qì Tāng* can activate the uterus and several other organs. It can improve the general body state, alleviate damage caused by radioactive rays and chemical drugs, and boost immunity. *Shēng má* and *chái hú* exert a significant synergic effect in this formula. Bidirectional regulation is also apparent; when intestinal peristalsis is hyperactive, it acts to inhibit, and when intestinal tension decreases, it functions to activate. *Huáng qí* has similar properties in the regulation of sex hormones and is able to stimulate the central nervous system. If it is combined with *rén shēn*, the body will be robustly strengthened and organ functions rectified. *Dāng guī* can improve blood circulation and is beneficial to the restoration of organ functions.

Treatment reference

Bǔ Zhōng Yì Qì Tāng is widely used in the clinic, and is applicable to all kinds of diseases within the realm of the qi deficiency with sagging qi pattern, such as internal diseases (gastroptosis, nephroptosis, ulcers, chronic enteritis, rectal prolapse, inguinal hernia, chyluria, etc.), gynecological diseases (uterine prolapse, postpartum urinary retention or during pregnancy, a bulging bladder and vagina, vaginal bleeding or other kinds of bleeding, profuse leukorrhea, etc.), and ophthalmological diseases (paralytic strabismus and ptosis). Moreover, this formula has favorable effects on boosting qi and eliminating heat, so it is used to treat deficiency–heat due to spleen–stomach weakness, namely relieving fever with sweet–warm medicinals.

In practice, proper modification is required. If only *rén shēn, huáng qí, zhì gān cǎo, shēng má*, and *bái zhú* are used for decoction, it becomes *Jǔ Yáng Jiāng* (Yang-Lifting Decoction), which is indicated for sinking qi due to deficiency or yang qi desertion presenting profuse uterine bleeding, profuse sweating, and extreme weakness. In the formula, *rén shēn* and *huáng qí* are applied in large doses. If *cāng zhú* and *mù xiāng* are added to *Bǔ Zhōng Yì Qì Tāng*, it becomes *Tiáo Zhōng Yì Qì Tāng* (Center-Rectifying and Qi-Boosting Decoction), which is indicated for qi deficiency with damp–turbidity obstruction in the middle. For headaches caused by clear yang failing to ascend due to center qi deficiency, add *bái sháo, xì xīn, chuān xiōng*, and *màn jīng zǐ*. For sinking qi deficiency due to yang deficiency presenting symptoms of cold, add *ròu guì, fù zǐ*, and *gān jiāng*. For serious diarrhea or profuse sweating, add *wū méi, wǔ bèi zǐ*, and *hē zǐ*. For gastroptosis, add *fú líng, yù jīn, zhǐ qiào, shān zhā, jī nèi jīn, shān yào, dà zǎo*, and others medicinals to fortify the spleen and boost qi as well as assist digestion. For postpartum urinary retention, add *fú líng* and *dōng kuí zǐ*. For infantile diarrhea in the autumn, if it is complicated by food accumulation, add *shén qū* and *shān zhā*; if it is complicated by sensations of incomplete defecation and mucus in the stool, add *mù xiāng* and *huáng lián*; if it is complicated by heat pathogens impairing yin, add *hú huáng lián* and *bái sháo*; and if it is complicated by rectal prolapse, add *yīng sù qiào, hē zǐ, ér chá*, and so on.

Cautions

As *Bǔ Zhōng Yì Qì Tāng* is warm-natured and travels upward, it is not appropriate for treating a flushed face, a bitter taste in the mouth, dizziness, and a dry mouth and throat caused by up-flaming of deficiency–fire, and nausea, vomiting, and stomach distention caused by ascending counterflow of qi movement.

Daily Exercises

1. What is the center deficiency with sinking qi pattern? What are the clinical manifestations of this formula?

2. What are the ingredients of *Bǔ Zhōng Yì Qì Tāng*? What are the main characteristics of this formula combination?
3. Ms. Chen is a 34-year-old female. Tall and thin, she tends to be afflicted with illnesses. Her clinical report indicates fatigue, a lack of strength, a poor appetite, abdominal distention and discomfort after meals, frequent belching, loose stool, a pale red, bulgy, and tender tongue with a white coating, and a thin and weak pulse. A physical examination shows gastroptosis and uterine prolapse. Please prescribe a Chinese medicinal formula for this case.

Additional Formulae

Jǔ Yáng Jiāng (Yang-Lifting Decoction)

Rén shēn (Radix et Rhizoma Ginseng) 12 g; *zhì huáng qí* (Radix Astragali Praeparata cum Melle) 12 g; *zhì gān cǎo* (Radix et Rhizoma Glycyrrhizae Praeparata cum Melle) 5 g; *shēng má* (Rhizoma Cimicifugae) 3 g; *bái zhú* (Rhizoma Atractylodis Macrocephalae) 5 g. Add water to decoct.

Actions

Boosting qi and lifting the sunken.

Indications

Sinking qi due to deficiency, profuse uterine bleeding, blood desertion, and yang collapse.

Tiáo Zhōng Yì Qì Tāng (Center-Rectifying and Qi-Boosting Decoction)

Rén shēn (Radix et Rhizoma Ginseng) 9 g; *huáng qí* (Radix Astragali) 12 g; *gān cǎo* (Radix et Rhizoma Glycyrrhizae) 4 g; *chén pí* (Pericarpium Citri Reticulatae) 6 g; *shēng má* (Rhizoma Cimicifugae) 4 g; *chái hú* (Radix Bupleuri) 6 g; *cāng zhú* (Rhizoma Atractylodis) 6 g; *mù xiāng* (Radix Aucklandiae) 4 g. Add water to decoct.

Actions

Boosting qi and lifting the sunken; drying dampness and fortifying the spleen.

Indications

Spleen and stomach qi deficiency with encumbering dampness.

DAY THREE

The Deficiency of Both Qi and Yin Pattern

The deficiency of both qi and yin pattern results in a disease pattern involving deficiency of both qi and body fluids, mainly qi–yin deficiency of the heart and lung. All the organs of the human body have both yin and yang, and cases of deficiency of both yin and yang are quite common. For example, the stomach, kidney, liver, heart, and lung often have patterns of deficiency of both yin and yang. However, the deficiency of both qi and yin pattern mainly lies in the fluid and qi deficiencies of the heart and lung. With regards to the disease causes, some are derived from exuberant interior heat driving fluids outward and impairing qi and yin of the heart and lung in the course of externally contracted febrile diseases, while others are resulted from a persistent cough due to lung deficiency that renders qi and yin deficiencies of the lung. Yet, others are due to anxiety and overstrain that cause the heart and yin to be consumed and damaged. This pattern is commonly seen in internal diseases of chronic lung diseases (pneumosilicosis, lung cancer, and tuberculosis), rheumatic heart disease, myocarditis, and coronary disease, as well as acute febrile diseases with profuse sweating and weakness, heart failure, and shock.

Diagnosis

The main symptoms and signs of this pattern are fatigue, a lack of strength, shortness of breath, a dry mouth with thirst, and sweating. Other clinical manifestations may include thirst with a desire for drinking, an irritable cough with scant phlegm, a dry and red or dry and pale tongue with a thin coating, and a deficient and thin, deficient and rapid, or scattered, large, and weak pulse.

Insufficiency of heart and lung qi causes fatigue, a lack of strength, shortness of breath, and even panting. Profuse sweating not only consumes body fluids, but also eats away at qi. Insufficient body fluids of the heart and lung manifest as a dry mouth, thirst, and a dry tongue coating. Consumption of qi further worsens symptoms of qi deficiency. An irritable cough with scant phlegm is caused by lung yin deficiency and ascending counterflow of lung qi. A deficient and weak pulse is a reflection of healthy qi deficiency.

If this pattern occurs in externally contracted febrile diseases, extreme deficient qi and body fluids will be in a state of desertion, and symptoms of profuse sweating and a drastic drop of high fever may be observed. A reduction in blood pressure can also be detected via a physical examination. If this pattern worsens, desertion will occur due to persistent sweating and overconsumption of qi and body fluids.

Treatment method

Supplementing yin and qi.

Formula and Ingredients: Shēng Mài Sǎn (Pulse-Engendering Powder)

Rén shēn (Radix et Rhizoma Ginseng) 10 g; *mài dōng* (Radix Ophiopogonis) 10 g; *wǔ wèi zǐ* (Fructus Schisandrae Chinensis) 6 g.

Formula verse

Shēng Mài applies *mài wèi* and *rén shēn*, urgently needed for deficiency of both qi and yin.

Usage

Add 800 mL of water to decoct until 300 mL are left. Remove the dregs and take the decoction warm at any time of the day. *Rén shēn* in the formula can be replaced by *dǎng shēn* (Radix Codonopsis), but the latter's effect is relatively inferior.

Analysis

This formula is also called *Shēng Mài Yǐn* (Pulse-Engendering Decoction). It uses *rén shēn* as the chief ingredient, whose property is sweet and warm, and is a powerful medicinal for supplementing qi, generating fluids, and nourishing yin. Sweet and cold *mài dōng* is combined to nourish yin (especially heart yin) and produce fluids. *Wǔ wèi zǐ* is sour, and able to check sweating, astringe the lung, and relieve coughing and panting. Therefore, the whole formula can supplement qi and yin of both the lung and heart, promote fluid production, nourish the heart, boost the lung, and astringe the lung.

According to modern pharmacological researches, when *Shēng Mài Sǎn* is applied to treat coronary disease and shock, it is able to strengthen the contraction of heart muscles, improve blood circulation (especially in the coronary arteries), stimulate endocrine secretion, rectify the general state of the body, and increase blood pressure, and has lasting beneficial effects on fortifying the heart. This formula can also regulate the immune system. All in all, it exerts a wide range of effects on the human body.

Treatment reference

Shēng Mài Sǎn is applicable to both acute and critical diseases and to many chronic diseases, being a commonly used qi–yin-nourishing formula by practitioners. Aside from treating qi–yin deficiency of both the heart and lung, it can also be applied to treat other organs with both qi and yin deficiency. Clinically, it can be used singly, or with other medicinals. Nowadays, preparation forms of oral fluids and injection have been made for convenience of use. It can be used to treat many heart and lung diseases, heart failure, and shock.

In practice, proper modification is required. For the desertion of both yin and yang pattern of acute febrile diseases presenting profuse sweating, dispiritedness, cold sensations in the four extremities, and a fine pulse, add *fù zǐ, ròu guì, gān jiāng*, and so on. For extreme deficiency of heart and lung qi presenting spontaneous sweating and palpitations, add *huáng qí* and *zhì gān cǎo*. For thin patients with prolonged coughing, a lack of appetite, and restlessness in sleep, add *huái shān yào, fú líng, lián zǐ*, and *bái zhú*. For heart yin insufficiency presenting insomnia and sweating, add *fú shén*, *dān shēn*, *lóng gǔ*, and *mǔ lì*. For tachycardia, add *fú shén*, *lóng chǐ*, *cí shí*, *suān zǎo rén*, *shēng dì*, *zhì gān cǎo*, and so on.

Cautions

This is a formula for supplementing deficiency. It should not be prescribed to treat profuse sweating and extreme thirst caused by exuberant heat in the interior. This formula was prescribed for summer heat syndrome in the past, but its purpose was to treat summer heat consuming qi and yin rather than to clear summer heat.

Daily Exercises

1. How is the diagnosis of the deficiency of both qi and yin pattern carried out? Is it an acute disease pattern or a chronic one?
2. What are the ingredients of *Shēng Mài Sǎn?* What are its indications?
3. Ms. Wang is a 63-year-old female. She was hospitalized due to heart failure secondary to chronic bronchitis complicated by pneumonia. She has been treated by antibiotics, diuretics, and cardiotonics. Last night, her complexion turned pale all of a sudden, and she experienced fatigue, a lack of strength, profuse sweating, chest oppression, shortness of breath, nausea, vomiting, and had a dry mouth with thirst, a dry and red tongue, and a thin and moderate pulse (46 beats per minute). Her blood pressure was recorded as 75/20 mmHg. Please prescribe a Chinese medicinal formula for this case.

DAY FOUR

The Blood Deficiency Pattern

The blood deficiency pattern is a pattern of weakness due to blood insufficiency. It can be resulted from the dysfunctional generation and conversion of food due to spleen–stomach weakness, profuse bleeding, or blood consumption due to chronic illness. This pattern is commonly seen in anemia, the recovery stage after an illness, and many gynecological diseases.

Diagnosis

The main symptoms and signs of this pattern are a sallow complexion, pale lips and nails, headaches, dizziness, and a pale tongue. Other indications may include palpitations, insomnia, scant menses, amenorrhea, postpartum oligogalactia, infertility, and a thin pulse.

The main function of blood is to nourish organs and the body. Blood deficiency almost definitely causes weakness of organs, which is especially significant to the heart and liver. As the blood fails to reach the head and eyes, the complexion turns sallow and lips become pale, together with symptoms of dizziness, vertigo, and a pale tongue. Heart blood insufficiency leads to the chaos of the heart spirit, hence palpitations, insomnia, and anemia are common. Blood insufficiency also leads to menstruation without a stable source of blood, hence bleeding is scant, delayed, or even absent. As blood fails to be converted into breast milk due to deficiency, postpartum oligogalactia or even a lack of milk secretion may occur. Blood deficiency also leads to empty vessels, which is reflected by a thin pulse.

Treatment method

Supplementing the blood.

Formula and ingredients: Sì Wù Tāng (Four Substances Decoction)

Wine-soaked before being fried *dāng guī* (Radix Angelicae Sinensis) 10 g; *chuān xiōng* (Rhizoma Chuanxiong) 10 g; *bái sháo* (Radix Paeoniae Alba) 10 g; steamed with wine spray *shú dì huáng* (Radix Rehmanniae Praeparata) 10 g.

Formula verse

Sì Wù contains *guī dì sháo* and *xiōng*, being the fundamental formula for yin and blood insufficiencies.

Usage

Grind the above ingredients into a crude powder. Decoct 9 g with 400 mL of water until 200 mL are left. Remove the dregs and take the decoction warm on an empty stomach, 3 times a day in the morning, afternoon, and evening.

Analysis

In the formula, *dāng guī*, being able to supplement and stimulate blood, and *shú dì huáng*, being able to supplement and nourish blood with its warm and sweet natures, are used as the chief ingredients of this formula. *Chuān xiōng* is pungent and unblocks and rectifies qi and blood, adding a blood-invigorating dimension to this formula. *Bái sháo* is acidic and supplements yin and blood, and acts to astringe. Therefore, all the ingredients as a whole ensures this formula supplements blood without stagnation, and moves blood without breaking it up, termed "dissipation in supplementation and astringency in dissipation." It is the fundamental formula for supplementing blood.

Sì Wù Tāng can improve blood circulation and promote the production of red blood cells. *In vitro* tests have provided evidence that this formula can improve cellular and fluidal immunity. All studies have indicated that it can not only ameliorate anemia, but also rectify multiple functions of the whole body.

Treatment reference

Sì Wù Tāng is a commonly used formula for supplementing blood and rectifying menstruation in gynecology. Aside from anemia and weakness after illness, it is also applicable to many gynecological diseases, such as menstrual irregularities, dysmenorrhea, amenorrhea, abdominal pain during pregnancy, an unborn or a dead fetus, and life-threatening abortions.

In practice, there are many kinds of formula modifications. For blood deficiency with cold exuberance in the lower *jiao* presenting abnormal cold pain, scant and light-colored menses, and delayed menstruation, add *ài yè* and *ē jiāo*, becoming *Jiāo Ài Sì Wù Tāng* (Artemisiae and Donkey Hide Four Substances Decoction). For blood deficiency with static blood presenting the stagnation of blood, purplish and sticky menses with blood clots, and abdominal pain, add *táo rén* and *hóng huā*, becoming *Táo Hóng Sì Wù Tāng* (Peach Kernel and Carthamus Four Substances Decoction). For blood deficiency with qi failing to control blood due to deficiency presenting early menstruation in profuse amounts and pale in color, add *rén shēn* and *huáng qí*, becoming *Shèng Yù Tāng* (Saint Recovery

Decoction). For blood deficiency with constrained heat, add *huáng qín*, *dì gǔ pí*, and *mǔ dān pí*, and replace *shú dì huáng* with *shēng dì*. By adding *jú huā*, *bái jí lí*, and so on, this formula is applicable in treating hypertension due to blood deficiency stirring wind. For various urticarial diseases, add *chán tuì*, *jiāng cán*, *kǔ shēn*, *mǔ dān pí*, and *zhī zǐ* accordingly. In addition, modified *Sì Wù Tāng* is indicated for many other diseases, such as allergic purpura, nosebleeds, nervous headaches, pertusis, and angioneurotic edema.

Cautions

The ingredients of this formula are nourishing, but greasy or sour and astringent, which are inappropriate for patients with exuberant pathogenic factors or with spleen–stomach weakness and dyspepsia. Both *shú dì huáng* and *dāng guī* in this formula can relax bowels, so they are not appropriate for patients with loose stool.

Daily Exercises

1. How can the blood deficiency pattern be diagnosed?
2. What are the ingredients of the *Sì Wù Tāng*? List at least three modified formulae based on the strength of *Sì Wù Tāng*.
3. Ms. Shi is a 26-year-old female. She had menarche at the age of 17. Since then, her menstruation is always scant and light in color. Her cycle averages 45–50 days. When her period arrives, she feels cold abdominal pain and her complexion turns sallow, with occasional headaches, palpitations, a pale tongue with a scant coating, and a thin and weak pulse. Please prescribe a Chinese medicinal formula for this case.

Additional Formulae

Jiāo Ài Sì Wù Tāng (Artemisiae and Donkey Hide Four Substances Decoction)

Ingredients of *Sì Wù Tāng* together with *ē jiāo* (Colla Corii Asini) 8 g and *ài yè* (Folium Artemisiae Argyi) 10 g.

Decoct the ingredients with water and remove the dregs. Dissolve *ē jiāo* in the decoction and take it warm.

Actions

Nourishing blood and stopping bleeding; rectifying menstruation and calming the fetus.

Indications

Flooding and spotting (*bēng lòu*; 崩漏) in females presenting profuse menstruation, persistent postpartum bleeding or after abortion, or bleeding during pregnancy, and abdominal pain.

Táo Hóng Sì Wù Tāng (Peach Kernel and Carthamus Four Substances Decoction)

Ingredients of *Sì Wù Tāng* together with *táo rén* (Semen Persicae) 6 g and *hóng huā* (Flos Carthami) 4 g. Add water to decoct.

Actions

Supplementing and invigorating blood, and resolving stasis.

Indications

Early menstruation in females in profuse amounts, purplish and sticky menses, or menses with blood clots, and abdominal pain and distention.

Shèng Yù Tāng (Saint Recovery Decoction)

Shú dì huáng (Radix Rehmanniae Praeparata) 20 g; wine-stirred *bái sháo* (Radix Paeoniae Alba) 15 g; *chuān xiōng* (Rhizoma Chuanxiong) 9 g; *rén shēn* (Radix et Rhizoma Ginseng) 15 g; wine-washed *dāng guī* (Radix Angelicae Sinensis) 12 g; *zhì huáng qí* (Radix Astragali Praeparata cum Melle) 12 g. Add water to decoct.

Actions

Boosting qi and supplementing and controlling blood.

Indications

Early menstruation in large amounts in females (light in color), mental fatigue, and a lack of strength.

DAY FIVE

The Deficiency of Both Qi and Blood Pattern

Evidently from its name, this is a weakness pattern with deficiency of both qi and blood; it can either be derived from qi deficiency or from blood deficiency. It is commonly seen in anemic disorders, poor nursing after recovery from disease, neurosis, many heart diseases, malnutrition, chronic consumptive diseases, and gynecological diseases.

Diagnosis

The main symptoms and signs of this pattern are fatigue, a lack of strength, a lusterless complexion, headaches, palpitations, a pale tongue, and a thin and weak pulse. Other manifestations may include weak breathing, a reluctance to speak, spontaneous sweating, dizziness, insomnia, amnesia, scant menses or amenorrhea in females, and uterine bleeding.

This pattern has symptoms of both qi deficiency and blood deficiency. It is clinically manifested as the deterioration of functions and lack of nourishment of the *zang–fu* organs. It occurs more commonly in the heart and spleen, because these two organs are closely related to the production and transportation of qi and blood. Due to qi deficiency, fatigue, the loss of strength, weak breathing, and a reluctance to speak are often presented. As qi fails to secure the exterior due to deficiency, there is spontaneous sweating. The deprivation of nourishment of the head and face from blood and qi leads to headaches, dizziness, a pale or sallow complexion without rosiness, and a pale tongue and lips. In addition, the lack of self-nourishment of blood causes palpitations, insomnia, and amnesia. As qi and blood are insufficient, blood vessels are partially filled or even completely unfilled and blood flow is inefficient, manifesting as a thin and weak pulse.

The deficiency of both qi and blood pattern is usually associated with the heart and spleen, thus it is also sometimes called the heart–spleen deficiency pattern. This is different from the deficiency of both qi and yin pattern, which is mainly related to the heart and lung.

Treatment method

Boosting qi and supplementing blood.

Formula and ingredients: *Guī Pí Tāng (Spleen-Restoring Decoction)*

Bái zhú (Rhizoma Atractylodis Macrocephalae) 30 g; *fú shén* (Sclerotium Poriae Pararadicis) 30 g; *huáng qí* (Radix Astragali) 30 g; *lóng yǎn ròu* (Arillus Longan) 30 g; dry-fried *suān zǎo rén* (Semen Ziziphi Spinosae) without shell 30 g; *rén shēn* (Radix et Rhizoma Ginseng) 15 g; *mù xiāng* (Radix Aucklandiae) 15 g; *zhì gān cǎo* (Radix et Rhizoma Glycyrrhizae Praeparata cum Melle) 8 g; *dāng guī* (Radix Angelicae Sinensis) 3 g; honey-fried *yuǎn zhì* (Radix Polygalae) 3 g.

Formula verse

Guī Pí Tāng contains *zhú shēn qí*, *guīcǎo*, *fú shén*, *suān zǎomù xiāng*, and *lóng yǎn ròu*. To be decocted with ginger and jujubes, it is beneficial to the heart and spleen.

Usage

Grind the above ingredients into a crude powder and decoct 12 g each time with 500 mL of water, 5 pieces of ginger, and 1 piece of jujube until 300 mL are left. Remove the dregs and take the decoction warm at any time of the day. Alternatively, decoct 1/3 of the original dosages of all ingredients with water, 5 g of ginger, and 3 pieces of jujube. Another common method is to make honey pills in similar doses, weighing 15 g each or in the size of firmiana seeds, called *Guī Pí Wán* (Spleen-Restoring Pill). Take 1 pill or 9 g each on an empty stomach with warm water, 3 times a day.

Analysis

In this formula, *rén shēn*, *huáng qí*, *bái zhú*, *gān cǎo*, *shēng jiāng*, and *dà zǎo* are sweet and warm and can supplement qi. *Dāng guī* and *lóng yǎn ròu* are able to nourish yin and blood. Therefore, the effect of supplementing both qi and blood is implied in this formula. *Rén shēn*, *huáng qí*, and *dāng guī* are the chief ingredients for this purpose. Specifically targeting the symptoms of palpitations, insomnia, and amnesia, which are due to insufficient heart blood, *fú shén* and *suān zǎo rén* are used to nourish the heart and calm the mind. *Yuǎn zhì* is added to anchor the mind. *Mù xiāng* rectifies qi, fortifies the spleen, assists in food transportation and conversion, and prevents cloying qi- and blood-supplementing medicinals from hindering qi movement and spleen–stomach functions. Overall, this formula is excellent in supplementing qi and blood, and especially effective in fortifying the spleen and nourishing the heart. As the spleen partly manages blood flow, severe spleen qi deficiency may lead to extensive bleeding symptoms, such as spitting of blood and bloody stool. As for women, uterine bleeding may occur. Profuse bleeding further aggravates the degree of deficiency of qi and blood. This formula strengthens the spleen's blood-managing function by boosting the heart and the spleen. This formula is thus named *Guī Pí Wán* according to its action of nourishing blood by restoring the function of the spleen.

Guī Pí Wán is able to increase blood sugar, resist shock due to scalding, increase hemoglobin production, and improve coagulatory functions. These properties are related to complex pharmacological functions of *rén shēn*, *dāng guī*, and *huáng qí* on strengthening the body, activating the nervous system, and improving endocrine functions.

Treatment reference

Guī Pí Wán is a commonly used formula for deficiencies of both heart–spleen and qi and blood. Indications of this formula range from amnesia and palpitations caused by excessive anxiety or overstrain that impairs the heart and spleen, to qi and blood deficiency and various bleeding disorders due to the loss of function of the spleen to manage blood. In modern clinical practice, this formula is further applied to treat leukorrhea caused by damp–turbidity pouring downward due to spleen deficiency, night sweat, neurosis, thrombopenic purpura, functional uterine bleeding, multiple erythema, allergic reactions, post-traumatic brain syndrome, heart disease, chronic heart failure, and so on.

The qi and blood deficiency pattern is quite commonplace, but as its manifestations are widespread, modification of the formula is done in many ways. For severe blood deficiency, add *shú dì huáng* and *gǒu qǐ zǐ*. For massive bloody stool, add *ē jiāo zhū*, *xuè yú tàn*, *ǒu jié*, and so on. For menopausal syndrome, add *lóng gǔ* and *mǔ lì*. For accompanying symptoms of a flushed face and vexing heat in the five centers (chest, palms, and soles) due to deficiency–heat, add *dì gǔ pí* and *mǔ dān pí*. If there is a presence of edema, add *fú líng*, *zé xiè*, and so on. Currently, clinicians are often spoilt for choice in selecting qi- and blood-supplementing formulae, examples of which include *Shèng Yù Tāng* mentioned in the previous section, which is a formula both for qi and blood supplementation. *Bā Zhēn Tāng* (Eight-Gem Decoction), a combination of *Sì Jūn Zǐ Tāng* and *Sì Wù Tāng*, is another general formula for qi and blood deficiency. For deficient yang desertion due to qi and blood insufficiency presenting fever, a flushed face, vexation, thirst with a desire for drinking, a large, surging, and deficient pulse, or fever and headaches due to blood deficiency during menstruation, prescribe a large dose of *huáng qí* together with *dāng guī* to supplement and nourish the qi and blood, becoming *Dāng Guī Bǔ Xuè Tāng* (Chinese Angelica Blood-Supplementing Decoction).

Cautions

Although the nature of this formula is mild, it is not applicable to cases with the sinking of center qi or lingering pathogenic factors. If the spleen and stomach of the patient are functioning poorly and he has a poor appetite and loose stool, the doctor should be cautious when prescribing this formula, because it may interfere with the functions of the spleen and stomach because of its enriching and cloying properties.

Daily Exercises

1. What are the clinical manifestations of the deficiency of both qi and blood pattern?
2. What are the ingredients of *Guī Pí Tāng*? What are its indications?
3. Ms. Zhao is a 22-year-old female. She has a pale complexion, and experiences fatigue, a lack of strength, vertigo, palpitations, a poor appetite, profuse and light red menses, occasional bleeding from the teeth, frequent purple macules in the skin, a pale tongue, and a thin and weak pulse. Her platelet count is recorded as $42 \times 10^9/L$. Please prescribe a Chinese medicinal formula for this case.

Additional Formulae

Bā Zhēn Tāng (*Eight-Gem Decoction*)

Wine-stirred *dāng guī* (Radix Angelicae Sinensis) 9 g; *chuān xiōng* (Rhizoma Chuanxiong) 6 g; *bái sháo* (Radix Paeoniae Alba) 9 g; wine-stirred *shú dì huáng* (Radix Rehmanniae Praeparata) 12 g; *rén shēn* (Radix et Rhizoma Ginseng) 6 g; dry-fried *bái zhú* (Rhizoma Atractylodis Macrocephalae) 9 g; *fú líng* (Poria) 6 g; *zhì gān cǎo* (Radix et Rhizoma Glycyrrhizae Praeparata cum Melle) 3 g. Add 3 pieces of ginger and 2 pieces of jujube for decoction in water.

Actions

Supplementing qi and blood.

Indications

Qi and blood deficiency presenting a pale or sallow complexion, vertigo, dizzy vision, fatigue, shortness of breath, a reluctance to speak, (severe) palpitations, a poor appetite, a pale tongue, and a thin and weak pulse.

Dāng Guī Bǔ Xuè Tāng (*Chinese Angelica Blood-Supplementing Decoction*)

Huáng qí (Radix Astragali) 30 g; wine-washed *dāng guī* (Radix Angelicae Sinensis) 6 g. Add water to decoct.

Actions

Boosting qi and generating blood.

Indications

Blood deficiency presenting fever, hot sensations in the muscles, a flushed face, vexing thirst with a desire to drink, a large, surging, and deficient pulse, headaches during menstruation or after delivery, or lingering ulcers and sores.

CHAPTER 14

The Complex Pattern

DAY SIX

In previous chapters, we have learnt about the diagnosis, treatment methods, and corresponding formulae of the exterior pattern, interior pattern, cold pattern, heat pattern, deficiency pattern, and excess pattern originating from different sources. However, clinically, the nature of disease does not exist in a single form, but in various permutations, such as diseases involving both the exterior and interior, cold and heat, and deficiency and excess. Such combinatorial natures make up the complex pattern. The disease can also be complicated by pathogenic factors, such as dampness, rheum, phlegm, qi stagnation, and food accumulation, but the complex pattern discussed here refers to the co-existence of two opposing aspects of the eight principles in a disease.

Features of the Complex Pattern

With the presence of symptoms of two opposing natures in the complex pattern, its clinical profile is thus much more complicated. In particular, this pattern can either be of the exterior–interior complex, cold–heat complex, deficiency–excess complex, or of many other circumstances, hence it is extremely challenging to pinpoint any uniform clinical features due to its vast scope. For diagnosis, the key point lies in the presence of symptoms of the specific patterns involved in the disease. Therefore, precise judgment can only be made on the basis of the thorough understanding of the clinical manifestations of the exterior, interior, cold, heat, deficiency, and excess patterns.

Categories of the Complex Pattern

The complex pattern can be generally classified into diseases encompassing both the exterior and interior, the cold–heat complex, and the deficiency–excess complex. Delving further according to different pathogenic natures and locations, there are many more explicit patterns, such as exterior cold and interior heat, exterior heat and interior cold, upper heat and lower cold, lower heat and upper cold, qi deficiency with stagnation, blood deficiency with stasis, yang deficiency and exterior cold, yin deficiency and bowel excess, spleen deficiency and dampness obstruction, liver hyperactivity and spleen weakness, and internal block and external desertions. In this chapter, we will focus on the diagnosis and treatment of the yang deficiency and exterior cold pattern, the exterior cold with fluid retention pattern, and the cold–heat complex in the middle *jiao* pattern. Some of the other cases have already been discussed in the previous chapters while the rest will not be included in this book.

Treatment Methods of the Complex Pattern

Treatment methods must be tailored to the strength of healthy qi and the nature of pathogenic pathogens, while the medicinals administered are often opposing in nature. For diseases involving both the exterior and interior, the main technique is to relieve the exterior and clear the interior (or relieve the exterior by purgation, or relieve the exterior and warm yang). For the cold–heat complex, heat-clearing and cold-expelling methods are applied simultaneously. For the deficiency–excess complex, supplementing the deficiency and expelling the pathogens are critical, and are effected via supplementing and moving qi, supplementing qi and resolving stasis, supplementing qi and promoting digestion, supplementing qi and removing dampness, supplementing blood and moving stasis, enriching yin and relaxing bowels, and so on.

The diagnosis and treatment of the complex pattern are fairly complicated and difficult, but it is very common in clinic, especially for cases of deficiency and excess in complex. For this, several aspects should be kept in mind. First, the key concept, i.e., discerning the main symptoms of the exterior, interior, cold, heat, deficiency, and excess patterns from the complicated clinical manifestations, especially for some paradoxical symptoms. Only through this manner, treatment methods can then be determined. In addition, the various natures should be prioritized. In a complex pattern, the level of importance of differently natured or completely opposing pathogenic aspects are unequal and one of them is more significant. For example, in diseases involving both the exterior and interior, the dominant pattern can be the exterior or interior. Likewise, for the cold–heat complex, the cold may be more severe than the heat, or vice versa, and for the deficiency–excess complex, healthy qi in deficiency may be primary concern or pathogenic excess may be more significant. Therefore, priority levels must be appropriately assigned before establishing the treatment method. Next, after prioritization, although one nature may be less significant, there is still a need to consider its contribution to the disease. What does this mean? As there is co-existence of opposing pathological changes in the complex pattern, it implies it is different from the pattern of a single pathogen and thus, the application of treatment methods and medicinals should be given more attention so as to prevent further complications involving the minor nature while treating its major counterpart. For example, when exterior cold-releasing medicinals are prescribed for the treatment of the exterior cold and interior heat pattern, dispersion by acrid–warm medicinals should never be applied in excess, or the interior heat will be boosted. As for the cold–heat complex pattern, cold and cool medicinals should not be used excessively in case of assisting the cold pathogen, and similarly, large doses of warm- and heat-natured ingredients should be avoided. For the deficiency–excess complex, excessive supplementing medicinals are discouraged as they may retain pathogens and increase the difficulty in treatment. Also, pathogens should not be intensely targeted, in case of the further impairment of healthy qi.

Daily Exercises

1. What is the complex pattern? What are its general categories?
2. When attending to a patient with the complex pattern, how are accurate diagnosis and judgment performed?
3. What are the treatment methods for the complex pattern? What aspects are noteworthy when diagnosing and treating the complex pattern?

THE 13TH WEEK

DAY ONE

The Yang Deficiency and Exterior Cold Pattern

This is a disease pattern involving both the exterior and interior in which the patient with yang qi deficiency is further affected by wind–cold. This pattern is commonly seen in several special types of the common cold or at the initial stage of other infectious diseases. It also exists in nephritis, Keshan disease, and at the acute stage of vascular headaches. With regards to the disease nature, this pattern involves both the exterior and interior, and is also accompanied by both deficiency and excess.

Diagnosis

The main symptoms and signs of this pattern are fever, an aversion to cold, an absence of sweat, cold limbs, and a deep pulse. Other indications may include headaches, mental fatigue, a lusterless complexion, and a pale tongue with a white and moist coating.

This pattern is a complex of internal deficiency of yang qi and attack of wind–cold at the exterior. As *wei* yang is lacking, it fails to expel the wind–cold pathogens in the exterior. In addition, the wind–cold pathogens further hinder and damage the yang qi in the exterior. As a result, this pattern is more severe than general cases of the exterior wind–cold pattern. Wind–cold attacking the exterior is deemed as a *taiyang* disease, while internal deficiency of yang qi is a *shaoyin* disease, so this pattern is also termed the *taiyang–shaoyin* complex or direct cold attack on the *shaoyin* channel. Wind–cold in the exterior is manifested as fever, an aversion to cold, an absence of sweat, and headaches, while yang qi deficiency is reflected by cold limbs, a lusterless complexion, mental fatigue, and a pale tongue. As yang qi is usually too weak to invigorate the body, the fever is usually mild.

The main difference between this pattern and the exterior wind–cold pattern lies in the presence of cold limbs and a deep pulse, which are important indicators of yang qi deficiency.

Treatment method

Warming yang and promoting sweating.

Formula and ingredients: *Má Huáng Fù Zǐ Xì Xīn Tāng (Ephedra, Aconite, and Asarum Decoction)*

Má huáng (Herba Ephedrae) without knots 5 g; blast-fried *fù zǐ* (Radix Aconiti Lateralis Praeparata) without skin 3 g; *xì xīn* (Radix et Rhizoma Asari) 3 g.

Formula verse

Má Huáng Fù Zǐ Xì Xīn Tāng is the best formula for warming channels and relieving the exterior.

Usage

Add 2 L of water to decoct with *má huáng* first until 1.6 L are left. Remove the foam and add the other ingredients until 600 mL are left. Remove the dregs and take the decoction warm, 200 mL at a time, 2 times a day.

Analysis

This formula is also called *Má Fù Xì Xīn Tāng*. *Má huáng* is applied to induce sweating and relieve the exterior. *Fù zǐ* serves to warm and supplement yang qi of the heart and kidney, eliminating pathogens by invigorating yang. *Xì xīn* is able to disperse wind–cold by warming and unblocking channels. For patients with serious yang qi deficiency and further affected by wind–cold, if only acrid–warm and dispersing medicinals are administered, the yang qi will be too weak to invigorate, resulting in failure to remove pathogens by inducing sweat. If the sweat-inducing method is applied erroneously, the weak yang qi will be further consumed, contributing to yang collapse in severe cases. Therefore, *fù zǐ* is added to assist yang qi so that the exterior can be relieved without impairing yang.

According to modern pharmacological researches, *fù zǐ* can strengthen heart muscles, so in cases of heart failure or heart insufficiency, it improves general blood circulation. When patients with the exterior wind–cold pattern have signs of yang deterioration, it indicates dysfunction of peripheral circulation or heart dysfunction, so it is extermely critical to use *fù zǐ*. Additionally, *má huáng* and *xì xīn* can not only induce sweating and disperse heat, but also dilate blood vessels to assist *fù zǐ* in improving blood circulation.

Treatment reference

Má Huáng Fù Zǐ Xì Xīn Tāng is indicated for the yang deficiency and exterior cold pattern caused by contraction of wind–cold on the basis of constitutional yang qi weakness or from certain chronic diseases, such as heart disease, pulmonary infection, and nephritis. It is also applicable to the sudden loss of voice presented with a pale tongue but without obvious reddish swelling in the throat after contraction of wind–cold. It is effective in treating acute occurrences of nephritis presenting exterior excess and interior deficiency symptoms. For headaches penetrating to the brain after the contraction of wind–cold, also previously regarded as cold contraction in the *shaoyin* channel, this formula can also be used together with *chuān xiōng* and *shēng jiāng* to strengthen the dispersing and unblocking effects of acrid–warm medicinals.

Clinically, if the exterior wind–cold symptoms are mild while yang qi deficiency is severe, *xì xīn* is removed from this formula and *gān cǎo* is added, becoming *Má Huáng Fù Zǐ Gān Cǎo Tāng* (Ephedra, Aconite, and Licorice Decoction), which reduces the potency of inducing sweat with its mild nature. For constitutional yang qi deficiency with the contraction of external cold, *Zài Zào Sǎn* (Renewal Powder) formulated according to *Mā Huáng Fù Zǐ Xìn Xīn Tāng*, can be applied. It can warm and stimulate yang, as well as boost qi, being more comprehensive.

Cautions

If yang qi is extremely deficient and there are signs of yang collapse, such as diarrhea with fluids and indigested food and a feeble pulse, first apply suitable formulae to restore yang and rescue from desertion, but not acrid and dispersing ingredients like *má huáng* and *xì xīn*.

Daily Exercises

1. What is the yang deficiency and exterior cold pattern? What are its main symptoms and signs?

2. What are the functions of *Má Huáng Fù Zǐ Xì Xīn Tāng*? What are its indications?

3. Ms. Zhang is a 42-year-old female. One night, she contracted a cold on night duty. The next day, she experienced an aversion to cold with fever, sweating, a hoarse voice, insignificant redness and swelling in the throat, a bland taste in the mouth, an absence of thirst, a sallow complexion, a pale tongue with a thin coating, and a deep and thin pulse. After such an occurrence, she constantly fears the cold and her limbs often lack warmth. Please prescribe a Chinese medicinal formula for this case.

Additional Formulae

Má Huáng Fù Zǐ Gān Cǎo Tāng (Ephedra, Aconite, and Licorice Decoction)

Má huáng (Herba Ephedrae) 6 g; *zhì gān cǎo* (Radix et Rhizoma Glycyrrhizae Praeparata cum Melle) 6 g; cooked *fù zǐ* (Radix Aconiti Lateralis Praeparata) 9 g. Add water to decoct.

Actions

Assisting yang and relieving cold.

Indications

Mild pattern of yang deficiency and external contraction of cold presenting a serious aversion to cold, mild fever, an absence of sweating, and a deep pulse.

Zài Zào Sǎn (Renewal Powder)

Fù zǐ (Radix Aconiti Lateralis Praeparata); *xì xīn* (Radix et Rhizoma Asari); *guì zhī* (Ramulus Cinnamomi); *sháo yào* (Radix Paeoniae); *shēng jiāng* (Rhizoma Zingiberis Recens); *dà zo* (Fructus Jujubae); *zhì gān cǎo* (Radix et Rhizoma Glycyrrhizae Praeparata cum Melle); *huáng qí* (Radix Astragali); *rén shēn* (Radix et Rhizoma Ginseng); *chuān xiōng* (Rhizoma Chuanxiong); *qiāng huó* (Rhizoma et Radix Notopterygii); *fáng fēng* (Radix Saposhnikoviae). Add water to decoct.

Actions

Boosting qi and assisting yang; dispersing cold and relieving the exterior.

Indications

Yang deficiency and external contraction of wind–cold presenting an aversion to cold with fever (relatively severe cold and mild fever), headaches, an absence of sweating, cold limbs, fatigue, somnolence, a pale a complexion, a low voice, a pale tongue with a white coating, and a deep and weak pulse.

DAY TWO

The Exterior Cold with Fluid Retention Pattern

This pattern commonly presents coughing and panting resulted from the external contraction of wind–cold due to internal water retention, which mainly refers to water accumulation in the lung and stomach, so-called "fluid below the heart" by the ancient Chinese. This pattern pertains to diseases involving both the exterior and interior and is commonly seen in many lung diseases, such as chronic bronchitis further affected by the common cold or flu, asthma, emphysema, and pertussis.

Diagnosis

The main symptoms and signs of this pattern are fever, an aversion to cold, an absence of sweating, coughing, panting, and spitting of clear and loose phlegm. Other indications may include headaches, body aches, vomiting, thirst with a desire for hot beverages, limb and facial edema, inhibited urination, lower abdominal distention and fullness, a thin, white, and moist tongue coating, and a floating or wiry pulse.

Exterior wind–cold is manifested as an aversion to cold with fever, an absence of sweating, headaches, and body aches. Internal fluid retention checks the flow of yang qi in the chest and back, so an aversion to cold is usually more significant in the back. Fluid retention with cold pathogens in the lung prevents lung qi from diffusing and flowing downward, hence triggering coughing and panting. Spitting clear and loose phlegm, as well as inhibited urination and lower abdominal distention, are signs of fluid retention. If fluids are retained in the muscle and skin, it will cause edema in the limbs and face. If there is fluid retention in the stomach, stomach qi will tend to flow upward, resulting in vomiting. The patient may also feel thirsty with a compulsion to drink hot beverages, and a thin and moist tongue coating is indicative of internal cold retention.

Clinically, the diagnosis of this pattern should mainly focus on the coughing, panting, and clear and loose or foamy phlegm. Fever is not a definite symptom. As for the aversion to cold, it can either exist in the exterior pattern, or in cases of fluid retention obstructing yang qi without the exterior pattern. Therefore, this pattern can be seen in both externally contracted diseases and diseases of chronic internal damage. It is not necessary limited within the scope of diseases involving both the exterior and interior.

Treatment method

Relieving wind–cold in the exterior and removing fluid retention in the interior.

Formula and ingredients: Xiǎo Qīng Lóng Tāng (Minor Green Dragon Decoction)

Má huáng (Herba Ephedrae) without knots 9 g; *sháo yào* (Radix Paeoniae) 9 g; *xì xīn* (Radix et Rhizoma Asari) 3 g; *gān jiāng* (Rhizoma Zingiberis) 3 g; *zhì gān cǎo* (Radix et Rhizoma Glycyrrhizae Praeparata cum Melle) 6 g; skinless *guì zhī* (Ramulus Cinnamomi) 6 g; washed *bàn xià* (Rhizoma Pinelliae) 9 g; *wǔ wèi zǐ* (Fructus Schisandrae Chinensis) 3 g.

Formula verse

Xiǎo Qīng Lóng Tāng contains *guì sháo mú, gān jiāng xīn cǎo xià*, and *wèi*. For external wind–cold and internal fluid retention, it is also good for releasing the exterior and resolving rheum.

Usage

Add 2 L of water first to decoct *má huáng* until 1.6 L are left. Remove the foam and add the other ingredients to decoct until 600 mL are left. Remove the dregs and take the decoction warm, 200 mL each time.

Analysis

In this formula, *má huáng* and *guì zhī* are applied to induce sweating and relieve the exterior. Once the exterior is relieved, lung qi tends to diffuse and ventilate, which is beneficial in relieving coughing and calming panting, hence these two ingredients are chief in *Xiǎo Qīng Lóng Tāng*. *Xì xīn* and *gān jiāng* are addded to assist *má huáng* and *guì zhī* to eliminate external wind–cold. In addition, their warm and unblocking natures can be used to warm the lung and resolve fluid retention. At the same time when applying the above acrid dispersing medicinals that can diffuse the lung, sour and astringent *wǔ wèi zǐ* and *sháo yào* are administered. With regards to formula properties, it is both opening and closing, dispersing and astringing, and is good for the restoration of lung's diffusing and lowering functions. *Bàn xià* warms and removes phlegm–rheum to harmonize the stomach, while *zhì gān cǎo* boosts qi to harmonize the actions of other medicinals. Therefore, this formula can not only disperse exterior cold, but also diffuse and lower lung qi to relieve coughing and calm panting. Aside from the exterior cold with fluid retention pattern, this formula is applicable only if the disease has symptoms of coughing, panting, and spitting of clear loose and foamy phlegm caused by fluid retention affecting the lung.

Xiǎo Qīng Lóng Tāng is a formula proven to be able to relax bronchial smooth muscles and resist histamine effects. The combination of *má huáng* and *sháo yào* can relieve bronchial spasms. *Bàn xià*, *má huáng*, and *gān cǎo* can dispel phlegm and relieve coughing. *Guì zhī* can improve blood circulation. *Wǔ wèi zǐ* can also relieve coughing and strengthen the functions of the adrenal cortex.

Treatment reference

Xiǎo Qīng Lóng Tāng is mainly applied to treat coughing and panting induced by internal phlegm–rheum and contraction of wind–cold.

Clinically, it is indicated for chronic bronchitis, asthma, emphysema, and pulmonary heart disease complicated by external pathogenic contraction, or cases with spitting of loose and clear phlegm, an aversion to cold in the back, and an absence of thirst without external contraction.

The ingredients of the formula can be modified under different circumstances. For exterior excess without sweating, use raw *má huáng* and remove *sháo yào* from the formula. For exterior deficiency with sweating, use honey-fried *má huáng* and apply *sháo yào*. For the presence of coughing and panting without fever, apply honey-fried *má huáng* and remove *guì zhī*. For cold lungs with severe fluid retention, the dose of *gān jiāng* should be twice as large as *wǔ wèi zǐ*. For chronic lung qi deficiency with coughing, the dose of *wǔ wèi zǐ* should be large or even two times more than *gān jiāng*. For lung deficiency, use honey-fried *gān jiāng*.

For chronic fluid retention that is transformed into heat, presenting thirst, yellow and sticky phlegm, a yellow tongue coating, and a rapid pulse, add *shí gāo*, becoming *Xiǎo Qīng Lóng Jiā Shí Gāo Tāng* (Minor Blue Green Dragon Decoction plus Gypsum). For the constraint of fluid retention with an insignificant exterior pattern, remove *sháo yào*, *guì zhī*, *gān jiāng*, and *gān cǎo*, and add *shè gān*, *shēng jiāng*, *zǐ wǎn*, *kuǎn dōng huā*, and *dà zǎo*, becoming *Shè Gān Má Huáng Tāng* (Belamcanda and Ephedra Decoction). For fluid retention with severe coldness that causes dysphagia, add *fù zǐ*. For internal obstruction due to fluid retention presenting lower abdominal fullness and inhibited urination, add *fú líng*.

Cautions

If this pattern does not present the symptom of thirst, but it occurs after taking the decoction of this formula, it indicates that fluid retention will soon be resolved and is not necessarily a sign of being transformed into heat.

Daily Exercises

1. What are the clinical manifestations of the exterior cold with fluid retention pattern?
2. What are the ingredients of *Xiǎo Qīng Lóng Tāng*? What are its indications?

3. Mr. Zheng is a 54-year-old male. He has been afflicated with coughing and panting for more than 10 years, which are especially severe in
   winter. This winter, the coughing and panting have relapsed and he
   was unable to lie flat on his back in the evening. Other clinical manifestations include an aversion to cold especially in the back, spitting
   of massive amounts of loose phlegm, a thin, white, and slightly greasy
   tongue coating, and a wiry and tight pulse. Please prescribe a Chinese
   medicinal formula for this case.

Additional Formulae

Xiǎo Qīng Lóng Jiā Shí Gāo Tāng (Minor Blue Green Dragon Decoction plus Gypsum)

Ingredients of *Xiǎo Qīng Lóng Tāng* together with *shí gāo* (Gypsum
Fibrosum) 6 g. Add water to decoct.

Actions

Relieving the exterior, removing fluid retention, clearing heat, and
relieving vexation.

Indications

Fluid retention below the heart presenting coughing, panting, vexation, a
dry mouth, and a floating pulse.

Shè Gān Má Huáng Tāng (Belamcanda and Ephedra Decoction)

Shè gān (Rhizoma Belamcandae) 6 g; *má huáng* (Herba Ephedrae) 9 g;
shēng jiāng (Rhizoma Zingiberis Recens) 9 g; *xì xīn* (Radix et Rhizoma
Asari) 3 g; *zǐ wǎn* (Radix et Rhizoma Asteris) 6 g; *kuǎn dōng huā* (Flos
Farfarae) 6 g; *bàn xià* (Rhizoma Pinelliae) 9 g; *wǔ wèi zǐ* (Fructus
Schisandrae Chinensis) 3 g; jujube 2 pieces. Add water to decoct.

Actions

Diffusing the lung, dissolving phlegm, relieving coughing, and calming
panting.

Indications

Coughing and panting with a gurgling sound.

DAY THREE

The Cold–Heat Complex in the Middle *Jiao* Pattern

This is a disease pattern involving the failure of the spleen and stomach to ascend and descend, with the cold–heat complex in the middle *jiao*, caused by spleen and stomach yang qi insufficiency, internal production of deficiency–cold, and pathogenic heat attacking the spleen and stomach by exploiting their weakness in function. This pattern may occur in the course of externally contracted febrile diseases when the patient's spleen–stomach yang qi is weak or purgation is erroneously applied as a treatment such that spleen–stomach yang is impaired and the organs are further attacked by pathogenic heat. It may also occur in diseases of internal damage when the spleen and stomach yang qi are deficient and there is constrained heat in the middle *jiao*. This pattern is commonly seen together with the relapse of gastrointestinal diseases, various acute and chronic gastritis or enteritis, ulcers, chronic hepatitis, chronic cholecystitis, gastrointestinal neurosis, and many more.

Diagnosis

The main symptoms and signs of this pattern are gastric distention, fullness, and discomfort, belching or vomiting, borborygmus, diarrhea, and a slippery and greasy tongue coating. Other indications may include softness and tenderness in the stomach region, and a wiry and rapid pulse.

Spleen–stomach yang deficiency and pathogenic heat obstruction in the middle lead to inhibited qi movement, causing distention, fullness, and discomfort in the stomach. But as there is no internal obstruction of substantial pathogens, such as phlegm–rheum, static blood, and food stagnation, the abdomen is soft and not tender when pressed. Spleen–stomach weakness renders diminished function of food transportation and conversion, and together with the influence of heat pathogens in the spleen and stomach, the affected organs are unable to ascend and descend normally, and thus stomach qi ascends reversely, manifesting as belching or vomiting. Since food cannot be transported and converted, it travels downward to trigger borborygmus and diarrhea. In the course of diagnosis, attention should be paid to symptoms of diarrhea, gastric distention and fullness, and loud borborygmus, which are key pathological features of the cold–heat complex pattern. In terms of the disease nature, this pattern not only comprises the cold–heat complex, but it is also a complex of deficiency and excess — healthy qi deficiency and pathogenic excess.

Treatment method

Warming the middle, discharging heat, and harmonizing the intestines and stomach.

Formula and ingredients: Bàn Xià Xiè Xīn Tang (Pinellia Heart-Draining Decoction)

Washed *bàn xià* (Rhizoma Pinelliae) 9 g; *huáng qín* (Radix Scutellariae) 6 g; *gān jiāng* (Rhizoma Zingiberis) 6 g; *rén shēn* (Radix et Rhizoma Ginseng) 6 g; *zhì gān cǎo* (Radix et Rhizoma Glycyrrhizae Praeparata cum Melle) 6 g; *huáng lián* (Rhizoma Coptidis) 3 g; *dà zǎo* (Fructus Jujubae) 4 pieces.

Formula verse

Bàn Xià Xiè Xīn contains *huáng lián qín*, *gān jiāng zǎo cǎo*, and *rén shēn*. Acrid, bitter, sweet, and warm, it disperses distention in the middle and is indicated for vomiting, diarrhea, and borborygmus.

Usage

Add 2 L of water to decoct until 1.2 L are left. Remove the dregs and decoct the fluid until 600 mL are left. Take the decoction warm, 200 mL each time, 3 times a day. Alternatively, add water to decoct the ingredients 2 times and take it 2 times a day.

Analysis

This formula contains bitter and cold *huáng lián* and *huáng qín*, which can remove pathogenic heat or constrained heat in the middle *jiao*. Acrid–warm *gān jiāng* and *bàn xià* are added to disperse cold by warming spleen and stomach yang qi. Sweet and warm *rén shēn*, *gān cǎo*, and *dà zǎo* are used to supplement spleen and stomach qi. In this formula, both cold- and heat-natured medicinals are used to supplement qi and harmonize the middle. Particularly, acrid and bitter ingredients are applied, so-called "acrid medicinals open and bitter medicinals promote descent," which is best at rectifying the ascending and descending functions of the spleen and stomach. Since acrid and bitter medicinals can dry dampness, and bitter and cold medicinals can clear heat, this formula can be used to remove damp–heat. The method of "acrid medicinals opening and bitter medicinals promoting descent" is also the treatment method for the middle *jiao* damp–heat pattern.

Bàn xià has the proven function of relieving vomiting and dispelling phlegm. *Huáng lián* has broad-spectrum antibiotic effects and can inhibit viruses, and also activates the smooth muscles of the intestines and stomach. *Huáng qín* inhibits bacteria and resists allergy. It can also promote gallbladder functions and strengthen body immunity, similar to the actions of *huáng lián*. Both *rén shēn* and *gān cǎo* can fortify the body. Judging from all these properties, this formula is able to rectify digestion and absorption in multiple ways.

Treatment reference

The application of *Bàn Xià Xiè Xīn Tang* is not necessarily limited to the cold–heat complex. However, it takes effect only if the disease pattern presents spleen–stomach weakness with organic lesions of the stomach and intestines, functional disorder, and damp–heat obstruction in the middle *jiao*. Clinically, this formula is widely applied to treat various digestive diseases, such as dyspepsia, acute gastroenteritis, chronic enteritis, chronic dysentery, chronic gastritis, digestive ulcers, chronic cholecystitis, chronic hepatitis, and gastrointestinal neurosis. It is also applicable to mouth and tongue aphtha, and trilogy of the eye, mouth, and genitals due to damp–heat.

This is a representative formula of "acrid medicinals opening and bitter medicinals promoting descent." In practice, proper modification is required. If *gān jiāng* is removed from the formula and *shēng jiāng* is added, it becomes *Shēng Jiāng Xiè Xīn Tāng* (Fresh Ginger Heart-Draining Decoction), which has high efficacy in removing water retention in the intestines and stomach through warming. If a dose of *gān cǎo* is added, it becomes *Gān Cǎo Xiè Xīn Tāng* (Licorice Heart-Draining Decoction), which is strong at boosting qi in the middle *jiao*. If *huáng qín* is removed and a dose of *huáng lián* is added with some *guì zhī*, it becomes *Huáng Lián Tāng* (Coptis Decoction), which is able to clear heat from the chest and dispel cold from the stomach.

Cautions

As this formula contains both cold- and heat-natured medicinals, a large part of it can be modified according to the state of spleen–stomach yang and the strength of pathogenic heat or constrained heat. For the treatment of the middle *jiao* damp–heat pattern, if middle deficiency is not severe, sweet and warm ingredients such as *rén shēn*, *gān cǎo*, and *dà zǎo* can be removed to prevent pathogens from lingering, which will otherwise increase the difficulty in treatment.

Daily Exercises

1. What are the clinical manifestations of the cold–heat complex in the middle *jiao* pattern?
2. What are the ingredients of *Bàn Xià Xiè Xīn Tang*? What are its indications? What is meant by "acrid medicinals open and bitter medicinals promote descent?"
3. Mr. Chen is a 38-year-old male. His chief complaint is recurring gastric distress and pain for 4–5 years. In the past month, the pain have aggravated, but he responded favorably to warmth and pressure in that region. Other clinical manifestations are occasional vomiting of clear fluids, frequent vomiting in the evening, a bitter taste in the mouth, chest oppression, a lack of appetite, general fatigue, a luster-less complexion, a slightly yellow and greasy tongue coating, and a

thin and weak pulse. Please prescribe a Chinese medicinal formula for this case.

Additional Formulae

Shēng Jiāng Xiè Xīn Tāng (Fresh Ginger Heart-Draining Decoction)

Ingredients of *Bàn Xià Xiè Xīn Tang* with *gān jiāng* reduced to 4 g and *shēng jiāng* (Rhizoma Zingiberis Recens) 12 g. Add water to decoct.

Actions

Harmonizing the stomach and relieving distention; dispersing mass and eliminating fluid retention.

Indications

Middle deficiency with fluid retention and heat obstruction in the middle, presenting distention and hardness below the heart, belching with a musty odor, borborygmus in the abdomen, and diarrhea.

Gān Cǎo Xiè Xīn Tāng (Licorice Heart-Draining Decoction)

Ingredients of *Bàn Xià Xiè Xīn Tang* with *gān cǎo* increased to 9 g. Add water to decoct.

Actions

Boosting qi and harmonizing the stomach; relieving distention and checking vomiting.

Indications

Stomach qi weakness presenting borborygmus, diarrhea with the presence of indigested food, distention and fullness below the heart region, belching, and vexation.

Huáng Lián Tāng (Coptis Decoction)

Huáng lián (Rhizoma Coptidis) 6 g; *zhì gān cǎo* (Radix et Rhizoma Glycyrrhizae Praeparata cum Melle) 6 g; *gān jiāng* (*Rhizoma Zingiberis*) 6 g; *guì zhī* (Ramulus Cinnamomi) 6 g; *rén shēn* (Radix et Rhizoma Ginseng) 3 g; washed *bàn xià* (Rhizoma Pinelliae) 9 g; crushed *dà zǎo* (Fructus Jujubae) 4 pieces. Add water to decoct.

Actions

Rectifying cold and heat and keeping them in balance, harmonizing the stomach, and directing counterflow downward.

Indications

Heat in the chest and coldness in the stomach presenting vexation and distress in the chest, nausea, abdominal pain, borborygmus, diarrhea, a white and slippery tongue coating, and a wiry pulse.

CHAPTER 15

Formulae for Diseases of the Respiratory System

DAY FOUR

In the previous chapters, the diagnoses, treatments, and formulae for several representative patterns of exterior, interior, heat, cold, deficiency, and excess have been introduced and discussed. At this last stage of the book, we will review and summarize a number of formulae presented earlier for the convenience of clinical application, and simultaneously, we will incorporate other commonly used formulae for the different systems of the body.

In Chinese medicine, the respiratory system is mainly associated with the lung, but it generally includes the trachea, bronchi, throat, and nose as well. The lung governs qi of the body, controls respiration, acts to diffuse, purify, and descend, distributes food essences, and free and regulate water-conducting pathways. Consequently, pathological changes of the lung largely lie in its failure to diffuse and govern descent, inability to free and regulate the water-conducting pathways, and loss of control in enlarging or reducing pores connected to sweat glands. Related diseases can either be deficient or excess. The excess pattern is essentially caused by six exogenous pathogenic factors attacking the lung, fluid retention, or phlegm and damp obstruction in the lung, while the deficiency pattern is due to lung qi deficiency or lung yin deficiency. Clinical manifestations include coughing, panting, hemoptysis, a sore and swollen throat, and nasal inflammation or bleeding.

Coughing

Coughing is a common symptom caused by the ascending counterflow of lung qi. Various factors may contribute to coughing, such as the six externally contracted pathogenic factors, up-flaming of fire, internal obstruction by phlegm–damp, fluid retention attacking the upper part of the body, and lung qi deficiency. Among the formulae given in previous chapters, some of them can be applied to treat coughs. If the disease involves wind–cold invading the lung, *Má Huáng Tāng* or *Sān Ào Tāng* is used. If it pertains to wind–heat invading the lung, apply *Yín Qiào Sǎn* or *Sāng Jú Yǐn*. If it is caused by obstruction of the lung by phlegm–damp, prescribe *Èr Chén Tāng* together with *Píng Wèi Sǎn*. For exuberant lung heat, apply *Má Xìng Shí Gān Tāng*. For exterior cold with fluid retention, prescribe *Xiǎo Qīng Lóng Tāng*. For lung yin deficiency, use *Shā Shēn Mài Dōng Tāng*. For deficiency of both qi and yin of the lung, apply *Shēng Mài Sǎn*. In the following, we will introduce another formula for coughing caused by external pathogenic contraction.

Formula and ingredients: Zhǐ Sòu Sǎn (Cough-Stopping Powder)

Dry-fried *jié gěng* (Radix Platycodonis) 10 g; *jīng jiè* (Herba Schizonepetae) 10 g; dry-fried *zǐ wǎn* (Radix et Rhizoma Asteris) 10 g; dry-fried *bǎi bù* (Radix Stemonae) 10 g; *bái qián* (Rhizoma et Radix Cynanchi Stauntonii) 10 g; *zhì gān cǎo* (Radix et Rhizoma Glycyrrhizae Praeparata cum Melle) 3.5 g; *chén pí* (Pericarpium Citri Reticulatae) 5 g.

Formula verse

Zhǐ Sòu Sǎn contains *jié gěng* and *zǐ wǎn jīng jiè bǎi bù chén*, and the powder of *bái qián* and *gān cǎo*, excellent at dissolving phlegm and relieving coughing.

Usage

Grind the ingredients into a fine powder and take 9 g each time orally with warm water. If the disease occurs soon after catching wind–cold, take the powder with ginger soup. Alternatively, serve it as a decoction.

Actions

Relieving cough and dissolving phlegm; scattering the exterior and diffusing the lung.

Indications

Coughing, an itchy throat, coughing up of white phlegm, and a thin and white tongue coating after contracting external pathogens.

Treatment reference

This formula is originally applied to treat coughs caused by external contraction of wind–cold, but after appropriate modification, it can be used to treat coughs induced by other pathogens. For external contraction of wind–heat presenting coughing, an itchy throat, thick phlegm, a red tongue with a yellow coating, add *jīn yín huā, lián qiào, niú bàng zǐ*, and *lú gēn*. For external contraction of wind–cold with a significant exterior pattern, add *zǐ sū yè, xìng rén, fáng fēng*, and so on. For external contraction of summer heat presenting body and head heaviness, coughing, chest and gastric distention and fullness, vexation, and a white and greasy tongue coating, add *huò xiāng, pèi lán*, and *dà dòu juǎn*. For the presence of an aversion to cold, an absence of sweating, and body pain and cramps, add *xiāng rú*. For pathogenic dryness invading the lung presenting frequent coughing, add *guā lóu pí, pí pá yè, bèi mǔ*, pear skin, and so on.

Panting

Panting is a symptom caused by the failure of the lung to diffuse and govern descent. It is associated with shortness and difficulty in breath, which is different from wheezing. Both of these symptoms can occur simultaneously. For instance, wheezing is definitely accompanied by panting, but panting does not necessarily appear with wheezing. Panting can be caused by many factors, but they all fall within that of contraction of external pathogens, pathogenic obstruction in the lung, lung qi deficiency, and so on. Generally, the initial occurrence is usually triggered by external contraction, which chiefly pertains to pathogenic obstruction in the lung.

Chronic illness often relates to internal damage or internal damage caused by external contraction, which is mostly due to healthy qi deficiency and phlegm obstruction in the lung. Panting can also be purely triggered by extreme deficiency of the lung and kidney. As the pathogenesis and treatment method of panting are comparable to coughing, the formulae applied are also similar. If the disease is due to wind–cold, use *Má Huáng Tāng* or *Sān Ào Tāng*. If it is resulted from lung heat, apply *Má Xìng Shí Gān Tāng*. For exterior cold with fluid retention, prescribe *Xiǎo Qīng Lóng Tāng*. If it is caused by phlegm–damp obstruction in the lung, use *Èr Chén Tāng* together with *Píng Wèi Sǎn*. For deficiency of both qi and yin of the lung, apply *Shēng Mài Sǎn*. In addition, if panting is induced by yang deficiency complicated with edema, apply *Zhēn Wǔ Tāng* or *Wǔ Líng Sǎn*. For deficiency of both the lung and kidney, apply *Shèn Qì Wán*. In the following, we will introduce a commonly used formula for panting.

Formula and ingredients: *Dìng Chuǎn Tāng* (*Arrest Wheezing Decoction*)

Shell-less, crushed, and dry-fried until yellow *bái guǒ* (Semen Ginkgo) 9 g; *má huáng* (Herba Ephedrae) 9 g; *zǐ sū zǐ* (Fructus Perillae) 6 g; *gān cǎo* (Radix et Rhizoma Glycyrrhizae) 3 g; *kuǎn dōng huā* (Flos Farfarae) 9 g; *xìng rén* (Semen Armeniacae Amarum) 9 g; *sāng bái pí* (Cortex Mori) 9 g; *huáng qín* (Radix Scutellariae) 6 g; *bàn xià* (Rhizoma Pinelliae) 9 g.

Formula verse

Dìng Chuǎn contains *bái guǒ* and *má huáng*, *kuǎn dōng bàn xià bái pí sāng*; *sū zǐ huáng qín gān cǎo xìng*, applicable to panting caused by exterior cold and interior heat.

Usage

Add water to decoct.

Actions

Diffusing the lung and directing qi downward; calming panting and resolving phlegm.

Indications

Panting with sticky yellow phlegm, distention and oppression in the chest, a yellow and greasy tongue coating, and a slippery and rapid pulse.

Treatment reference

Dìng Chuǎn Tāng is most applicable to panting caused by lung qi obstruction due to the internal accumulation of phlegm–heat with further contraction of wind–cold. If the phlegm–heat is serious and manifests as spitting of sticky yellow phlegm, a dry and bitter taste in the mouth, and a red tongue, add *guā lóu, jīn qiáo mài, yú xīng cǎo, dōng guā zǐ*, and so on. If phlegm–damp is exuberant while heat signs are insignificant, remove *huáng qín* and *sāng bái pí*, and add *hòu pò* and *shè gān*.

Hemoptysis

Hemoptysis involves the coughing up of blood spilled from the lung or trachea. The direct cause of hemoptysis can be traced to the rupture of lung collaterals, which is often triggered by pathogenic fire and heat. Pathogenic fire is divided into excess–fire and deficiency–fire. The former refers to exuberant lung heat, such as heat exuberance in the lung, dry heat impairing the lung, and liver fire invading the lung. The latter refers to internal exuberance of deficiency–heat following lung yin insufficiency. Among the formulae in the previous chapters, some of them can be applied to treat hemoptysis. For hemoptysis caused by exuberant blood heat in the lung, use *Xī Jiǎo Dì Huáng Tāng*. For exuberant liver and gall-bladder fire invading the lung, apply *Lóng Dǎn Xiè Gān Tāng*. For lung yin insufficiency with deficiency fire, use *Shā Shēn Mài Dōng Tāng*. Clinically, it is advisable to add some medicinals that arrest bleeding, such as *bái máo gēn, ǒu jié, cè bǎi yè, xuè yú tàn*, and *sān qī*. In the following, we will introduce a commonly used formula for lung heat hemoptysis.

Formula and ingredients: *Kǎ Xuě Fāng (Treat Coughing of Blood Formula)*

Water-ground *qīng dài* (Indigo Naturalis) 6 g; *guā lóu rén* (Semen Trichosanthis) 9 g; *hē zǐ* (Fructus Chebulae) 6 g; *hǎi fú shí* (Pumex) 9 g; dry-fried until black *zhī zǐ* (Fructus Gardeniae) 9 g.

Formula verse

Kǎ Xuě Fāng contains *hē zǐ*, *hǎi shí zhī zǐ*, and *guā lóu*. *Qīng dài* purges the liver and cools blood. It is a good formula for the coughing up of blood-streaked phlegm.

Usage

Grind the ingredients into powder and make them into pills with honey and ginger juice. Melt the pills in the mouth, 9 g at a time. Alternatively, serve it as a decoction.

Actions

Clearing fire and arresting bleeding; dissolving phlegm and relieving coughing.

Indications

Coughing up of blood-streaked and sticky phlegm, non-gratifying spitting, vexation, thirst, flushed cheeks, constipation, a yellow tongue coating, and a wiry and rapid pulse.

Treatment reference

Kǎ Xuě Fāng is often applied to treat coughs due to lung heat or liver fire attacking the upper body. For exuberant lung heat presenting fever, coughing, and panting, add *jīn yín huā*, *lián qiào*, *yú xīng cǎo*, *hǔ zhàng*, and similar heat-clearing and toxin-resolving herbs. For acute coughs with scant phlegm that is difficult to be expectorated, add *xìng rén*, *zhè bèi mǔ*, *pí pá yè*, *tiān zhú huáng*, and *nán shā shēn*. If the disease is presented with impaired lung yin, add *běi shā shēn* and *mài dōng*. For chronic deficiency, add *bǎi hé* and *ē jiāo zhū*. For massive bleeding, add *bái jí* and *sān qī* or the *Yunnan* white medicinal powder commonly sold in Chinese drug stores, 1 g a time, 3 times a day.

Daily Exercises

1. Summarize the formulae for treating coughing and panting, and compare the differences among their indications.

2. What are the ingredients of *Zhǐ Sòu Sǎn?* What are its main functions?
3. What are the ingredients of *Dìng Chuǎn Tāng?* What are its indications?
4. What are the ingredients of *Kǎ Xuě Fāng?* What are its indications?

DAY FIVE

Lung Abscesses

Lung abscesses refer to sores in the lung that produce pus. The disease can be caused by either the contraction of wind–heat attacking the lung or phlegm–heat accumulation in the lung, which contributes to blood stasis and appearence of rotten flesh. Its clinical manifestations are fever, coughing, chest pain, and spitting of pus with a pungent fishy odor, blood, and turbid phlegm. At its onset, if it is due to pathogenic heat attacking the lung, apply *Yín Qiào Sǎn.* If the lung heat lingers and causes internal accumulation of phlegm–heat, which is an indicator for the formation of pus, it is a must to administer the following formula.

Formula and ingredients: *Wěi Jìng Tāng (Phragmites Stem Decoction)*

Lú gēn (Rhizoma Phragmitis) 60 g; *yì yǐ rén* (Semen Coicis) 15 g; *dōng guā zǐ* (Scmen Benincasae) 15 g; *táo rén* (Semen Persicae) 9 g.

Formula verse

Wěi Jìng táo yǐ dōng guā zǐ clears heat and dispels stasis, reducing the ease of formation of abscesses.

Usage

Decoct *lú gēn* with water first and then add the other ingredients to decoct. Take the decoction twice.

Actions

Clearing lung heat and dissolving phlegm, and expelling stasis and pus.

Indications

Lung abscesses with the accumulation of heat, stasis, and phlegm presenting spitting of pungent yellow phlegm with pus and blood, dull chest pain that are aggravated during coughing, fever, a dry mouth, vexation, a yellow and greasy tongue coating, and a slippery and rapid pulse.

Treatment reference

Wěi Jìng Tāng is good for treating lung abscesses; it dissipates the sores if pus has not been formed, and expels pus after it is. Clinically, for lung abscesses without pus or lobar pneumonia, add more heat-clearing and toxin-removing medicinals, such as *yú xīng cǎo*, *huáng lián*, *huáng bǎi*, *zhī zǐ*, *huáng qín*, *qiān nián jiàn*, *jīn qiáo mài*, and *bài jiàng cǎo*. If pus is produced and the patient suddenly coughs up pungent phlegm or massive amounts of phlegm with pus and blood, add *zhè bèi mǔ*, *jié gěng* (a large dose of above 10 g), *tíng lì zǐ*, and large doses of *bài jiàng cǎo* and *jīn qiáo mài* (above 30 g) to clear heat and expel pus. *Yú xīng cǎo* should not be decocted for a long time and alternatively, pound fresh pieces (60–90 g) to obtain their juice and add to the decoction for oral intake.

Rhinitis

Rhinitis can be acute or chronic, and chronic rhinitis is further classified into simple, hypertrophic, and allergic. It is usually induced by the contraction of external pathogens, lung qi deficiency–cold, or internal accumulation of phlegm–heat. Among the previous formulae presented, *Guì Zhī Tāng* can be applied to treat rhinitis due to external attack of wind–cold, *Yù Píng Fēng Sǎn* can be prescribed to treat allergic rhinitis due to weakness of the *wei* exterior, and *Yín Qiào Sǎn* is applicable in treating acute rhinitis due to wind–heat invading lung *wei*. In the following, we will introduce a commonly used formula for rhinitis and nasosinusitis due to the contraction of lung heat.

Formula and ingredients: *Cāng Ěr Zǐ Sǎn (Cocklebur Fruit Powder)*

Dry-fried *cāng ěr zǐ* (Fructus Xanthii) 8 g; *xīn yí* (Flos Magnoliae) 15 g; *bái zhǐ* (Radix Angelicae Dahuricae) 30 g; *bò he* (Herba Menthae) 1.5 g added later.

Formula verse

Cāng Ěr Zǐ Sǎn contains *xīn yí, bò he,* as well as *bái zhǐ.* To be made into powder, and then taken with shallot tea; effective for nasal congestion and discharge, and headaches.

Usage

Grind the ingredients into a fine powder and take 6 g each time with the decoction of shallot and tea after meals.

Actions

Dispelling wind and clearing heat, and unblocking the nasal orifices.

Indications

Nasal congestion, loss of sense of smell, yellow and turbid nasal discharge, and pain in the forehead.

Treatment reference

This formula is mainly indicated for the different types of chronic rhinitis and nasosinusitis caused by wind–heat accumulation in the upper part of the body. If pathogenic heat is strong, with nasal discharge that is as thick as pus, head distention, and severe pain in the forehead, add raw *shí gāo, lián qiào, huáng qín, jú huā,* and so on. If rhinitis is caused by the contraction of wind–cold with clear and loose nasal discharge that is aggravated after catching a cold, and a white tongue coating, remove *bò he* from the formula and add *zǐ sū yè, shēng má, fáng fēng, jīng jiè, xì xīn,* and so on.

Nosebleeds

Bleeding from nasal cavities is termed nosebleeds. They can be caused either by local lesions or by systemic diseases. Its patho-mechanism stems from exuberant fire heat driving blood flow out of vessels, the external contraction of fire–heat, or heat produced by visceral constrained heat or yin deficiency. Many formulae learnt previously can be applied to treat nosebleeds. For disorders triggered by wind–heat invading the lung, apply modified *Sāng Jú Yǐn.*

For exuberant up-flaming of stomach heat and impairment of collaterals, use *Bái Hǔ Tāng*. For exuberant blood heat, use *Xī Jiǎo Dì Huáng Tāng*. For up-flaming of liver fire, apply *Lóng Dǎn Xiè Gān Tāng*. For yin deficiency resulting in vigorous fire, prescribe *Zhī Bǎi Dì Huáng Tāng* (Anemarrhena, Phellodendron, and Rehmannia Decoction). For deficiency of qi and blood with the failure of blood flow management by the spleen, apply *Guī Pí Tāng*. In the following, we will introduce a commonly used formula for nosebleeds, which is also applicable to bleeding stemmed from other sources.

Formula and ingredients: *Shí Huī Sǎn (Ten Charred Substances Powder)*

Equal amounts of *dà jì* (Herba Cirsii Japonici); *xiǎo jì* (Herba Cirsii); *hé yè* (Folium Nelumbinis); *cè bǎi yè* (Cacumen Platycladi); *bái máo gēn* (Rhizoma Imperatae); *qiàn cǎo gēn* (Radix et Rhizoma Rubiae); *zhī zǐ* (Fructus Gardeniae); *dà huáng* (Radix et Rhizoma Rhei); *mǔ dān pí* (Cortex Moutan); *zōng lǚ pí* (Petiolus Trachycarpi).

Formula verse

Shí Huī Sǎn contains 10 kinds of ashes: *bǎi qiàn máo hé dān lǚ pí*; and *dà jì*, *xiǎo jì*, and *zhī huáng* are fried until blackened. It is a formula that is recommended for staunching bleeding by cooling.

Usage

Burn the ingredients into ashes and grind them into a very fine powder. Take the powder 9–15 g a time with lotus root juice or radish juice. Alternatively, prepare the ingredients into pills and take them 9 g each time with warm water. It can also be served as a decoction.

Actions

Cooling the blood and staunching bleeding.

Indications

Frenetic flow of blood presenting hematemesis, nosebleeds, and hemoptysis.

Treatment reference

Shí Huī Săn is effective for all kinds of bleeding due to blood heat. It is usually prepared for oral intake, but for nosebleeds, it can be used externally by blowing the powder into the nose. This formula is also good for staunching bleeding during emergencies. As it is primarily aimed at treating the branch, further treatment targeting the disease cause should be carried out to prevent repeated bleeding episodes.

Daily Exercises

1. Summarize the formulae for treating rhinitis and nosebleeds, and compare the differences among their indications.
2. What are the ingredients of *Wĕi Jìng Tāng*? What are its main functions?
3. What are the ingredients of *Cāng Ĕr Zĭ Săn*? What are the main modifications in clinical practice?
4. What are the ingredients of *Shí Huī Săn*? In practice, what aspects should be noted?

CHAPTER 16

Formulae for Diseases of the Digestive System

DAY SIX

In Chinese medicine, the digestive system mainly involves the spleen and stomach, but is also related to the small intestine, large intestine, and liver. The spleen governs transportation and conversion of food. After it transports food essences to the lung, they are distributed to the whole body. The spleen also manages blood. The stomach largely deals with the reception and digestion of food. Nevertheless, the digestion, absorption, and transportation of food require the assistance of intestinal conveyance and its function of raising the clear and directing the turbid downward, and the dredging function of the liver and gallbladder. Diseases of the digestive system generally involve disorders of transportation, transformation, descent, and ascent. The disease pattern can either be that of deficiency or of excess. The deficiency pattern includes qi deficiency, yang deficiency, and yin deficiency, while the excess pattern may involve pathogenic sources such as cold–damp, damp–heat, static blood, phlegm–rheum, and food stagnation. Clinical manifestations are usually abdominal distention and pain, stool morbidity, vomiting, belching, edema, a lack of appetite, and bloody stool.

Stomachaches

Disease causes of stomachache are extensive. The major ones include pathogenic cold attacking the stomach, food poisoning, anger damaging the liver, anxiety impairing the spleen, body weakness, and long periods of illness, all of which can lead to the constraint of stomach qi, malnourishment of the stomach, and ultimately, stomachaches. Some of the formulae introduced in the previous chapters can be applied to treat stom-achaches. For stomach cold causing pain, apply *Lǐ Zhōng Tāng* or *Wú Zhū Yú Tāng*. For cold–damp obstructing the stomach, prescribe *Huò Xiāng Zhèng Qì Sǎn*. For food stagnation blocking qi movement, use *Bǎo Hé Wán*. For the adverse effects of the constraint of the liver invading the stomach, apply *Sì Nì Sǎn* or *Chái Hú Shū Gān Sǎn*. For the cold–heat complex in the middle *jiao*, administer *Bàn Xià Xiè Xīn Tang*. For stomach yin insufficiency, apply *Shā Shēn Mài Dōng Tāng*. In the following, we will introduce another formula for stomachaches caused by dampness obstruction, congealing cold, and qi stagnation.

Formula and ingredients: Xiāng Shā Yǎng Wèi Wán (Aucklandia-Amomum Stomach-Nourishing Pill)

Bái zhú (Rhizoma Atractylodis Macrocephalae) 12 g; *xiāng fù* (Rhizoma Cyperi) 4 g; *shā rén* (Fructus Amomi) 4 g; *fú líng* (Poria) 4 g; *hòu pò* (Cortex Magnoliae Officinalis) 4 g; *zhǐ qiào* (Fructus Aurantii) 4 g; *huò xiāng* (Herba Agastachis) 4 g; *bàn xià* (Rhizoma Pinelliae) 4 g; *jú pí* (Pericarpium Citri Reticulatae) 2 g; *gān cǎo* (Radix et Rhizoma Glycyrrhizae) 2 g; *dòu kòu* (Fructus Amomi Rotundus) 2 g; *mù xiāng* (Radix Aucklandiae) 2 g; *dà zǎo* (Fructus Jujubae) 1.6 g; *shēng jiāng* (Rhizoma Zingiberis Recens) 0.4 g.

Formula verse

Xiāng Shā Yǎng Wèi contains *zhú xiāng fù*, *shā rén xià pò zhǐ qiào fú*; *jú pí hòu cǎo kòu mù xiāng*, especially for stomachaches, distention, and fullness.

Usage

The ingredients are made into pills the size of firmiana seeds. Take the pills orally 6–9 g at a time, 2 times a day. Alternatively, make the above ingredients into a decoction at the same dosages, but do not decoct them for too long.

Actions

Fortifying the spleen and strengthening the stomach; rectifying qi and removing dampness.

Indications

Dampness obstruction and qi stagnation or cold–damp and qi stagnation presenting gastric distention, fullness, and pain, and a lack of appetite.

Treatment reference

This formula is a combination of *Èr Chén Tāng* and *Zhǐ Zhú Wán*, together with some qi-rectifying, stomach-warming, and dampness-removing medicinals. This formula is favorable in treating many types of stomach-aches only if there are no obvious signs of heat and deficiency.

Hiccups

When qi counterflow rushes upward, frequent and short sounds in the throat are resulted. These are known as hiccups. The exact patho-mechanism of this occurrence is triggered by the ascending counterflow of stomach qi disrupting the diaphragm. The disease cause can be due to pathogenic cold invading the stomach, ascending counterflow of stomach fire, phlegm–damp obstruction in the middle, spleen–stomach yang deterioration, insufficiency of stomach yin, and many other reasons. For hiccups resulting from deficiency of spleen–stomach yang or insufficiency of stomach yin, apply *Lǐ Zhōng Tāng* or *Shā Shēn Mài Dōng Tāng*, respectively. If the hiccups are due to stomach qi weakness and phlegm–damp obstruction in the middle, the following formula can be applied.

Formula and ingredients: Xuán Fù Dài Zhě Tāng (Inula and Hematite Decoction)

Wrapped *xuán fù huā* (Flos Inulae) 9 g; *dài zhě shí* (Haematitum) 12 g; *rén shēn* (Radix et Rhizoma Ginseng) 6 g; *bàn xià* (Rhizoma Pinelliae) 9 g; *zhì gān cǎo* (Radix et Rhizoma Glycyrrhizae Praeparata cum Melle) 9 g; *shēng jiāng* (Rhizoma Zingiberis Recens) 15 g; *dà zǎo* (Fructus Jujubae) 4 pieces.

Formula verse

Xuán Fù Dài Zhě contains *gān cǎo*, *bàn xià rén shēn*, and *jiāng zǎo*. It is for hiccups and epigastric *pǐ*, checking qi counterflow, and dissolving phlegm.

Usage

Add water to decoct.

Actions

Directing counterflow downward and dissolving phlegm; boosting qi and harmonizing the stomach.

Indications

Hiccups with hardness and fullness at the region below the heart, vomiting, and a white and slippery or greasy tongue coating.

Treatment reference

Xuán Fù Dài Zhĕ Tāng is applicable to belching, hiccups, and vomiting due to stomach weakness or internal obstruction by phlegm–turbidity of nervous vomiting, cramps in the diaphragm, gastrectasis, incomplete pyloric obstruction, and other gastrointestinal diseases. In practice, if stomach qi is not weak, remove *rén shēn* and *dà zăo*. If there is epigastric distention and fullness due to severe phlegm–damp, add *fú líng*, *chuān pò*, and *chén pí*. If the disease complicated with pathogenic cold attacking the stomach and insufficient spleen–stomach yang qi, add *dīng xiāng*, *shì dì*, and *dāo dòu* and replace *shēng jiāng* with *gān jiāng*. For hiccups due to deficiency–heat in the stomach, add *zhú rú*, *lú gēn*, *shí hú* and other such medicinals to clear the stomach and relieve hiccups.

Daily Exercises

1. Summarize the formulae for treating stomachaches and vomiting, and compare the differences among their indications.
2. What are the ingredients of *Xiāng Shā Yăng Wèi Wán*? What are its functions?
3. What are the ingredients of *Xuán Fù Dài Zhĕ Tāng*? How can it be modified in clinical practice?

THE 14TH WEEK

DAY ONE

Painful Diarrhea

Diarrhea involves increased bowel movements with the discharge of loose or watery stool. It also includes dysentery in Chinese medicine, which is characterized by abdominal pain, tenesmus, and stool with red and white mucus. Many causes may be responsible for diarrhea, among which the major ones are related to the weak transportation function of the spleen and the prevalence of dampness. Functional disorder of the intestines, liver qi invading the spleen, and kidney yang insufficiency may also be connected to diarrhea. Among the formulae in the previous chapters, many of them can be applied to treat this widespread ailment. For diarrhea due to cold–damp, apply *Huò Xiāng Zhèng Qì Săn*. For diarrhea due to damp–heat, use *Gé Gēn Huáng Qín Huáng Lián Tāng*. For food poisoning, use *Bǎo Hé Wán*. For spleen deficiency, prescribe *Sì Jūn Zǐ Tāng* or *Shēn Líng Bái Zhú Săn*. For spleen yang deficiency, administer *Lǐ Zhōng Tāng* or *Fù Zǐ Lǐ Zhōng Tāng* (Aconite Center-Regulating Decoction). In the following, we will introduce a formula specially designed for abdominal pain and diarrhea due to liver qi invading the spleen.

Formula and ingredients: Tòng Xiè Yào Fāng (Important Formula for Painful Diarrhea)

Earth-fried *bái zhú* (Rhizoma Atractylodis Macrocephalae) 9 g; dry-fried *bái sháo* (Radix Paeoniae Alba) 6 g; dry-fried *chén pí* (Pericarpium Citri Reticulatae) 4.5 g; *fáng fēng* (Radix Saposhnikoviae) 6 g.

Formula verse

Tòng Xiè Yào Fāng contains *chén pí*, *zhú sháo*, and *fáng fēn*. For diarrhea with boborygmus and abdominal pain, it aims to purge the liver and fortify the spleen.

Usage

Grind the above ingredients into a crude powder and administer 9–15 g each time for decoction in water. Remove the dregs and take the decoction warm. Alternatively, decoct the above ingredients directly in water.

Actions

Purging the liver, fortifying the spleen, and relieving diarrhea.

Indications

Liver constraint and spleen deficiency presenting borborygmus, abdominal pain before episodes of diarrhea and alleviation after the episodes, a thin and white tongue coating, and a wiry and moderate pulse.

Treatment reference

This formula exerts favorable effects on diarrhea caused by acute and chronic enteritis, and nervous diarrhea with liver hyperactivity and spleen deficiency. If it is complicated by damp–heat, add *là liào* and *dì jǐn cǎo*.

Diarrhea Before Dawn

Diarrhea before dawn is due to kidney yang deficiency, which indicates that the kidneys fail to warm the earth energy of the spleen, leading to the weakness of the latter organ to transport and ultimately, diarrhea. It is usually presented as abdominal pain and diarrhea at the arrival of dawn, with remission after diarrhea. It is also called "kidney diarrhea" or "Fifth Night Watch diarrhea." There is a formula specially crafted for this disease by the ancient Chinese, called *Sì Shén Wán*.

Formula and ingredients: Sì Shén Wán (Four Spirits Pill)

Ròu dòu kòu (Semen Myristicae) 12 g; dry-fried *bǔ gǔ zhī* (Fructus Psoraleae) 4 g; *wǔ wèi zǐ* (Fructus Schisandrae Chinensis) 12 g; soaked and fried *wú zhū yú* (Fructus Evodiae) 3 g.

Formula verse

Sì Shén requires *gǔ zhī* and *wú yú*, *ròu kòu* and *wǔ wèi*. With *dà zǎo* and *shēng jiāng* for decoction, it is most applicable to diarrhea before dawn.

Usage

Grind the ingredients into a fine powder. Decoct 10 g of ginger and 10 pieces of jujubes with water. When the water has evaporated and jujubes cooked, remove the ginger and mix the flesh of the jujubes with medicinal powder to make into pills. Take 9–12 g each time on an empty stomach or with warm water. Alternatively, serve it as a decoction with the same dosages as above.

Actions

Warming the kidney and spleen, astringing the intestines, and arresting diarrhea.

Indications

Diarrhea before dawn or prolonged diarrhea, a lack of appetite, abdominal pain relieved by warmth, lumbar soreness, cold limbs, mental fatigue, a lack of strength, a light and bulgy tongue with a thin and white coating, and a deep, slow, and weak pulse.

Treatment reference

Pills of this formula are on sale in China. If it is served as a decoction, modification of the formula can be carried out according to specific symptoms. For exuberance of cold presenting severe lumbar soreness and cold limbs, add *fù zǐ* and *ròu guì*. For prolonged diarrhea causing prolapse of the rectum, add *huáng qí*, *shēng má*, and roasted *gé gēn*. For diarrhea caused by excess pathogens, do not prescribe this formula, otherwise it will boost the pathogen.

Dysentery

Dysentery is characterized by the defecation of stool containing red and white mucus due to the combination of damp–heat, food stagnation, and cold–damp pathogens with qi and blood in the intestines that leads to the impairment of the intestinal membrane and blood vessels, decaying as bloody or white pus. *Mù Xiāng Bīng Láng Wán* and *Zhǐ Shí Dǎo Zhì Wán* can be applied to treat dysentery due to damp–heat or food stagnation. *Huò Xiāng Zhèng Qì Sǎn* can be used to treat dysentery due to cold–damp. In the following, we will introduce a commonly used formula for damp–heat dysentery.

Formula and ingredients: Xiāng Lián Wán (Costus Root and Coptis Pill)

Huáng lián (Rhizoma Coptidis) 60 g (fried with *wú zhū yú* 30 g until brown and remove *wú zhū yú*); *mù xiāng* (Radix Aucklandiae) 13 g.

Formula verse

Xiāng Lián Wán treats damp–heat dysentery, effective for purulent bloody stool.

Usage

Grind the ingredients into a fine powder and add vinegar and some water to make into water pills. For every 100 g of powder, add 8 g of vinegar. Take the pills 3–6 g orally each time with warm water, 3 times a day. Alternatively, serve it as a decoction.

Actions

Clearing heat and drying dampness.

Indications

Damp–heat dysentery presenting purulent bloody stool, abdominal pain, and tenesmus.

Treatment reference

Xiāng Lián Wán is usually indicated for mild damp–heat dysentery. If the condition is serious, it can be applied with other medicinals such as *huáng qín*, *dà huáng*, *huáng bǎi*, *qín pí*, *kǔ shēn*, and so on. For severe food accumulation, add *lái fú zǐ*, *shān zhā*, *bīng láng*, etc. For frequent episodes of diarrhea, add *dì jǐn cǎo*, *là liào*, and *shí liú pí*.

Bloody Stool

Bloody stool can be present either before or after defecation, and as stool mixed with blood or the discharge of pure blood. The main causes of bloody stool include intestinal damp–heat, exuberant heat in blood, and inadequate management of blood by qi due to deficiency, and spleen–stomach deficiency–cold. *Xī Jiǎo Dì Huáng Tāng* can be prescribed to treat bloody stool due to blood heat and *Guī Pí Tāng* to treat bloody stool due to qi deficiency. In the following, we will introduce a formula for bloody stool due to damp–heat in the large intestine.

Formula and ingredients: Huái Huā Sǎn (Sophorae Powder)

Dry-fried *huái huā* (Flos Sophorae) 12 g; baked *cè bǎi yè* (Cacumen Platycladi) 12 g; dry-fried *jīng jiè suì* (Spica Schizonepetae) 6 g; bran-fried *zhǐ qiào* (Fructus Aurantii) 6 g.

Formula verse

Huái Huā Sǎn treats bloody stool, by the actions of *jīng suì zhǐ qiào* and *cè bǎi*.

Usage

Grind the ingredients into a fine powder and take 6 g each time orally with warm water or rice soup. Alternatively, serve it as a decoction.

Actions

Clearing the intestines and arresting bleeding, and scattering wind to rectify blood.

Indications

Intestinal wind and visceral toxin presenting bloody stool before or after defecation, stool containing bright or dark red blood, or hemorrhoids with bleeding.

Treatment reference

Intestinal wind in Chinese medicine refers to bloody stool before defecation, with the acute production of bright red blood. Visceral toxin refers
to bloody stool before or after defecation, where the blood is darkly
colored. *Huái Huā Sǎn* is applicable to all kinds of bloody stool with
signs of heat. In clinical practice, if intestinal heat is exuberant, add
huáng lián and *huáng bǎi* to clear the intestines and purge heat. If bleeding is in massive amounts, add *dì yú* and charred *qiàn cǎo* to arrest it. For
bloody stool due to qi deficiency or deficiency–cold, this formula is not
suitable.

Daily Exercises

1. Summarize the formulae for treating diarrhea and compare the differ-
    ences among their indications.
2. What are the ingredients of *Tòng Xiè Yào Fāng* and *Sì Shén Wán*?
    What are the differences in their indications?
3. How can *Xiāng Lián Wán* be modified in clinical practice?
4. What are the ingredients of *Huái Huā Sǎn*? What is it indicated for?

DAY TWO

Constipation

Constipation refers to the difficulty in defecation or infrequent defecation
(e.g., once in several days). Though externally contracted febrile diseases
can also cause constipation due to heat bind in the intestines, this ailment
generally exists in chronic internal diseases. The disease cause includes
dryness–heat accumulation in the intestines, intestinal constraint and stagnation of qi, weakness of the transportation function of the spleen due to
deficiency, intestines lacking nourishment due to blood deficiency, and
cold congealing in the large intestine. In the following, we will introduce
a formula for constipation due to dryness–heat in the intestines and
stomach.

Formula and ingredients: Má Zǐ Rén Wán (Cannabis Fruit Pill)

Má zǐ rén (Fructus Cannabis) 10 g; *sháo yào* (Radix Paeoniae) 5 g; liquid-fried *zhǐ qiào* (Fructus Aurantii) 5 g; *dà huáng* (Radix et Rhizoma Rhei) 10 g; liquid-fried *hòu pò* (Cortex Magnoliae Officinalis) 5 g; dry-fried *xìng rén* (Semen Armeniacae Amarum) without skin and tip 5 g.

Formula verse

Má Zǐ Rén Wán treats splenic constipation, by the actions of *zhǐ pò dà huáng xìng* and *sháo*; for constipation due to spleen dryness and fluid damage, it moistens the intestines and purges heat.

Usage

The ingredients are ground into a fine powder, fried with honey, and made into pills. Take 9 g of pills each time with warm water, 1–2 times a day. Alternatively, serve it as a decoction.

Actions

Moistening the intestines to promote defecation.

Indications

Dryness–heat in the intestines and stomach with insufficient fluids presenting hard stool and difficulty in defecation, or intestinal dryness and habitual constipation among the aged or after illness.

Treatment reference

The disease pattern indicated by this formula is known as splenic constipation, which means that the spleen is constrained by dryness–heat and fails to distribute fluids. Therefore, stool produced is dry, constipated, and difficult to be discharged. This formula is often prescribed as a patent medicine in clinical practice. If it is applied as a decoction, modification may be carried out. For severe fluidal damage, add *shā shēn*, *shēng dì*, *mài dōng*, and *xuán shēn*. If the stool produced is very hard and there is difficulty in defecation, add *xuán míng fěn*.

Jaundice

Jaundice is mainly characterized by yellow eyes, yellow skin, and yellow urine. The causes of jaundice are extensive. In Chinese medicine, it is associated with the accumulation of and steaming damp–heat, overflow of bile, cold–damp obstruction, and inactivated spleen yang. It can be seen in various types of hepatitis, leptospirosis, acute hemolysis, and biliary obstructions. In the following, we will introduce a commonly used formula for damp–heat jaundice.

Formula and ingredients: Yīn Chén Hāo Tāng (*Virgate Wormwood Decoction*)

Yīn chén (Herba Artemisiae Scopariae) 30 g; *zhī zǐ* (Fructus Gardeniae) 15 g; *dà huáng* (Radix et Rhizoma Rhei) 9 g.

Formula verse

Yīn Chén Hāo Tāng contains *dà huáng zhī*, effective for damp–heat yang jaundice.

Usage

Add water to decoct.

Actions

Clearing heat and draining dampness; treating jaundice.

Indications

Damp–heat jaundice presenting bright yellow body skin and eyes, slight abdominal fullness, thirst, deep yellow and inhibited urine, a yellow and greasy tongue coating, and a deep and excessive or slippery and rapid pulse.

Treatment reference

Yīn Chén Hāo Tāng is applicable to all kinds of jaundice with damp–heat signs. In practice, for severe pathogenic dampness, add *fú líng, zhū ling,* and *huá shí* to drain damp–heat or use *Yīn Chén Sì Líng Tāng* (Four Substances Powder with Poria plus Virgate Wormwood Decoction). For severe abdominal distention and fullness, add *qīng pí* and *yù jīn*. For nausea and vomiting, add *jú pí*, *zhú rú*, and *jiāng bàn xià*. For severe damp–turbidity, add *huò xiāng*, *bái dòu kòu*, and *pèi lán*. For the presence of rib-side pain, add *yán hú suǒ*, *chuān liàn zǐ*, raw *mài yá*, and *chì sháo*.

Biliary Ascariasis

Biliary ascariasis is described as sudden, acute, and paroxysmal pain under the xiphoid process or in the upper right abdomen due to roundworm obstruction in the biliary tract. In the following, we will introduce a commonly used formula for this disease.

Formula and ingredients: *Wū Méi Wán* (*Mume Pill*)

Wū méi (Fructus Mume) 10 g; *xì xīn* (Radix et Rhizoma Asari) 3 g; *gān jiāng* (Rhizoma Zingiberis) 6 g; *huáng lián* (Rhizoma Coptidis) 8 g; *dāng guī* (Radix Angelicae Sinens) 3 g; blast-fried *fù zǐ* (Radix Aconiti Lateralis Praeparata) without skin 3 g; *huā jiāo* (Pericarpium Zanthoxyli) fried with aroma 3 g; *guì zhī* (Ramulus Cinnamomi) 3 g; *rén shēn* (Radix et Rhizoma Ginseng) 3 g; *huáng bǎi* (Cortex Phellodendri Chinensis) 3 g.

Formula verse

Wū Méi Wán contains *xì xīn guì*, *huáng lián huáng bǎi*, *dāng guī*, as well as *rén shēn jiāo jiāng* and *fù zǐ*, warming organs, purging heat, and calming roundworms.

Usage

Grind into powder and make into pills with honey. Take the pills 9 g each time with warm water on an empty stomach, 1–3 times a day. Alternatvely, serve it as a decoction. Do not consume raw, cold, and greasy food during the medication period.

Actions

Warming viscera and calming roundworms to relieve pain.

Indications

Biliary ascariasis presenting acute and paroxysmal pain in the upper right abdomen or around the navel, vexation, vomiting or vomiting with round-worms, cold extremities, and a pulse alternating between weak and strong beats. It is also indicated for chronic diarrhea and dysentery.

Treatment reference

Aside from biliary ascariasis, *Wū Méi Wán* can treat pain in the abdomen and around the navel due to obstruction in the intestines due to round-worms. In addition, it can also be applied to treat diarrhea due to chronic gastroenteritis, chronic bacterial dysentery and functional bowel disorder, nervous vomiting, postgastrectomy syndrome, and uterine bleeding. If it is served as a decoction, modification may be performed. For the absence of cold signs, remove *guì zhī* and *fù zǐ*. If the patient has sufficient healthy qi, remove *rén shēn* and *dāng guī*. For severe abdominal pain, add *mù xiāng* and *yán hú* suǒ. For severe vomiting, add *jiāng bàn xià* and *wú zhū yú*. For roundworms in the biliary tract and intestines, a normal dose of Piperazine can be added.

Daily Exercises

1. What are the ingredients of *Má Zǐ Rén Wán?* What is it indicated for?
2. What are the ingredients and indications of *Yīn Chén Hāo Tāng*?
3. What are the ingredients and indications of *Wū Méi Wán*?
4. Summarize all the presented formulae for treating rib-side pain and abdominal pain.

Formulae for Diseases of the Cardiovascular System

DAY THREE

In Chinese medicine, the cardiovascular system mainly deals with the heart, but is also related to the liver, lungs, brain, and many more organs. The heart governs the blood and blood vessels, and pathological changes essentially lie in its lack of nourishment, morbid blood circulation, and obstruction of blood vessels. Diseases of the heart are classified into deficiency and excess. The excess pattern is often due to exogenous pathogens attacking the heart and vessels, qi stagnation, blood stasis, or phlegm obstruction, while the deficiency pattern is usually because of heart qi or heart yang insufficiency, and excessive consumption of heart yin or blood. Clinically, common symptoms of this system are agitation/fluster, precordium pain, chest oppression, insomnia, and bleeding.

Palpitations

Palpitations are an abnormality of heartbeat and are often the symptom of various heart disorders. The causes of palpitations can be due to either excess or deficiency. Deficient cases are resulted from the overconsumption of heart qi and blood, which may develop into heart yang depletion. Excess cases are caused by phlegm–fire, fluid–rheum, and static blood. Among the formulae presented in the previous chapters, some of them can be applied to treat palpitations. For palpitations due to both qi and blood deficiency and spleen–heart insufficiency, apply *Guī Pí Tāng*. For fluid retention affecting the heart, apply *Líng Guì Zhú Gān Tāng*. For heart blood stasis obstruction, prescribe *Táo Hóng Sì Wù Tāng* or *Xuè Fǔ Zhú Yū Tāng*. For inactivity of chest yang, apply *Guā Lóu Xiè Bái Bàn Xià Tāng*. For phlegm–fire harassment of the heart, apply *Huáng Lián Wēn Dǎn Tāng*. For heart qi insufficiency, apply *Sì Jūn Zǐ Tāng*. In the following, we will introduce a commonly used formula for palpitations caused by qi and yin deficiency.

Formula and ingredients: Zhì Gān Cǎo Tāng (Honey-Fried Licorice Decoction)

Zhì gān cǎo (Radix et Rhizoma Glycyrrhizae Praeparata cum Melle) 12 g; *shēng jiāng* (Rhizoma Zingiberis Recens) 9 g; *rén shēn* (Radix et Rhizoma Ginseng) 6 g; *shēng dì* (Radix Rehmanniae) 30 g; *guì zhī* (Ramulus Cinnamomi) 9 g; *ē jiāo* (Colla Corii Asini) 6 g; *mài mén dōng* (Radix Ophiopogonis) 9 g; *má rén* (Fructus Cannabis) 10 g; crushed *dà zǎo* (Fructus Jujubae) 5–10 pieces.

Formula verse

Zhì Gān Cǎo Tāng contains *shēn guì jiāng*, *mài dì jiāo*, and *má rén*; for palpitations as well as deficiency–consumption and lung atrophy.

Usage

Add water and 15 mL of yellow wine to decoct. Remove the dregs and add *ē jiāo* melted by hot water.

Actions

Boosting qi and nourishing blood; nourishing yin and restoring pulse.

Indications

Qi and yin insufficiencies presenting palpitations, body weakness, weak breathing, and intermittent pulse; deficiency–consumption and lung atrophy presenting dry coughing without phlegm or phlegm streaked with blood, emaciation, shortness of breath, spontaneous sweating, night sweat, a dry mouth and throat, and dry and constipated stool.

Treatment reference

Zhì Gān Cǎo Tāng is clinically used to treat all kinds of arrhythmia, coronary disease, rheumatic heart disease, and viral myocarditis with symptoms of palpitations, shortness of breath, and an irregular pulse due to insufficient qi and yin. In practice, if qi deficiency is severe, add *huáng qí*. For extreme blood deficiency, add *dāng guī* and *shú dì huáng*. If the patient appears overly flustered, add *suān zǎo rén*, *fú shén*, *wǔ wèi zǐ*, and *bǎi zǐ rén*. For complications with static blood, add *dān shēn*, *táo rén*, and *hóng huā*. For yang deficiency presenting sweating, a fear of cold, and a pale tongue, add cooked *fù zǐ*, *lóng gǔ*, *mǔ lì*, and *huáng qí*.

Coronary Disease

Coronary disease, abbreviated from coronary atherosclerotic heart disease, is characterized by sudden precordium pain or an oppressive feeling lasting for 3–5 min, an accompanying pallor complexion, fear, difficulty in breathing, and cold sweat. Among previously introduced formulae, *Xuè Fǔ Zhú Yū Tāng* can be applied to treat coronary disease due to obstruction by static blood, and *Guā Lóu Xiè Bái Bàn Xià Tāng* to treat coronary disease due to chest yang obstruction. In the following, we will present another formula for this disorder.

Formula and ingredients: *Guàng Xīn Sū Hé Wán* (*Coronary Storax Pill*)

Sū hé xiāng (Styrax) 50 g; *bīng piàn* (Borneolum Syntheticum) 105 g; prepared *rǔ xiāng* (Olibanum) 105 g; *tán xiāng* (Lignum Santali Albi) 210 g; *qīng mù xiāng* (Radix Aristolochiae) 210 g.

Formula verse

Sū Hé Wán contains *rǔ xiāng bīng*, qīng *mù xiāng*, and *tán xiāng*; for treatment of heart pain by opening the orifices with aromatics, especially for coronary disease.

Usage

The above ingredients are made into 1,000 pills. Take 1 pill a time, sucked or chewed, 1–3 times a day, before sleep or when the disease occurs.

Actions

Opening the orifices with aromatics and moving qi to relieve pain.

Indications

Coronary disease due to turbid phlegm and qi stagnation presenting angina, chest oppression, and difficulty in breathing.

Treatment reference

Besides coronary disease, this formula enjoys favorable effects in treating chest oppression and shortness of breath caused by qi stagnation and dampness obstruction in the chest. However, if the patient has a very high blood pressure or a physique of stomach coldness, be careful when applying this formula in case of elevating blood pressure levels and damaging the stomach due to its cold and cool natures.

Daily Exercises

1. Summarize the formulae for treating palpitations, and compare the differences among their indications.
2. What are the ingredients of *Zhì Gān Căo Tāng*? What are its indications?
3. What are the ingredients and functions of *Guàng Xīn Sū Hé Wán*?

CHAPTER 18

Formulae for Diseases
of the Urogenital System

DAY FOUR

The urogenital system in Chinese medicine mainly involves the kidney, but also includes the bladder and uterus, and is related to the functions of the lung, spleen, liver, and *sanjiao*. The kidney is the site of storage of essence, the source of growth, development, and reproduction, and it maintains the balance and discharge of body fluids. Diseases of the kidney are mainly caused by storage dysfunction, the loss of its warming and nourishing functions, and fluid consumption. Therefore, kidney disorders are often a deficiency pattern, but sometimes, they can be complicated by deficiency–fire, damp–turbidity, water retention, and static blood. Its clinical manifestations largely include edema, strangury, urine retention, lumbar pain, *xiāo kě* (wasting thirst, 消渴), seminal emission, impotence, white leukorrhea, and infertility.

Strangury

Strangury is characterized by frequent and dribbling urination with stabbing pain, scant urine, and lower abdominal cramps. Its disease causes include damp–heat obstruction in the bladder, obstruction by stones, qi constraint, stagnation of static blood, and storage dysfunction due to deficiency. Among the formulae in previous chapters, some of them can be applied to treat this disease. For strangury due to damp–heat pouring downward, apply *Lóng Dǎn Xiè Gān Tāng* or *Sān Miào Sǎn*. For static blood obstruction in the lower body, use *Shào Fǔ Zhú Yū Tāng*. For sinking of spleen qi, prescribe *Bǔ Zhōng Yì Qì Tāng*. In the following, we will introduce a commonly used formula for strangury caused by damp–heat obstruction in the lower body.

Formula and ingredients: *Bā Zhèng Sǎn (Eight Corrections Powder)*

Chē qián zǐ (Semen Plantaginis); *qú mài* (Herba Dianthi); *biǎn xù* (Herba Polygoni Avicularis); *huá shí* (Talcum); kernal of *zhī zǐ* (Fructus Gardeniae); *zhì gān cǎo* (Radix et Rhizoma Glycyrrhizae Praeparata cum Melle); *chuān mù tōng* (Caulis Clematidis Armandii); *dà huáng* (Radix et Rhizoma Rhei); 6 g each.

Formula verse

Bā Zhèng contains *mù tōng* and *chē qián*, *biǎn xù dà huáng zhī huá* powder; *gān cǎo qú mài* and *dēng xīn cǎo*, to be decocted for strangury due to damp–heat.

Usage

Grind the ingredients into a crude powder and decoct 6–9 g with *dēng xīn cǎo* (Medulla Junci) and water. Remove the dregs and take the decoction after meals or before sleep. Alternatively, decoct the above ingredients directly with water.

Actions

Clearing heat and purging fire; promoting urination and relieving strangury.

Indications

Damp–heat accumulation and obstruction in the bladder presenting frequent, painful, dribbling, or even blocked urination, lower abdominal distention and fullness, a dry mouth and throat, a red tongue with a yellow coating, and a rapid pulse.

Treatment reference

This formula is commonly used to treat different kinds of urinary system infections, such as pyelonephritis, cystitis, urethritis, prostatitis, and urinary stones. In clinical practice, for strangury with blood, add *xiǎo jì, bái máo gēn*, and raw *pú huáng*. For the presence of stones, add *jīn qián cǎo, hǎi jīn shā*, and so on. It is not indicated for body weakness after prolonged illness, absence of damp–heat in the lower *jiao*, and pregnant women.

Bloody Urine

Bloody urine is the production of urine mixed with blood or blood clots. It can be caused by either pathogenic heat impairing the vessels or the spleen and kidney failing to manage blood. For bloody urine due to blood–heat, apply *Xī Jiǎo Dì Huáng Tāng*. For kidney yin deficiency with flaming internal deficiency–fire, use *Zhī Bǎi Dì Huáng Tāng*. For the failure of blood management by the spleen, prescribe *Guī Pí Tāng*. In the following, we will introduce a formula for bloody urine due to heat exuberance in the lower *jiao*.

Formula and ingredients: Xiǎo Jì Yǐn Zǐ (Field Thistle Drink)

Shēng dì (Radix Rehmanniae) 24 g; *xiǎo jì* (Herba Cirsii) 3 g; *huá shí* (Talcum) 3 g; *chuān mù tōng* (Caulis Clematidis Armandii) 3 g; dry-fried *pú huáng* (Pollen Typhae) 3 g; *dàn zhú yè* (Herba Lophatheri) 3 g; *ǒu jié* (Nodus Nelumbinis Rhizomatis) 3 g; wine-soaked *dāng guī* (Radix Angelicae Sinensis) 3 g; dry-fried *zhī zǐ* (Fructus Gardeniae) 3 g; *zhì gān cǎo* (Radix et Rhizoma Glycyrrhizae Praeparata cum Melle) 3 g.

Formula verse

Xiǎo Jì Yǐn Zǐ contains *ǒu pú huáng, mù tōng huá shí*, and *shēng dì; guī cǎo zhī zǐ dàn zhú yè*, applicable to blood strangury and heat bind.

Usage

Grind the above ingredients into a crude powder and administer 12 g each time for decoction. Remove the dregs and take the decoction warm on an empty stomach. Alternatively, serve it as a decoction.

Actions

Cooling blood and staunching bleeding, promoting urination, and relieving strangury.

Indications

Blood strangury presenting bloody urine, frequent and painful urination, dark-colored urine, a red tongue, and a rapid pulse.

Treatment reference

This formula is widely used for treating acute infections of the urinary system, urinary tract calculi, renal tuberculosis, and acute nephritis with symptoms of bloody urine and painful urination. For exuberance of heat in the lower *jiao*, add *zhī mǔ*, *huáng bǎi*, and *hǔ zhàng*. For painful urination, add *hǔ pò* and *hǎi jīn shā*. For damage to both qi and yin due to prolonged illness, reduce the dosages of *huá shí* and *chuān mù tōng*, and add *huáng qí* and *ē jiāo*. If urine is bloody but not painful, there may be the possibility of urinary tumors and the patient should be advised to go for further examinations in a hospital.

Enuresis

Enuresis refers to urine incontinence (involuntary urination). Some cases occur in sleep, which is prevalent among young children, while others are resulted from kidney qi deficiency or an injured lumbar vertebra. *Shèn Qì Wán* learnt previously has moderate effects in treating enuresis due to kidney qi deficiency. In the following, we will introduce a commonly used formula for enuresis.

Formula and ingredients: Suō Quán Wán (Stream-Reducing Pill)

Equal amounts of *wū yào* (Radix Linderae); *yì zhì rén* (Fructus Alpiniae Oxyphyllae); *shān yào* (Rhizoma Dioscoreae).

Formula verse

Suō Quán Wán treats enuresis by the actions of *shān yào wū yào* and *yì zhì*.

Usage

Grind above ingredients into a fine powder and make it into small pills with wine-prepared *shān yào* powder. Take the pills 6–9 g orally each time with rice soup, 2–3 times a day. Alternatively, serve it as a decoction.

Actions

Warming the kidney and reducing urine production.

Indications

Frequent urination and enuresis.

Treatment reference

Pills of this formula are on sale in China. It is applicable to bed-wetting in children, senile frequent urination and urine incontinence, massive secretion of saliva, profuse nasal discharge, nervous frequent urination, and insipidus. If it is served as a decoction to treat more severe cases, add *tù sī zǐ, jīn yīng zǐ, sāng piāo xiāo, fù pén zǐ, bǔ gǔ zhī*, and so on.

Daily Exercises

1. Summarize the formulae for treating strangury and inhibited urination, and compare the differences among their indications.
2. What are the ingredients and indications of *Bā Zhèng Sǎn*?
3. What are the ingredients and indications of *Xiǎo Jì Yǐn Zǐ*?
4. What are the ingredients and indications of *Suō Quán Wán*?

DAY FIVE

Seminal Emission

Seminal emission refers to the unconscious discharge of semen without sexual intercourse. Some cases occur after sexually charged dreams, in which they are called nocturnal emission, while others happen without dreams or even at sober moments, which are termed spontaneous seminal emission. The causes of seminal emission include heart fire affecting the essence chamber, damp–heat pouring downward, the heart and spleen failing to control the production of semen due to qi deficiency, and the insecurity of the kidney due to deficiency. Among the formulae previously presented, *Lóng Dǎn Xiè Gān Tāng* and *Liù Wèi Dì Huáng Wán* can be respectively applied to treat seminal emission due to damp–heat pouring downward and insecurity of the kidney. In the following, we will introduce a commonly used formula for seminal emission due to kidney deficiency.

Formula and ingredients: Jīn Suǒ Gù Jīng Wán (Golden Lock Essence-Securing Pill)

Dry-fried *shā yuàn jí lí* (Semen Astragali Complanati) 12 g; steamed *qiàn shí* (Semen Euryales) 12 g; *lián xū* (Stamen Nelumbinis) 12 g; *lóng gǔ* (Os Draconis) 6 g; calcined *mǔ lì* (Concha Ostreae) 6 g.

Formula verse

Jīn Suǒ Gù Jīng contains *qiàn lián xū*, *lóng gǔ mǔ lì*, and *jí lí*; to be made into paste pills and taken with salty soup; it cures seminal emission.

Usage

The ingredients are ground into a fine powder and made into paste pills with the powder of lotus seeds. Take the pills 9 g at a time orally with salty soup at an empty stomach, 2–3 times a day. Alternatively, serve it as a decoction with similar doses.

Actions

Supplementing the kidney and securing essence.

Indications

Failure of storage by the kidney due to deficiency presenting seminal emission, efflux of diarrhea, lumbar soreness, tinnitus, mental fatigue, a lack of strength, a pale tongue, and a thin and weak pulse.

Treatment reference

This formula is not only applicable to frequent urination, seminal emission, and enuresis due to kidney deficiency failing to store essence, but also to chyluria, flooding and spotting (*bēng lòu*; 崩漏), leukorrhea, and chronic diarrhea due to kidney deficiency. In clinical practice, if the stool produced is dry and constipated, add *dāng guī* and *ròu cōng róng*. For thin and unformed stool, add *bǔ gǔ zhī* and *wǔ wèi zǐ*. For severe lumbar soreness and pain, add dry-fried *gǒu jǐ*, *dù zhòng*, and *sāng jì shēng*. For impotence, add *suǒ yáng*, *yín yáng huò*, and *tù sī zǐ*. This formula is not indicated for seminal emission due to heat exuberance and damp–heat.

Edema

Edema entails puffy swellings over the face, eyes, lower limbs, and even all over the body due to internal fluid retention. In severe cases, pleural effusion and ascites may also occur. Causes include the external contraction of wind–cold, water–dampness, food poisoning, exhaustion and fatigue, and qi stagnation, all of which will lead to the failure of the lung to free and regulate water-conducting pathways, the spleen unable to distribute, and the kidney incapable of transforming urine, inducing fluid accumulation and inhibited urine, and resulting in fluid overflow and edema. Among the formulae in previous chapters, some of them can be applied to treat these swellings. For edema caused by exogenous wind pathogens, apply *Yuè Bì Tāng*. For internal accumulation of water–dampness, prescribe *Wǔ Líng Sǎn*. For the inability of the spleen to transform dampness due to deficiency, use *Lǐ Zhōng Tāng* or *Shēn Líng Bái Zhú Sǎn*. If the kidney is unable to transform water–dampness due to deficiency, apply *Zhēn Wǔ Tāng* or *Shèn Qì Wán*. In the following, we will introduce a commonly used formula for edema caused by spleen deficiency with exuberance of dampness and qi stagnation with fluid retention.

Formula and ingredients: Wǔ Pí Yǐn (Five-Peel Beverage)

Shēng jiāng pí (Cortex Zingiberis Rhizomatis); *sāng bái pí* (Cortex Mori); *chén pí* (Pericarpium Citri Reticulatae); *dà fù pí* (Pericarpium Arecae); *fú líng pí* (Cutis Poriae); 9 g each.

Formula verse

Wǔ Pí Yǐn contains 5 kinds of skins, namely *chén líng jiāng sāng* and *dà fù*. Or replace *sāng bái* with *wǔ jiā pí*, applicable to spleen deficiency and abdominal distention.

Usage

Grind the above ingredients into a crude powder and administer 9–12 g each time for decoction. Remove the dregs and take the decoction warm, 2–3 times a day. Do not consumer raw, cold, greasy, and overly salty food during the medication period.

Treatment reference

Wǔ Pí Yǐn is commonly used in the clinic for treating edema. It has significant urination-promoting and edema-relieving effects for acute and chronic nephritis, edema of anemia, gestational edema, and many other kinds of edema. If it is accompanied by pain due to wind–damp encumbering the body surface, *sāng bái pí* in the formula can be replaced by *wǔ jiā pí*. In practice, for edema occurring largely in the upper part of the body, add *fáng fēng*, *qiāng huó*, *zǐ sū*, and *jīng jiè*. For edema mainly in the lower part of the body, add *zé xiè*, *fáng jǐ*, and *chē qián zǐ*. For the presence of cold signs, add *fù zǐ* and *gān jiāng*. For the presence of heat, add *huá shí* and *mù tōng*. For gestational edema, remove *sāng bái pí* and add *bái zhú*.

White Leukorrhea

White leukorrhea is the continuous discharge of white mucus from the vagina of a woman. It is primary caused by damp–turbidity pouring downward due to spleen deficiency, damp–heat of the liver channel pouring downward, the production of toxins due to damp–heat accumulation, or the kidney failing to secure due to deficiency. Among the previous formulae, *Lóng Dǎn Xiè Gān Tāng* and *Sān Miào Sǎn* can be applied to treat leukorrhea with damp–heat signs; *Bǔ Zhōng Yì Qì Tāng* to leukorrhea caused by spleen deficiency and qi sinking; and *Zhī*

Bǎi Dì Huáng Wán to kidney yin deficiency and the internal generation of deficiency heat. In the following, we will introduce a formula for white leukorrhea caused by damp–turbidity pouring downward due to spleen deficiency.

Formula and ingredients: *Wán Dài Tāng (Discharge-Ceasing Decoction)*

Earth-fried *bái zhú* (Rhizoma Atractylodis Macrocephalae) 30 g; dry-fried *shān yào* (Rhizoma Dioscoreae) 30 g; *rén shēn* (Radix et Rhizoma Ginseng) 6 g; wine-fried *bái sháo* (Radix Paeoniae Alba) 15 g; wine-fried and wrapped *chē qián zǐ* (Semen Plantaginis) 9 g; *cāng zhú* (Rhizoma Atractylodis) 9 g; *gān cǎo* (Radix et Rhizoma Glycyrrhizae) 3 g; *chén pí* (Pericarpium Citri Reticulatae) 1.5 g; *jīng jiè suì tàn* (Spica Schizonepetae Carbonisata) 1.5 g; *chái hú* (Radix Bupleuri) 1.8 g.

Formula verse

Wán Dài Tāng contains two *zhú* and *shēn cǎo chái shān yào*, as well as *bái sháo chē qián zǐ jīng jiè chén*, being beneficial to leukorrhea due to spleen deficiency.

Usage

Add water to decoct.

Actions

Boosting qi and fortifying the spleen; removing dampness and arresting vaginal discharge.

Indications

Damp–turbidity pouring downward due to spleen deficiency presenting white or light yellow loose vaginal discharge but with no odor, a pale complexion, fatigue, loose stool, a pale tongue with a white coating, and a moderate or soggy and weak pulse.

Treatment reference

Wán Dài Tāng is a typical formula used for leukorrhea in women. It is applicable to cases of deficiency without obvious damp–heat signs. Clinically, it is often used to treat leukorrhea due to chronic pelvic inflammatory disease, chronic cervicitis, and body weakness. If leukorrhea is massive or bleeding is present, add calcined *lóng gǔ*, *mǔ lì*, and *qiàn cǎo*. For severe kidney deficiency, add *shā yuàn jí lí*, *shú dì huáng*, *ròu cōng róng*, and *shān zhū yú*. For yellow, sticky, and pungent leukorrhea, which is a sign of damp–heat, add *huáng bǎi*, *chūn bái pí*, and *mǔ dān pí*. This formula is not indicated for leukorrhea with insignificant deficient signs, but instead with obvious damp–heat symptoms that is purulent or yellow-green and with a strong odor.

Daily Exercises

1. What are the ingredients of *Jīn Suǒ Gù Jīng Wán?* What are its indications?
2. What are the ingredients of *Wǔ Pí Yǐn*? What are its indications?
3. What are the ingredients and indications of *Wán Dài Tāng*? How can it be modified in clinical practice?
4. Summarize the formulae for treating edema.

CHAPTER 19

Formulae for Diseases of the Nervous System

DAY SIX

In Chinese medicine, the brain, heart, liver, and gallbladder are the key organs pertaining to the nervous system. The brain commands the innate spirit, the heart directs mental activity, and the liver and gallbladder control emotions and the uninhibited flow of qi. Nonetheless, the main functions reside in the heart and liver. Diseases of the nervous system can either be of deficiency or excess. Excess patterns are often resulted from phlegm–damp, phlegm–fire, static blood, and qi stagnation in the heart and liver, while its deficient patterns are caused by the deficiency of the heart, liver, kidney, or other organs. Its clinical manifestations include mental disorders, convulsions, vertigo, headaches, pain in other regions, paralysis, numbness, insomnia, abnormal sensations, and abnormal sweating. The prevalence of diseases occurring in the nervous system is fairly high. In the following, we will introduce several suitable formulae for selected disease patterns.

Insomnia

Insomnia refers to frequent reduced sleep, which includes difficulty in falling asleep and liability to wake and unable to easily fall asleep again (in mild cases), and the inability to fall asleep throughout the night (in severe cases). The causes of insomnia comprise the exuberance of heart fire, internal disturbance of liver fire, phlegm–heat affecting the heart, yin deficiency resulting in vigorous fire, the heart lacking nourishment due to its deficiency or weakness of the spleen, qi, and blood, and heart deficiency with the appearance of timidity. Many formulae in previous

437

chapters can be applied to treat this sleep disorder. For insomnia due to liver heat, apply *Lóng Dǎn Xiè Gān Tāng*. For phlegm–heat, use *Wēn Dǎn Tāng*. For yin deficiency resulting in vigorous fire, prescribe *Liù Wèi Dì Huáng Wán*. For deficiency of both the heart and spleen, prescribe *Guī Pí Tāng*. In the following, we will introduce a formula for liver blood deficiency and internal disturbance of deficiency–heat.

Formula and ingredients: Suān Zǎo Rén Tāng (Sour Jujube Decoction)

Suān zǎo rén (Semen ZiziphiSpinosae) 15 g; *fú líng* (Poria) 6 g; *zhī mǔ* (Rhizoma Anemarrhenae) 6 g; *chuān xiōng* (Rhizoma Chuanxiong) 6 g; *gān cǎo* (Radix et Rhizoma Glycyrrhizae) 3 g.

Formula verse

Suān Zǎo Rén Tāng is for insomnia, contains *chuān xiōng zhī cǎo* and *fú líng*. It nourishes blood, relieves vexation, and clears deficiency–heat, ensuring good quality sleep at night.

Usage

Add water to decoct.

Actions

Nourishing blood and calming the mind; clearing heat and relieving vexation.

Indications

Insomnia due to deficiency–consumption presenting palpitations, night sweat, dizziness, a dry mouth and throat, a red tongue, and a thin and wiry pulse.

Treatment reference

Suān Zǎo Rén Tāng is a common formula for insomnia of neurosis. It is also applicable to depression, anxiety, mild schizophrenia, and menopause. In order to strengthen the effect of calming the mind, use a large dose of *suān zǎo rén* (30–60 g). For severe deficiency–heat, remove *chuān xiōng* and add *shēng dì*, *bái sháo*, and *huáng lián*. For palpitations and dream-filled sleep, add *fú shén*, *lóng chǐ*, and *cí shí*.

Epilepsy

Epilepsy is a repeatedly occurring disease marked by sudden unconsciousness, saliva leakage from the mouth, up-turning of eyes, and cramps in the four extremities, but with spontaneous recovery after a while. It is associated with liver wind forcing phlegm–turbidity upward to cloud the brain, liver fire driving phlegm–heat to disrupt the heart, the impairment of the liver and kidney, and spleen–stomach weakness. Some previous formulae can be applied to treat epilepsy. For example, for epilepsy due to liver fire and phlegm–heat, *Lóng Dǎn Xiè Gān Tāng* can be used; for liver–kidney yin deficiency, *Jiā Jiǎn Fù Mài Tāng* is prescribed; while for spleen–stomach weakness, *Liù Jūn Zǐ Tāng* is applied. In the following, we will introduce a commonly used formula for epilepsy.

Formula and ingredients: Dìng Xián Wán (Convulsion-Settling Pill)

Tiān má (Rhizoma Gastrodiae) 30 g; *chuān bèi mǔ* (Bulbus Fritillariae Cirrhosae) 30 g; *jiāng bàn xià* (Rhizoma Pinelliae Praeparatum) 30 g; *fú líng* (Poria) 30 g; *fú shén* (Sclerotium Poriae Pararadicis) 30 g; wine-prepared *dǎn nán xīng* (Arisaema cum Bile) 15 g; *shí chāng pú* (Rhizoma Acori Tatarinowii) 15 g; *quán xiē* (Scorpion) without tail 15 g; fried *jiāng cán* (Bombyx Batryticatus) without mouth 15 g; *hǔ pò* (Succinum) 15 g; *dēng xīn cǎo* (Succinum) 15 g; *chén pí* (Pericarpium Citri Reticulatae) 21 g; *yuǎn zhì* (Radix Polygalae) without core 21 g; wine-steamed *dān shēn* (Radix et Rhizoma Salviae Miltiorrhizae) 60 g; *mài dōng* (Radix Ophiopogonis) 60 g; finely ground with water *zhū shā* (Cinnabaris) 9 g.

Formula verse

Dìng Xián contains two *fú and tiān má, dān mài chén yuǎn pú bàn xià*; *nán xīng xiē cán pò xīn shā*, applicable to epilepsy.

Usage

Grind the ingredients into a fine powder and add a small bowl of bamboo sap and a cup of ginger juice to boil into paste with 120 g of *gān căo* (Radix et Rhizoma Glycyrrhizae). Then, make the paste into pills the size of marbles and coat them with *zhū shā*. Take the pills orally 6 g at a time with warm water, 2 times a day.

Actions

Extinguishing wind and dissolving phlegm; opening the orifices and calming the mind.

Indications

Epilepsy causing sudden falling, unconsciousness, cramps, deviation of the eyes and mouth, leakage of saliva, and a "baa" sound. It is also applicable to schizophrenia.

Treatment reference

This formula is usually prepared beforehand for patients with frequent episodes of epilepsy. However, as this disorder is usually related to the factors of liver wind, phlegm–fire, yin deficiency, spleen–stomach qi deficiency, and qi deficiency and blood stasis, it is important to remove these factors and improve the patient's physique at the remission stage. Wind-extinguishing and heavy sedative medicinals should not be administered blindly. When served as a decoction, modification of this formula can be done. For profuse leakage of sticky phlegm, add *guā lóu*. For severe phlegm–heat, add alum-fried *yù jīn* and *gān jiāng*. For the production of loose and clear phlegm, add *gān jiāng* and *xì xīn*. For a chronic disease course and frequent occurrences, add *rén shēn*.

Night Sweat

Abnormal sweating generally includes spontaneous sweating and night sweat. The first refers to frequent sweating regardless of the influence of external factors and aggravation after exertion, while the second involves sweating in sleep, but stops after waking. *Guì Zhī Tāng* can be used to treat spontaneous sweating due to disharmony between *ying* and *wei* qi; *Yù Píng Fēng Sǎn* to treat spontaneous sweating due to exterior deficiency and lung *wei* insecurity; *Guī Pí Tāng* to treat spontaneous sweating and night sweat due to insufficiency of blood and qi, and a heart lacking nourishment; *Lóng Dǎn Xiè Gān Tāng* to treat spontaneous sweating and night sweat due to interior heat leading to steaming and driving of fluids outward by the liver and gallbladder. In the following, we will introduce a formula for night sweat due to yin deficiency and fire disturbance.

Formula and ingredients: Dāng Guī Liù Huáng Tāng (Chinese Angelica Six Yellow Decoction)

Equal doses of *dāng guī* (Radix Angelicae Sinensis); *shēng dì* (Radix Rehmanniae); *shú dì huáng* (Radix Rehmanniae Praeparata); *huáng qín* (Radix Scutellariae); *huáng bǎi* (Cortex Phellodendri Chinensis); *huáng lián* (Rhizoma Coptidis); and a doubled dose of *huáng qí* (Radix Astragali).

Formula verse

Liù Huáng Tāng is for yin deficiency night sweat, which contains *guī bǎi qín lián* and two *dì huáng*; doubled dose of *huáng qí* is to secure the exterior, being strong at nourishing yin, clearing heat, and astringing sweat.

Usage

Grind the above ingredients into a crude powder and administer 15 g each time for decoction. For children, the doses should be halved. Alternatively, serve it as a decoction.

Actions

Nourishing yin and clearing heat; consolidating the exterior and arresting sweating.

Indications

Night sweat due to yin deficiency and fire disturbance, presenting vexing heat in the five centers, flushed cheeks, a dry mouth and lips, difficulty in urination, dark-colored urine, a red tongue, and a thin and rapid pulse.

Treatment reference

This formula is specially designed for night sweat with signs of deficiency–heat. If sweating is profuse, add *fú xiǎo mài*, *mǔ lì*, *nuò dào gēn xū*, and *bì táo gān* (Fructus Amygdali Lmmaturi). If deficiency–heat is severe or there is mild lingering fever, add *qín jiāo*, *yín chái hú*, *dì gǔ pí*, and *bái wēi*. If signs of yin deficiency are significant, while those of deficiency–heat are not, this formula can be replaced by *Liù Wèi Dì Huáng Wán*, combined with *mài dōng* and *wǔ wèi zǐ*.

Daily Exercises

1. What are the ingredients and indications of *Suān Zǎo Rén Tāng*?
2. What are the ingredients of *Dìng Xián Wán*? How can it be modified if it is served as a decoction?
3. What are the ingredients of *Dāng Guī Liù Huáng Tāng*? What are its indications? How can it be modified according to different disease patterns?
4. Summarize the formulae for treating abnormal sweating, and compare the differences among their indications.

Formula Index

Subject Index